Keratoconjunctivitis Sicca and Filamentary Keratopathy

Helena M. Tabery

Keratoconjunctivitis Sicca and Filamentary Keratopathy

In Vivo Morphology in the Human Cornea and Conjunctiva

Springer

Helena M. Tabery, M.D.
helena.tabery@telia.com

Formerly
Ögonkliniken UMAS
205 02 Malmö
Sweden

ISBN 978-3-642-31027-0 ISBN 978-3-642-31028-7 (eBook)
DOI 10.1007/978-3-642-31028-7
Springer Heidelberg New York Dordrecht London

Library of Congress Control Number: 2012949320

Printed on acid-free paper

Springer is part of Springer Science+Business Media (www.springer.com)

Preface

This book is dedicated to keratoconjunctivitis sicca (KCS, also termed dry eye) (Part I), an extremely common ocular surface disease affecting millions of people worldwide, and to filamentary keratopathy (Part II), per se an unspecific and relatively rare phenomenon the most common underlying condition of which is KCS.

The in vivo captured high-magnification images show in detail the appearance of the ocular surface and of the mucus component discernible in the tear film. KCS is treated as a group with no ambition to grade the severity of the disease or to attribute the individual phenomena to any particular underlying cause. Although the majority of the images originate in patients with Sjögren's syndrome, I believe that they fairly represent the broad spectrum of ocular surface changes occurring in KCS. Included are long-term observations, less common KCS cases and images showing iatrogenic epithelial damage; a separate chapter treats four patients with corneal epitheliopathy occurring as sequela of herpes zoster ophthalmicus.

Filamentary keratopathy is a painful condition characterised by variously large ocular surface appendices termed filaments. The high-magnification in vivo images captured in KCS and some other surface conditions reveal their components which, in conjunction with their dynamics, offer a reasonable explanation of mechanisms behind their formation.

This book differs from current textbooks in that it shows ocular surface changes captured in vivo at a higher magnification level than used in standard slit lamp photography. The photographs show phenomena captured in various illumination modes, before and after staining with diagnostic dyes, and the photographic sequences illustrate their dynamics. The images reflect the in vivo situation, and the advantage is that once aware of the various phenomena, anyone working with a standard diagnostic equipment – the slit lamp and the diagnostic dyes – can easily detect almost all of them.

I hope that the reader dealing with ocular surface diseases, whether a general practitioner, a medical eye specialist, an ocular surgeon, an optometrist, an optician, or a rheumatologist, will find the images presented in this book helpful in estimations of the ocular surface condition, be for diagnostic or research purposes, be before interventions such as contact lens fitting or surgery.

Malmö, Sweden

Helena M. Tabery

Contents

About This Book

The photographs in this book have been chosen to show

Part I

- The in vivo morphology of preocular tear film mucus in KCS (Chap. 1)
- The in vivo morphology of corneal surface changes in KCS (Chap. 2)
- The in vivo morphology of conjunctival surface changes in KCS (Chap. 3)
- Clinical applications (Chap. 4)
- The in vivo morphology of corneal epitheliopathy after herpes zoster ophthalmicus (Chap. 5)

Part II

- The in vivo morphology and dynamics of filamentary keratopathy (Chap. 6)
- Clinical applications (Chap. 7)

The photographs were taken by *non-contact* in vivo *photomicrography*, a method that requires neither contact with the epithelium nor the use of anaesthetics. By this method are visualized structures that optically differ from their regularly organized surroundings; a normal corneal epithelium or stromal cells cannot be discerned. As there is no contact with the ocular surface, the architecture of epithelial changes is not disturbed by the examination, and there is no risk of spreading infections. The technique allows the use of various illumination modes to complement each other and a free application of *diagnostic dyes* to expand the information, e.g., 1 % fluorescein sodium and 1 % rose bengal (preservative-free solutions). These dyes are commonly used in clinical practice.

The KCS *diagnosis* was based on three tests: tear break-up time (BUT) $\leq$ 10 s, Schirmer 1 test $\leq$ 5 mm wetting/ 5 min and rose bengal score (RBS) $\geq$4, in one or both eyes (two pathological results of three, Copenhagen Criteria).

The *term KCS is used in all cases of dry eye irrespective of possible causes*.

The *bars indicate 200μm throughout the book*.

Abbreviations

BUT	break-up time
Fluorescein	fluorescein sodium
HSV	herpes simplex virus
HZ	herpes zoster
HZO	herpes zoster ophthalmicus
KCS	keratoconjunctivitis sicca
RBS	rose bengal score
SS	Sjögren's syndrome

Part I

Keratoconjunctivitis Sicca

About Keratoconjunctivitis Sicca (KCS)

KCS is a very common ocular surface disease causing a variety of *symptoms* such as ocular discomfort, burning, scratching, grittiness, sandy or foreign body sensation, stinging, eyestrain, tired eyes and blurred vision; sometimes itching, feeling of dryness or, conversely, tearing episodes. The *clinical findings* concern the eyelids and lid margins, the preocular tear film (excess of mucus) and the ocular surface proper (epithelial changes, mucus adherence, and disruptions of surface integrity). The *severity of symptoms and findings* varies largely, and they are poorly correlated; it is well known that in patients with pronounced symptoms findings may be minimal, or, conversely, severe findings may be accompanied by minimal symptoms.

There is a general agreement on that KCS is a *multifactorial disease* including an inflammatory component, and that surface changes occur concurrently with and are related to disturbances of the preocular *tear film*: lack of tears due to diminished production or increased evaporation caused by malfunction of fat-producing glands, or tears of poor quality for other reasons, have been implicated.

The clinical *diagnosis* is usually based on the extent of surface staining with diagnostic dyes and on tests aiming at measurements of some properties of the tear film. Frequently used *tests* are the tear break-up time (BUT) (the time elapsed between the last blink and the appearance of dark 'holes' in the tear film stained green with fluorescein sodium), the Schirmer 1 test (the length of wetting in mm of a standardised filter paper strip placed for 5 min in the lower fornix, without anaesthetics) and the van Bijsterveldt (rose bengal) score (the sum of rose bengal staining within the interpalpebral area divided into three parts – temporal and nasal conjunctiva, and cornea – each estimated on a scale 1–3). Less widespread are estimations of fluorescein sodium staining and staining with lissamine green dye instead of rose bengal. At present, there is no consensus on diagnostic criteria but there seems to be an agreement on the cut-off values of these tests (BUT ≤ 10, Schirmer 1 test ≤5 mm/5 min, van Bijsterveldt score ≥4).

The findings in *this book* refer to KCS diagnosis meeting the latter three criteria (two pathological results of three in one or both eyes, Copenhagen Criteria). Almost all patients had Sjögren's syndrome (SS) but attention was paid to other diseases that might have been involved (such as atopy, rosacea, psoriasis, autoimmune diseases other than SS, diabetes); if present, supplementary information is given.

The exact *mechanisms* behind KCS surface changes remain elusive and so does the question whether KCS is one disease or whether it should be subdivided depending on causes. Whatever, one should be aware of the possibility of an underlying autoimmune disease such as, for example, Sjögren's syndrome, an autoimmune multisystem exocrinopathy with dry eye and dry mouth as cardinal symptoms.

At present, there is no curative treatment. Artificial tears, also named tear substitutes or lubricating eye drops, have been the mainstay for many years now, but there have been also other modalities changing with time. This book on morphology contains no treatment recommendations but treatment is mentioned as a factor involved in Case Reports.

1 The Mucus in the Preocular Tear Film

In KCS, with the slit lamp, are often visible floating particles moving with blinks; such particles are usually termed tear film *debris*. This debris contains two components: mucus and cell debris/fragments.

The component interpreted as mucus shows two varieties, one with definite formes and one amorphous. The *formed mucus* appears as (a) thin and weakly light-reflecting sheet-like structures, some showing emanating strands and rounded holes and others folded or collapsed and (b) as variously thick and long, optically dense and light-reflecting strands or threads, and fine fibres. The *amorphous material* appears as variously shaped lumps often containing entrapped air bubbles. Both varieties may be present per se but mostly in combinations and often with addition of granular *cell debris*. Some rose bengal staining is visible almost always except for the very fine fibres in which it is beyond resolution.

The tear film debris treated in this chapter was apparently moving freely upon the surface but in some cases surface adherence could not be excluded. The composed structures implied that mucus moving on a deranged KCS surface has a sticky property ultimately serving a cleansing function. Mucus adherent to the surface, and its dynamics, is treated in the context of corneal surface changes (Chap. 2).

H.M. Tabery, *Keratoconjunctivitis Sicca and Filamentary Keratopathy*,
DOI 10.1007/978-3-642-31028-7_1, © Springer-Verlag Berlin Heidelberg 2012

Amorphous Material (1)

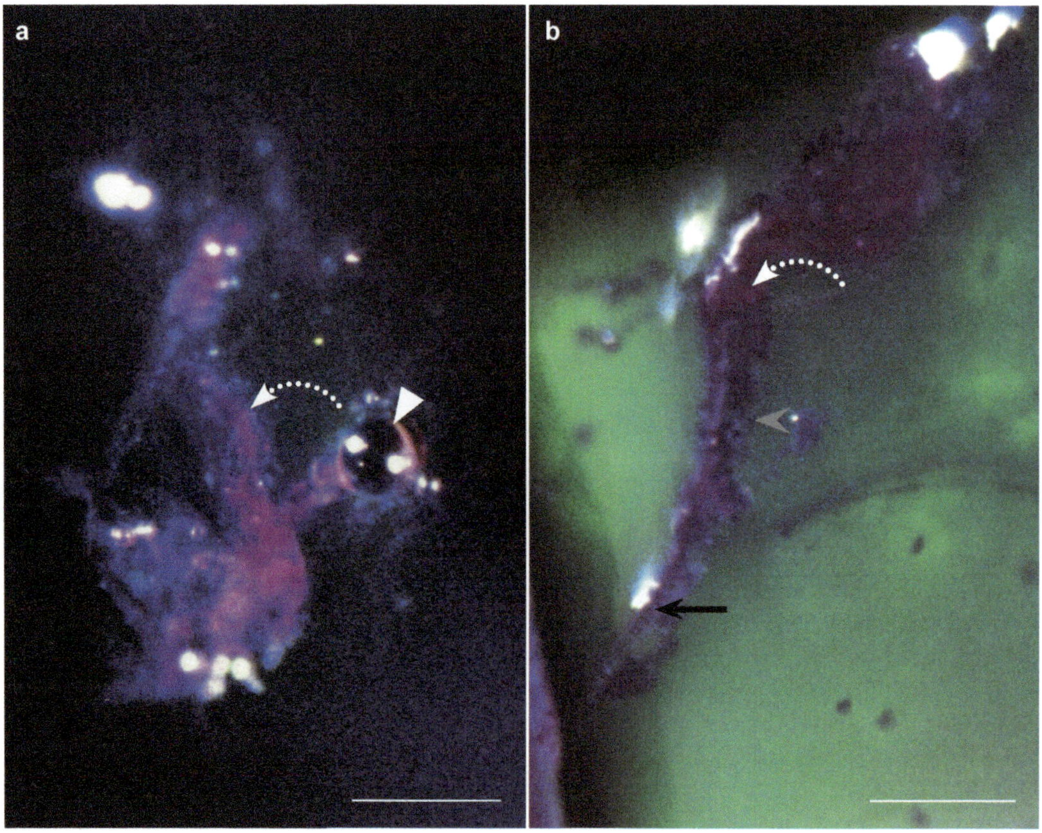

Fig. 1.1 The precorneal tear film shows (**a**) a piece of amorphous material (*bowed arrow*) with incorporated rose bengal dye and an air bubble (*arrowhead*) and (**b**) a complex structure containing cell debris (*arrowhead*), seemingly enmeshed in amorphous material (*bowed arrow*) and attached to a thread (*straight arrow*); this structure probably represents a torn-off bit of a filament (cf. Part II) (Adapted from [3])

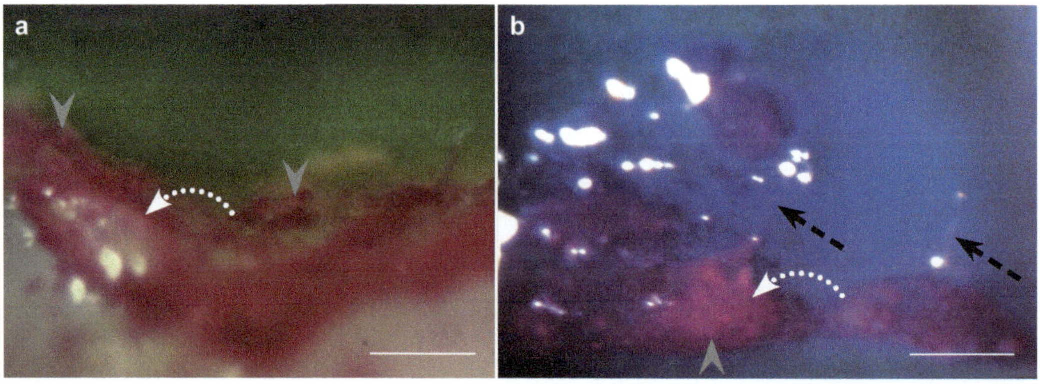

Fig. 1.2 (**a**) Rose bengal stained amorphous material (*arrow*) with little discernible debris (*arrowheads*) lying on the lower lid margo. (**b**) Another bit of amorphous material (*bowed arrow*) staining red with rose bengal; it is slightly granular (*arrowhead*) and in places seemingly sticking to the surface (*straight arrows*)

Amorphous Material (2)

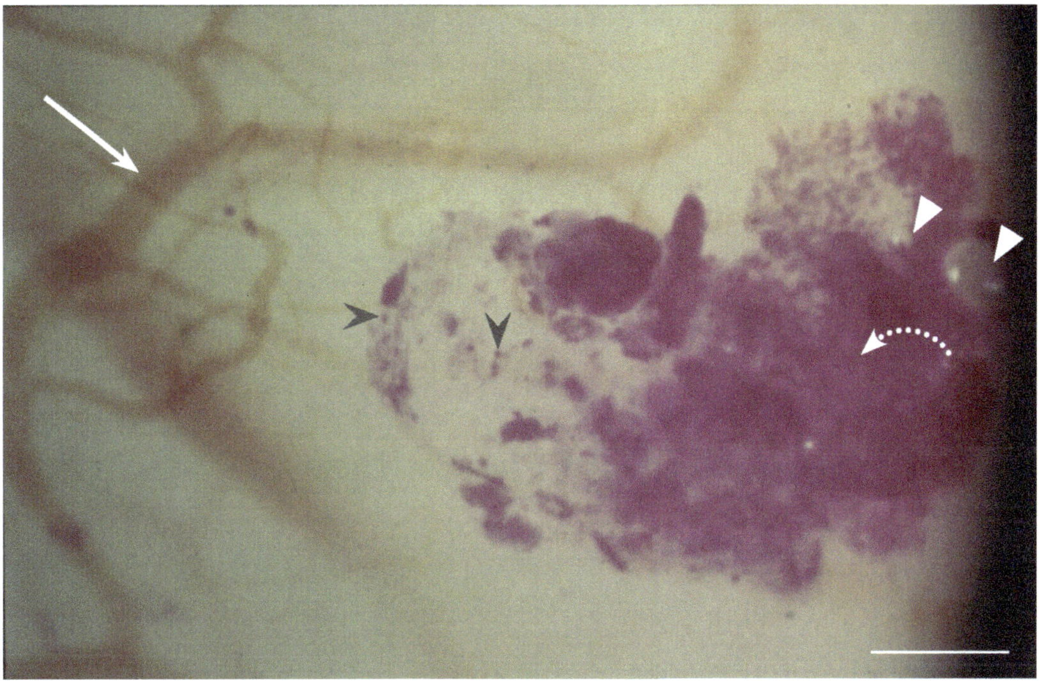

Fig. 1.3 An inhomogeneous rose bengal stained lump of amorphous material (*bowed arrow*) moving in the preconjunctival tear film; it contains granular debris (*grey arrowheads*) and air bubbles (*white arrowheads*). The *straight arrow* indicates a conjunctival vessel

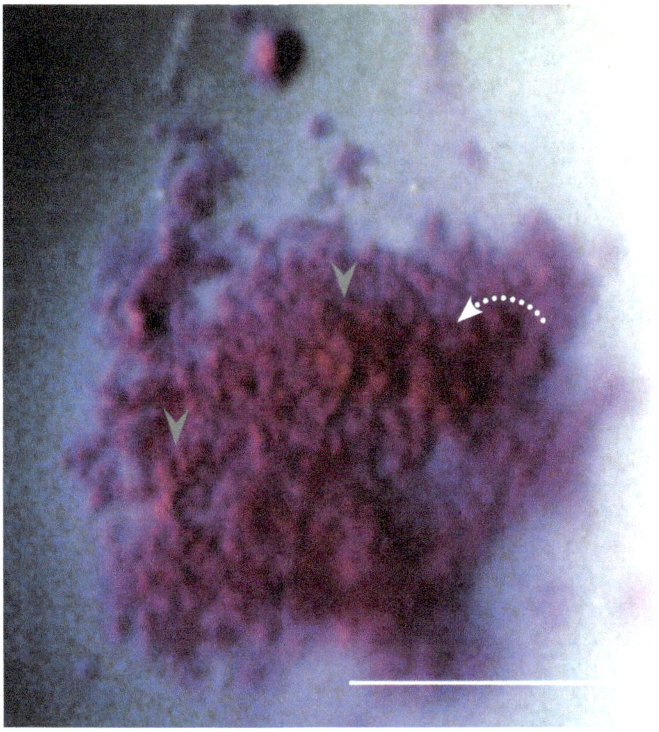

Fig. 1.4 A rose bengal stained lump (*arrow*) of granular debris (*arrowheads*) cemented together, possibly enmeshed in amorphous material (cf. Fig. 1.17) (Adapted from [3])

Mucus Sheets, Strands and Threads (1)

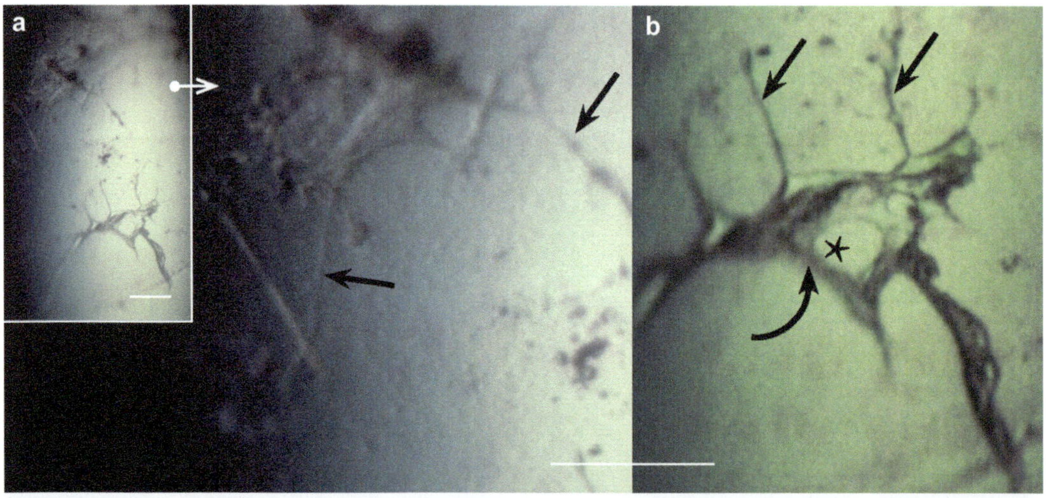

Fig. 1.5 *Inset*: Survey. (**a**) The left upper part shows intertwined thicker and thinner threads or strands (*arrows*), possibly adhering to the surface, and (**b**) the lower part an apparently free partly collapsed sheet (*bowed arrow*) with a central hole (*asterisk*) and with strands (*straight arrows*) emanating from the sheet (**b** Adapted from [3])

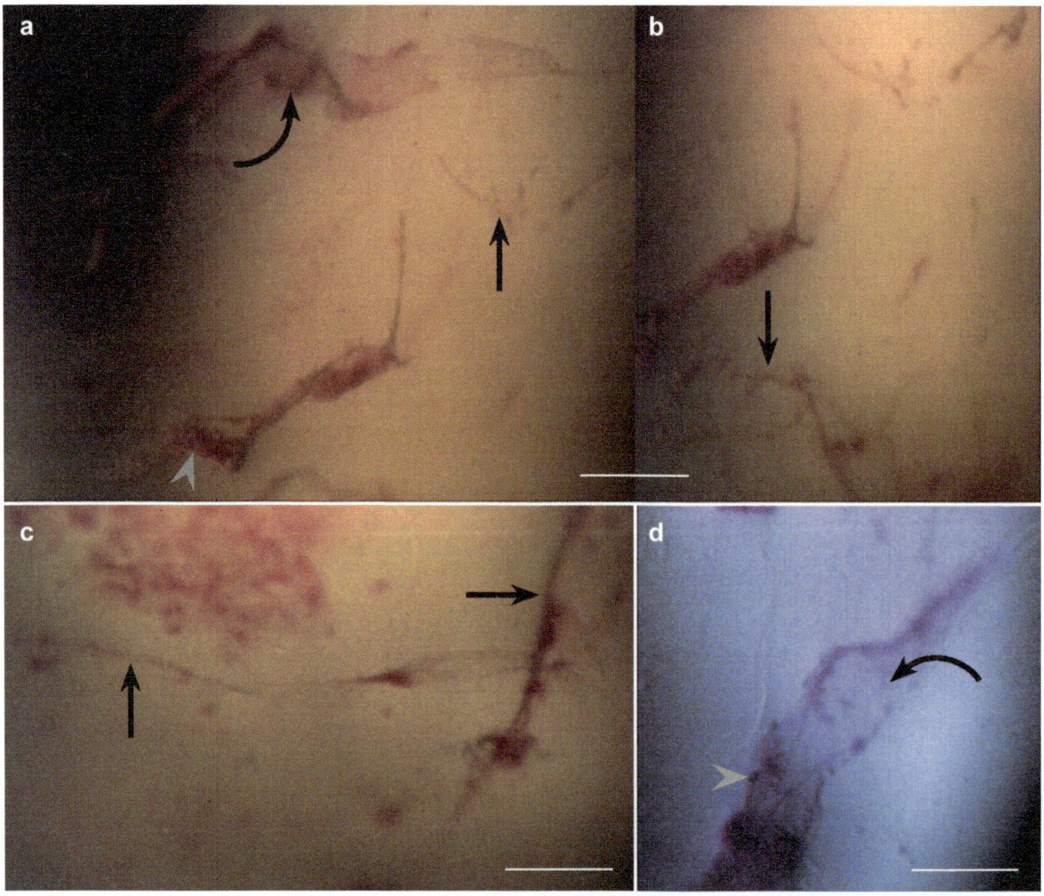

Mucus Sheets, Strands and Threads (2)

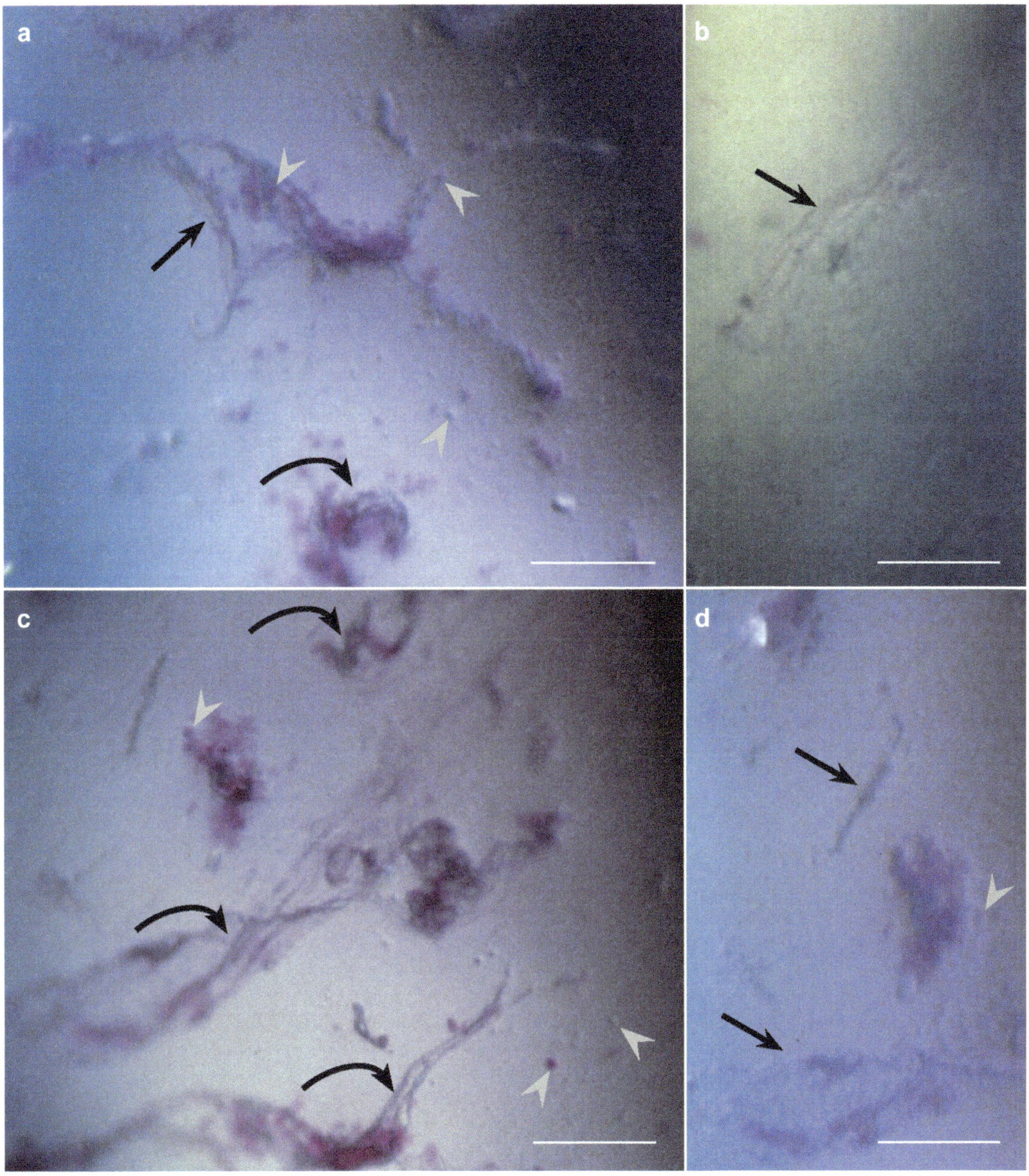

Fig. 1.7 (a–d) Strands (*straight arrows*), larger or smaller pieces of twisted, folded or crumpled sheets (*bowed arrows*) carrying rose bengal stained or unstained granulae (*arrowheads*); such granulae are also visible outside them (*arrowheads*)

Fig. 1.6 (a, b) Two consecutive photographs capturing (a) a crumpled sheet (*bowed arrow*) of which the right part seems torn off, a complex structure implying a crumpled or twisted sheet enveloping a partly granular cell debris (*arrowhead*) and some finer threads (*straight arrow*); in (b) are visible additional threads (*arrow*). (c) shows variously thick threads (*arrows*) carrying a small amount of stained material, and (d) a part of a crumpled sheet (*arrow*) with cell debris (*arrowhead*). Cf. Fig. 1.7. (Rose bengal)

Mucus Sheets, Strands and Threads (3)

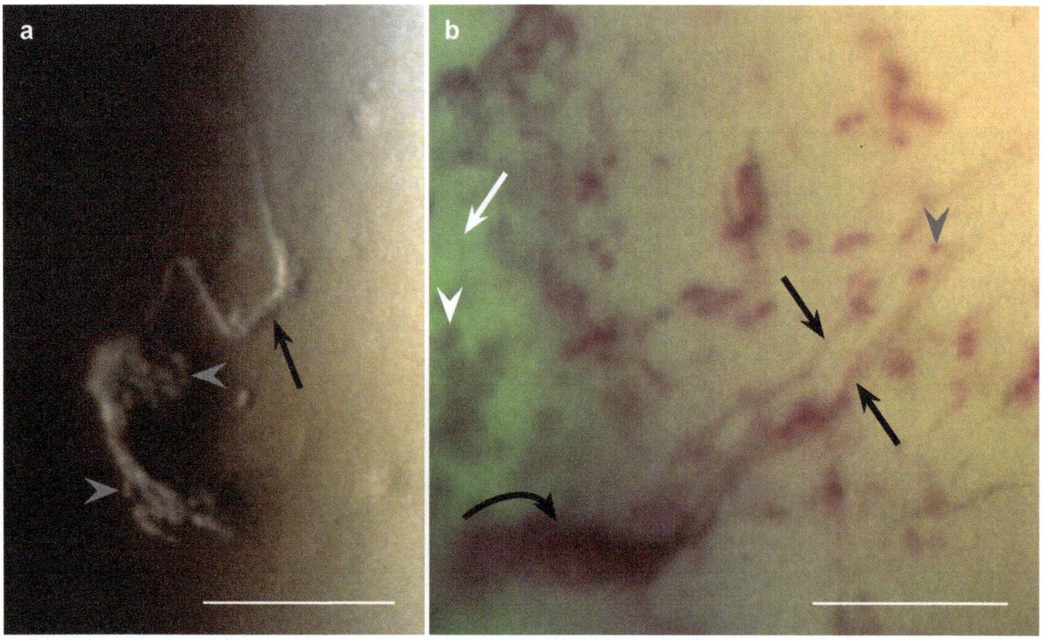

Fig. 1.8 (a) A crumpled strand (*arrow*) carrying granular material (*arrowheads*). In (b) is visible a clump of rose bengal stained material (*bowed arrow*) and threads (*arrows*) emanating from it; in the background is visible rose bengal staining of surface cells (*white arrowhead*) and cell debris (*grey arrowhead*); the *white arrow* indicates fluorescein diffusion into the tissues (green)

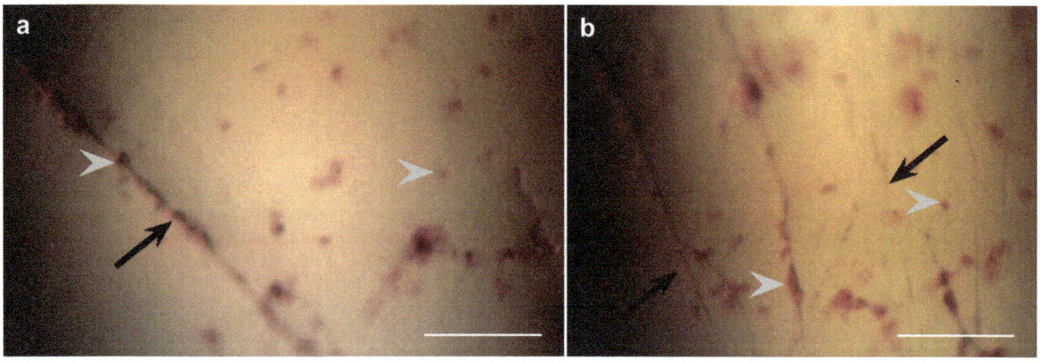

Fig. 1.9 (a, b) Rose bengal stained granular cell debris (*arrowheads*) lying on the surface or attached to thicker and thinner threads (*arrows*)

Fig. 1.11 (a, b) shows a long and thick strand (*arrows*), probably a result of a collapsed sheet, which has changed orientation while moving on the surface with blinks (a Adapted from [4])

Dynamics of Mucus Sheets, Strands and Threads

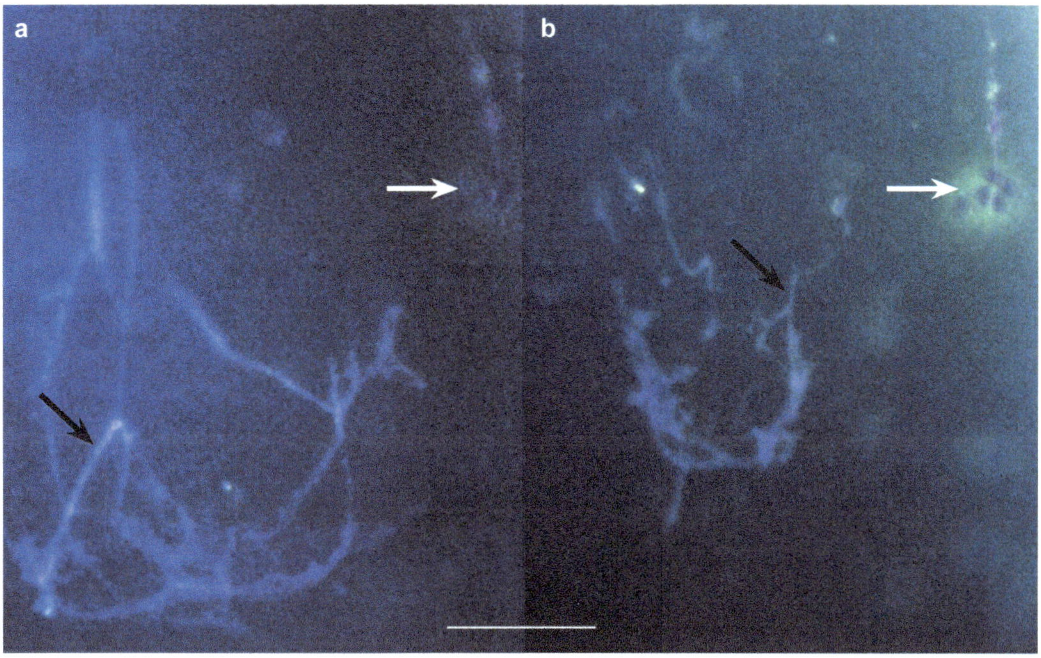

Fig. 1.10 (a, b) A figure consisting of light-reflecting intertwined strands (*black arrows*); it has (b) collapsed after a blink. The *white arrows* indicate a small green fleck with an attached minifilament (cf. Part II). (The white arrows are placed in corresponding locations; fluorescein and rose bengal)

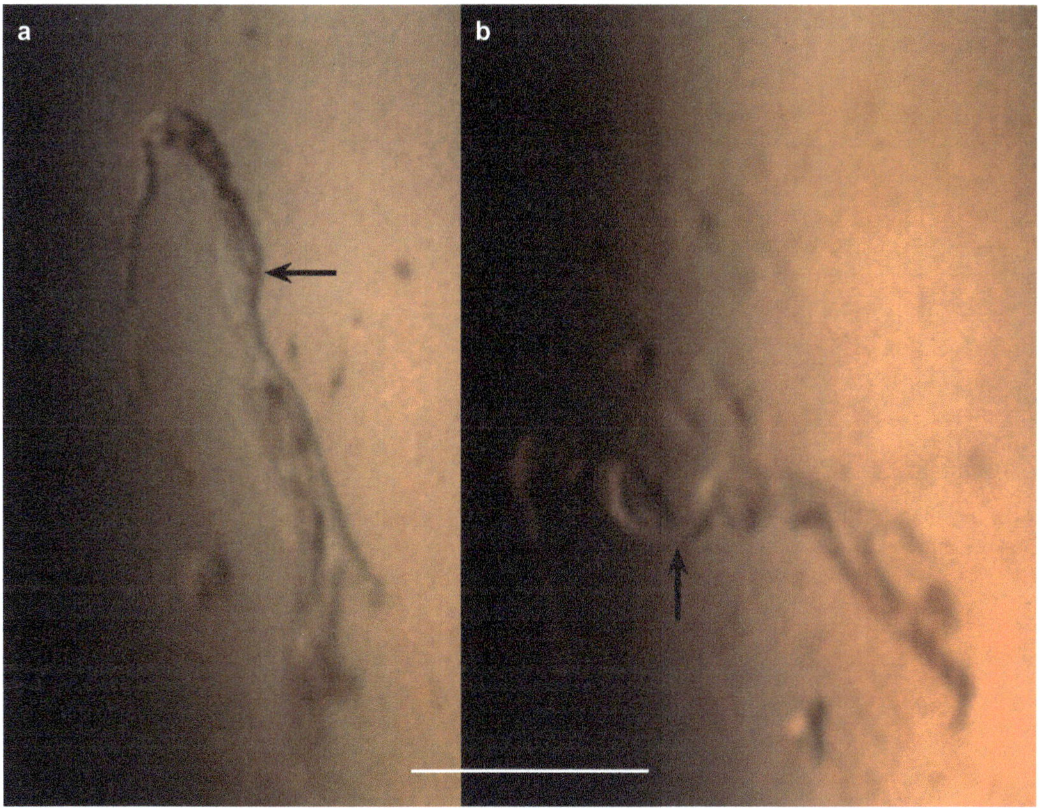

Complex Figures (1)

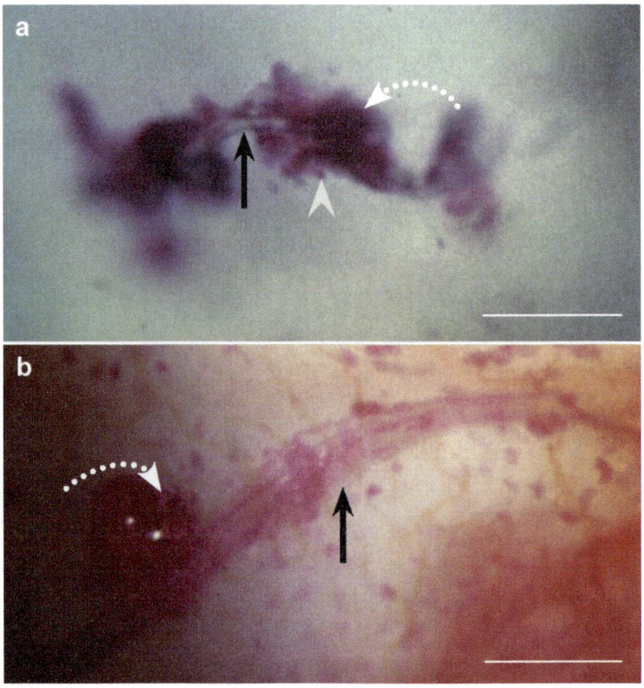

Fig. 1.12 (**a**) A thread (*straight arrow*) with adhering granular debris (*arrowhead*) enmeshed in amorphous material (*bowed arrow*). (**b**) Several parallel threads or a crumpled mucus sheet (*straight arrow*) with an attached lump of amorphous material (*bowed arrow*). (Rose bengal)

Fig. 1.13 (**a**) The *inset* shows a survey of the figure; in the left part is visible its light-reflecting property. (**a–d**) Mucus strands and threads (*straight arrows*) with attached amorphous material (*bowed arrows*); the *arrowheads* indicate air bubbles. (Fluorescein and rose bengal)

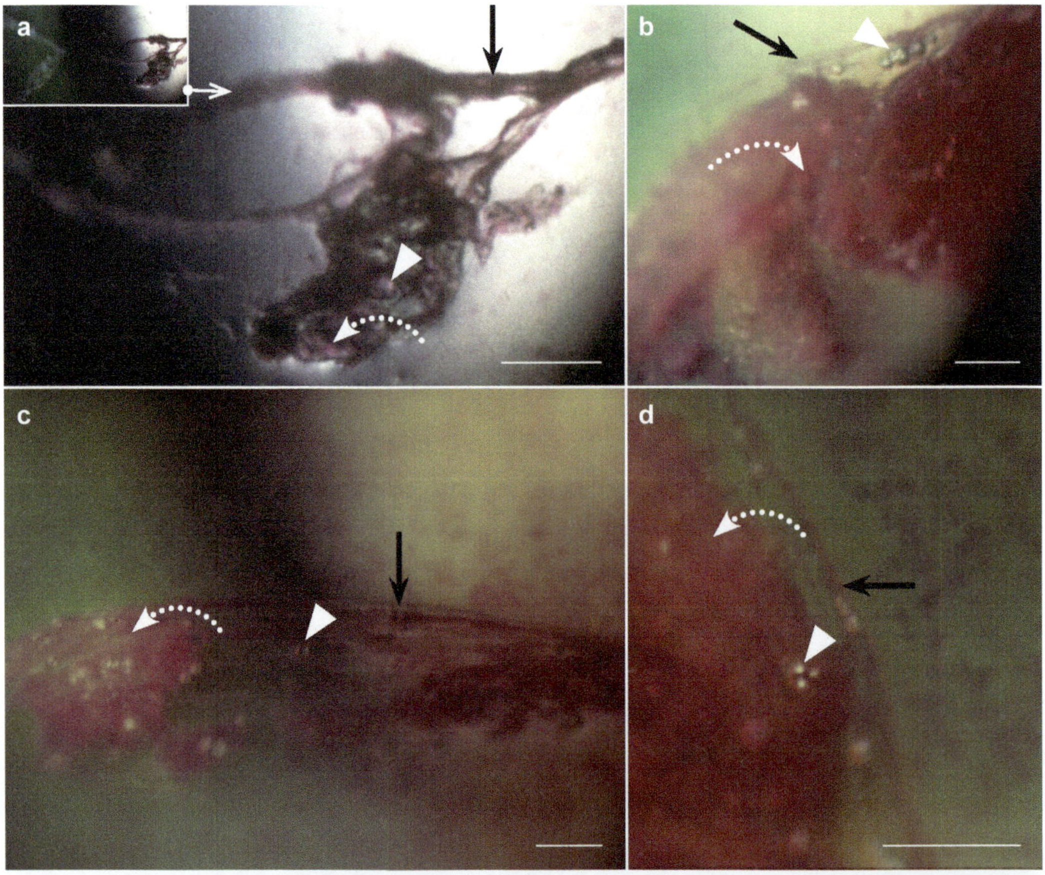

Complex Figures (2)

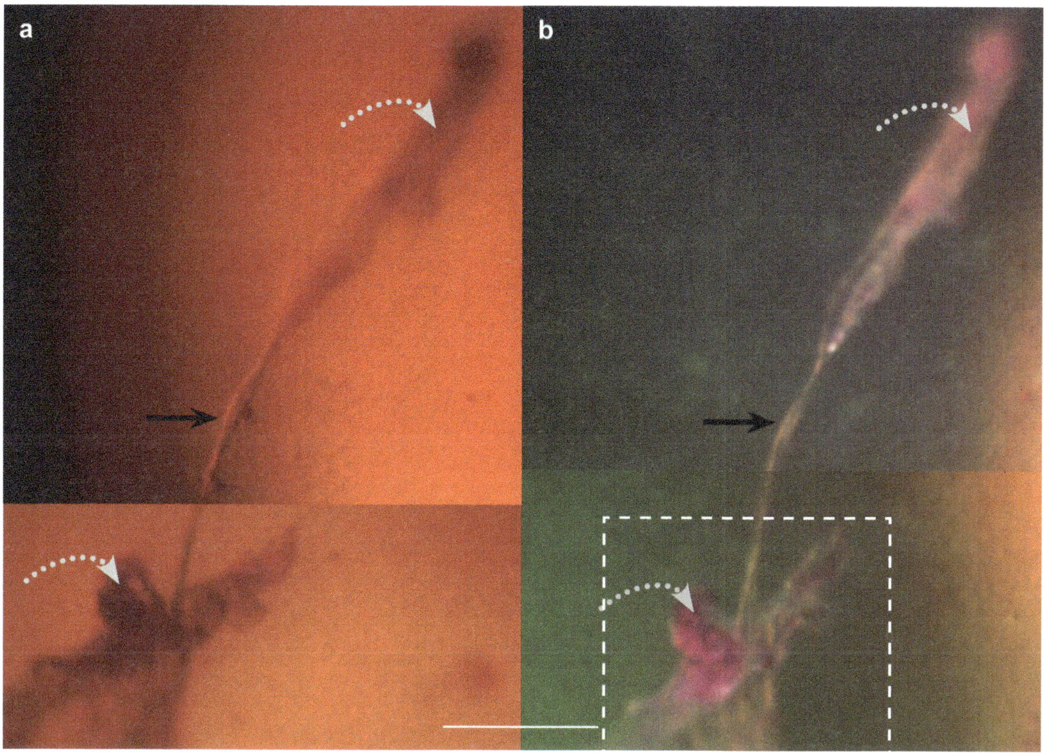

Fig. 1.14 (a, b) The long thread (*straight arrows*) with attached red stained material (*bowed arrows*) is the upper part of a large figure. The area in *frame* is shown in Fig. 1.15a. (Composed photographs; fluorescein and rose bengal)

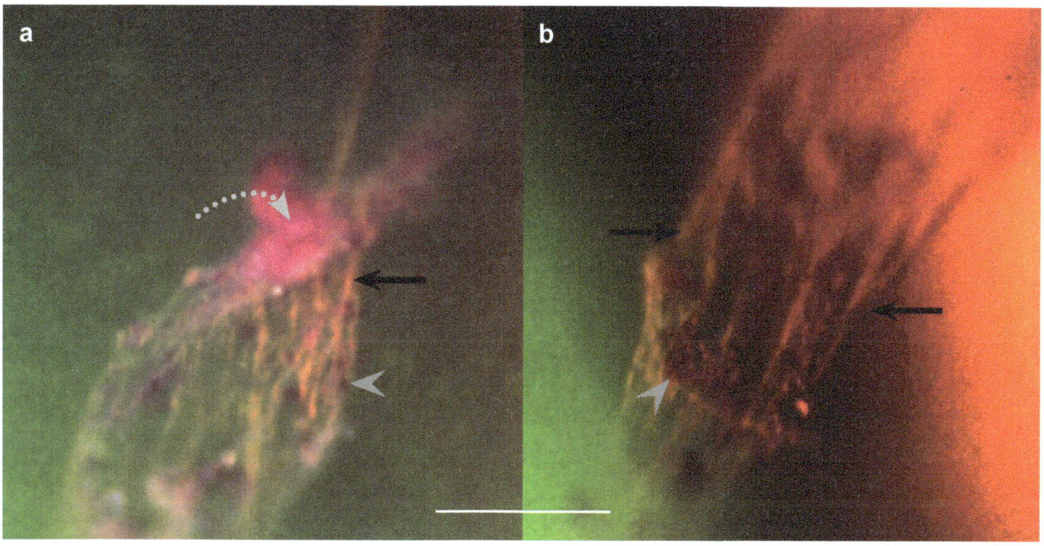

Fig. 1.15 (a) In the area indicated by frame in Fig. 1.14b are visible threads (*straight arrow*) granular debris (*arrowhead*) and a red stained lump of attached material; the pinkish hue of rose bengal is due to the material's light-reflecting property. (b) The lower part of the figure shows threads (*arrows*) and granular debris (*arrowhead*)

Tear Film Mucus and Ocular Surface (1)

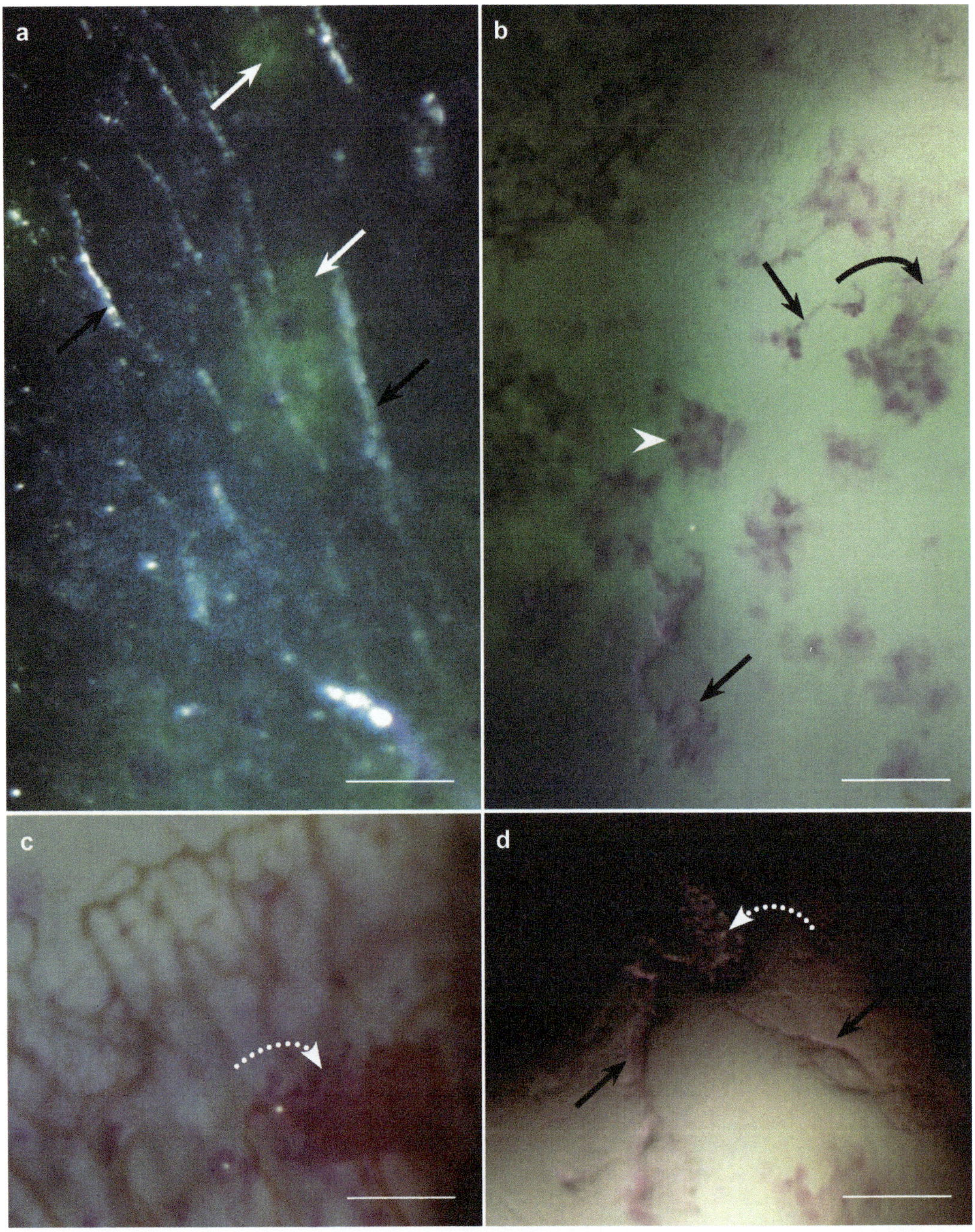

Fig. 1.16 Tear film mucus captured at the same occasion: (a) Light-reflecting threads (*black arrows*) lying upon a surface which shows fluorescein stained flecks (green, *white arrows*). (b) Threads (*straight arrows*) and a piece of a crumpled sheet (*bowed arrow*) visible against green background caused by fluorescein diffusion into the tissues; the surface shows rose bengal stained cells (*arrowhead*). (c) A lump of amorphous material (*arrow*) at the corneal limbus. (d) A lump with granular appearance (*bowed arrow*) and long threads (*straight arrows*)

Tear Film Mucus and Ocular Surface (2)

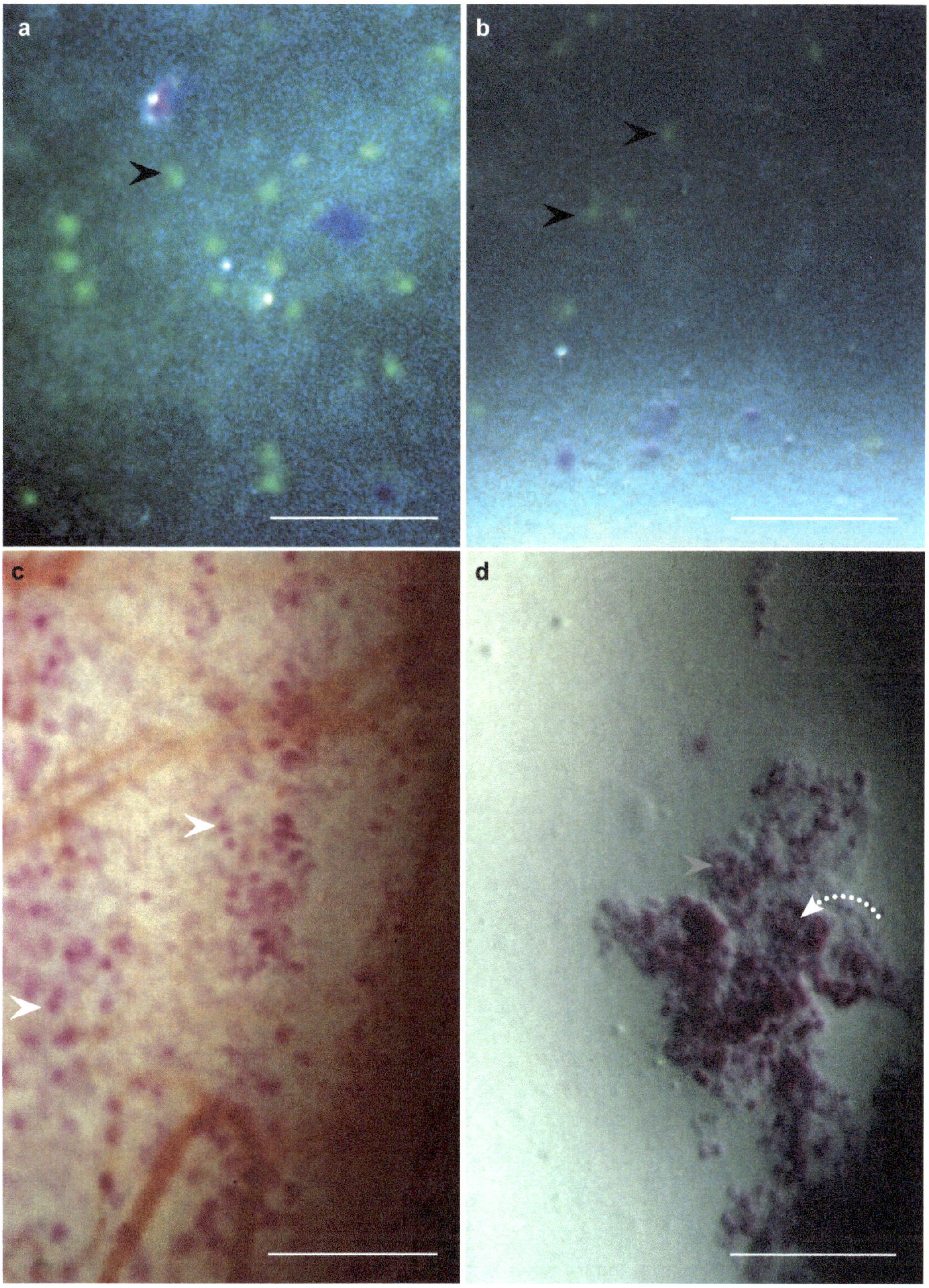

Fig. 1.17 In this patient, the cornea (a, b) shows fluorescein stained dots (green, *arrowheads*) but very little rose bengal staining. (c) On the conjunctiva are visible many rose bengal stained surface cells (*arrowheads*); some of the deeply red stained dots might represent cell nuclei. (d) A lump (*arrow*) in the precorneal tear film containing many red stained granulae (*arrowhead*)

The Corneal Surface 2

Surface phenomena captured in KCS indicate diseased surface cells, epithelial oedema, mucus adherence, and disruptions of surface integrity. Of these, some or all may be present at the same time. The changes are usually most pronounced in the interpalpebral area but the whole surface may be involved.

Before staining are visible greyish surface cells, either spread over the surface or in rows and groups; cystic spaces; strongly light-reflecting mucus adhering to the surface; and filaments.

Fluorescein sodium shows a *dual staining property,* a non-fluorescent and a fluorescent one. The *punctate non-fluorescent* staining (yellow-brown) reveals diseased surface cells. The *fluorescent* (green) one reveals penetration of fluid into: (1) *circumscript spaces* – the resulting *punctate fluorescent staining* visualises diseased surface cells (probably by penetration below them) and cystic spaces; and (2) the *tissues* – the resulting *flecks* indicate surface disruptions. *Rose bengal* stains diseased surface cells red.

Hence, with the two dyes, *diseased surface cells* are visualised in three modes: as *yellow-brown dots* (with non-fluorescent fluorescein), as *green dots* (with fluorescent fluorescein) and as *red dots* (with rose bengal). Basically, all reveal the same cells but with the green dots it might be difficult to distinguish surface cells from other cystic spaces (such as those due to epithelial oedema) visualised at the same time. With non-fluorescent fluorescein, the cells show various staining densities but no further details (an exception are brighter dots surrounded by a narrow brownish rim, captured only in two patients in connection with impaired corneal sensitivity). Also rose bengal shows various staining densities; additionally, the dye visualizes some cell details such as deeply stained dots interpreted as cell nuclei; also cell borders and cell fragments are easier to discern with rose bengal. The stained cells, whether with non-fluorescent fluorescein or rose bengal, may be present individually or in rows and groups, and the staining may be confluent. They measure about 30 μm in diameter, often less (about 15–20 μm, exceptionally more (about 45 μm)). The non-fluorescent staining is relatively short-lived and usually transforms into the fluorescent one; this phenomenon is difficult or impossible to observe against a green background caused by fluorescein diffusion. Rose bengal staining persists much longer, and occasionally some cells become displaced or disappear after the application of the dye.

Epithelial oedema manifests as cystic spaces of which many stain brilliantly green with fluorescein.

Mucus adhering to the surface appears as more or less strongly light-reflecting dots, lumps, and patches; smaller or larger sheets, some showing holes, rolled-up edges, and emanating strands; and thinner or thicker threads, often intertwined. With fluorescein, it appears yellow. With rose bengal, strongly light-reflecting mucus shows a brightly red or pinkish hue in focal illumination; its dark appearance in retroillumination indicates a light-obstructing property. Occasionally, some strands seem not to stain (see also Part II).

H.M. Tabery, *Keratoconjunctivitis Sicca and Filamentary Keratopathy*,
DOI 10.1007/978-3-642-31028-7_2, © Springer-Verlag Berlin Heidelberg 2012

Disruptions of surface integrity are visualised with fluorescein as *green flecks*. With the slit lamp, their development after the application of fluorescein can often be predicted by the presence of patches of greyish surface cells but they appear also in inconspicuous areas. There may be only a few, developing slowly, or many, developing rapidly. Flecks situated close to each other may rapidly float together with large green areas with diffuse, often undulating borders as a result. The flecks show surface cells staining with non-fluorescent fluorescein and rose bengal. Larger flecks may show many small cells with prominent nuclei and often also patches of surface-adherent mucus; small flecks sometimes show small filaments attached to them.

The flecks show also *rounded bodies*, measuring about 9–12 μm, and similar bodies are often present also outside them. Only rarely such rounded bodies were captured concentrated in small areas reminiscent of infiltrates occurring in the acute stage of adenovirus epithelial keratitis or Thygeson's superficial punctate keratitis but lacking the strong light-reflecting property. Their nature is unclear as with the present method cells with altered membranes, incipient cell swelling, invading inflammatory cells (and in KCS perhaps also epithelial oedema with small intercellular cystic spaces, cell and mucus fragments) would appear similar. For these reasons, I have chosen to term them 'rounded bodies' throughout (see also 'Final Remark').

The application of fluorescein is painless, and the dye has no known *adverse effects* on the corneal epithelium. Rose bengal has a stinging property, and after its application in eyes preinstalled with fluorescein appear myriads of green dots in corneae previously appearing normal or showing only a few green dots. This striking effect is probably caused by disruption of intercellular junctions allowing the green fluid to penetrate below the cells. (There is one more phenomenon occurring after the application of rose bengal – an appearance of rounded bodies the nature of which is unclear.)

Included in this chapter are also some sources of possible diagnostic errors: surface staining appearing in areas of *damage unrelated to KCS* (such as in trichiasis) or in *iatrogenic* damage caused by the paper strip used in the Schirmer test; green flecks showing similarity to those occurring in *herpes simplex* (but morphology observed before the application of the dye usually prevents confusion); and larger 'mucus plaques' in *herpes zoster ophthalmicus* epithelial keratitis (which differ from adhering mucus in KCS in that they do not show threads or strands).

Before Staining (1)

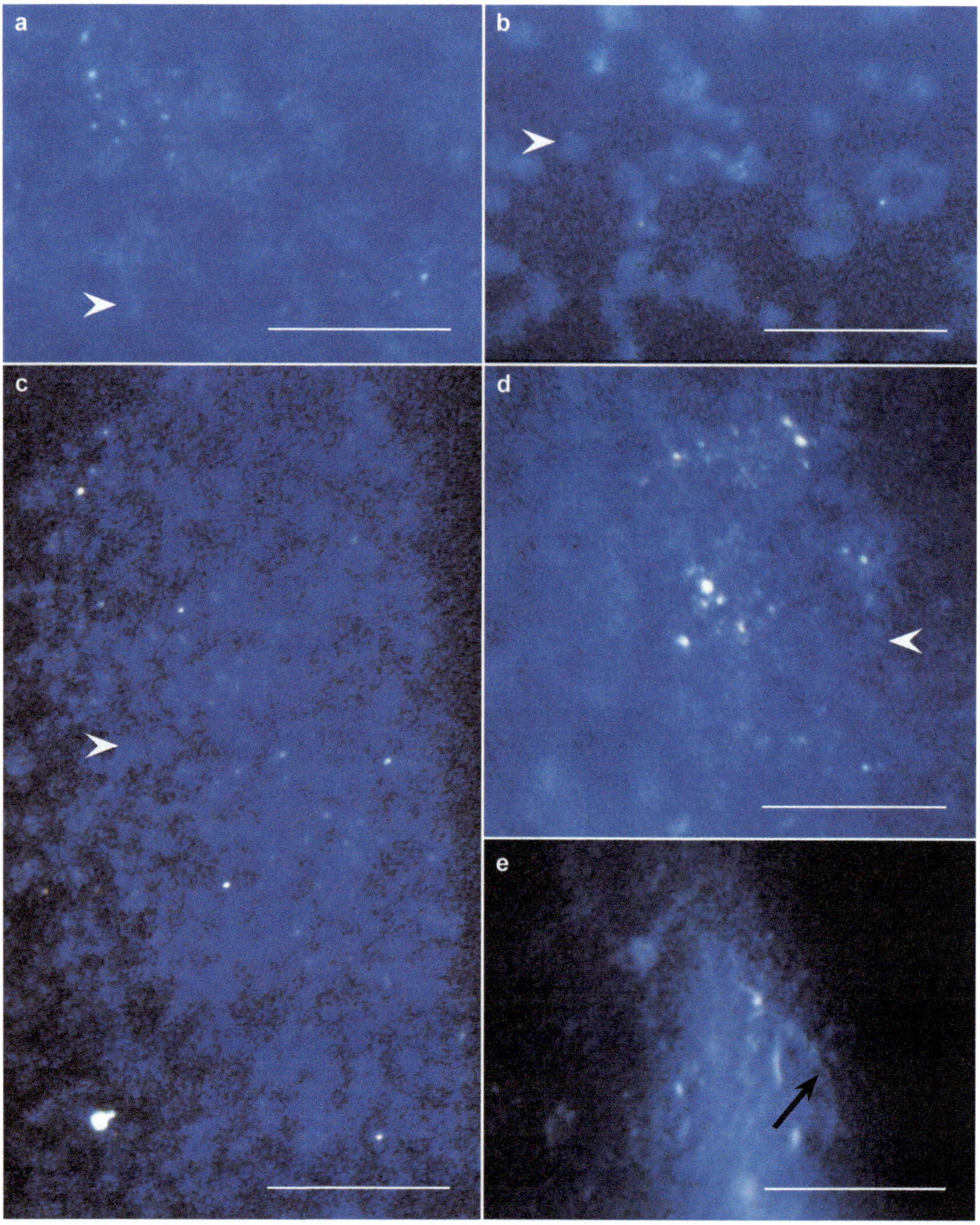

Fig. 2.1 (a–d) The epithelium shows many greyish surface cells (*arrowheads*), individual, in groups and rows, or confluent. In (e) is visible a mucus strand possibly adhering to the surface (*arrow*). The origin of the light-reflecting bright dots visible in all photographs is uncertain (cf. Fig. 4.20)

Before Staining (2)

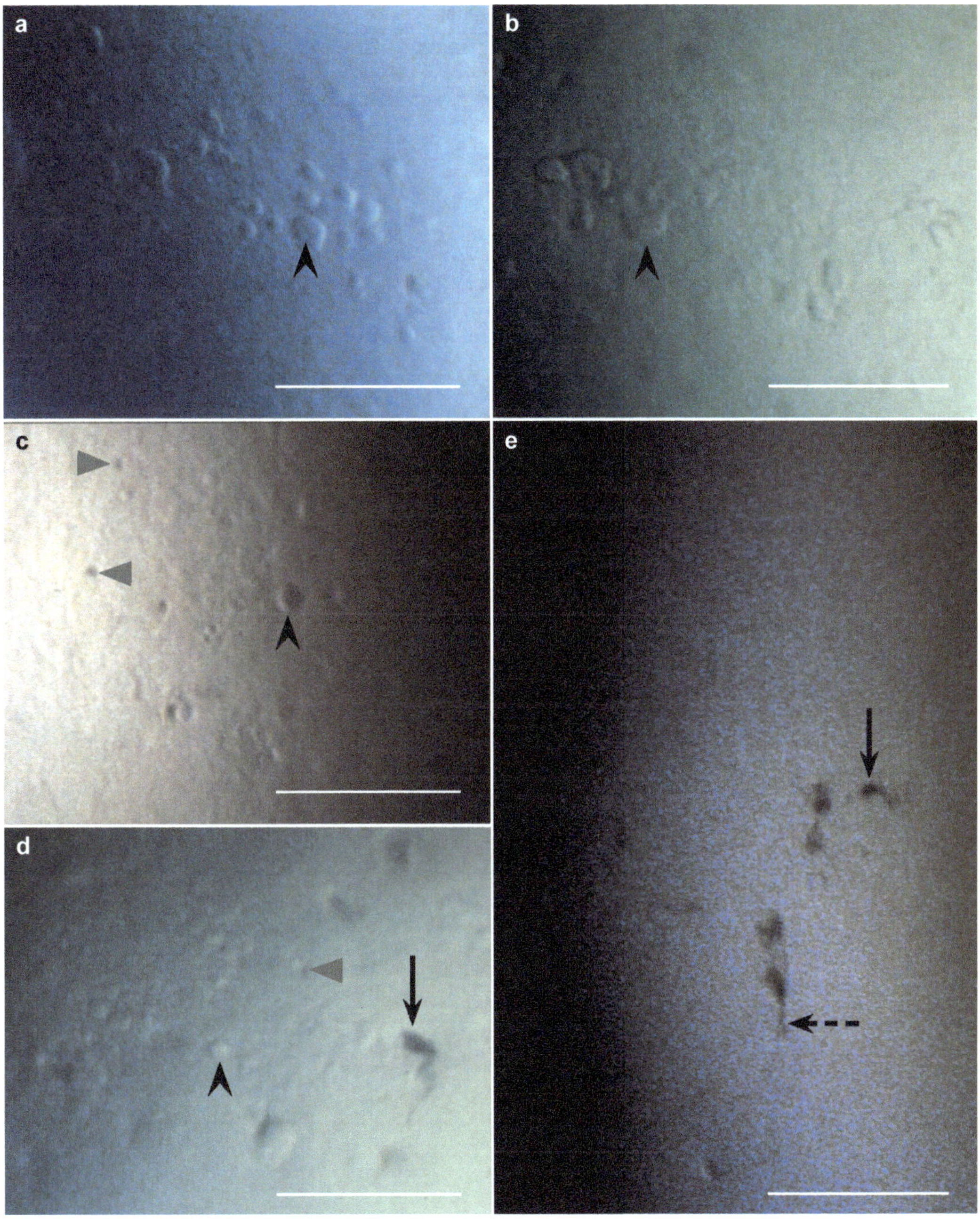

Fig. 2.2 (a–d) Larger and smaller epithelial cystic spaces (*black arrowheads*) and rounded bodies (c, d, *grey arrowheads*). In (d, e) are visible larger pieces of mucus (*plain arrows*); the *dashed arrow* in (e) indicates attachment point of a small filament (cf. Part II)

Punctate Non-fluorescent and Fluorescent Fluorescein Staining

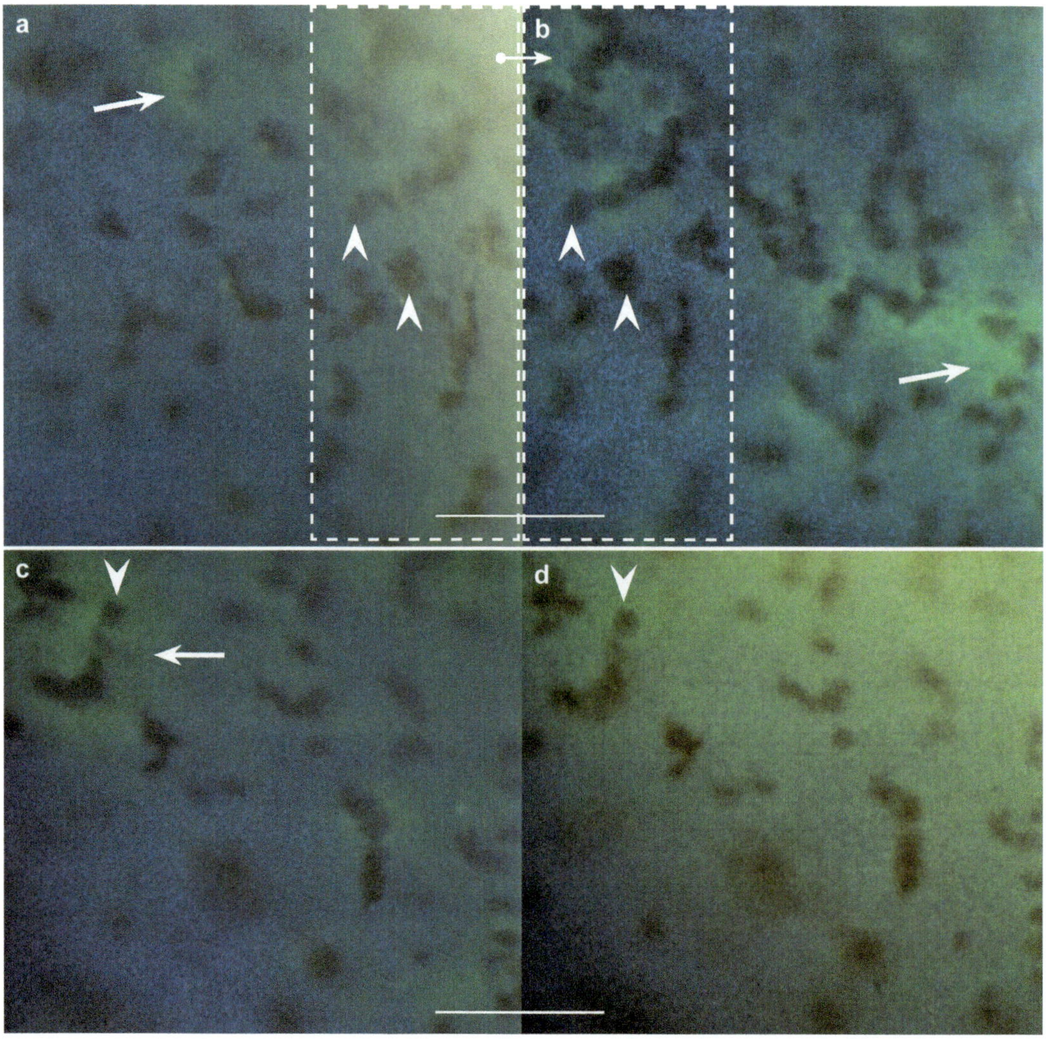

Fig. 2.3 Non-fluorescent fluorescein staining of diseased surface cells *(arrowheads)*, individual, in groups and rows. Depending on illumination, the hue varies between brownish and yellowish (cf. a, b, the area in *frame*, and c, d; the arrowheads are placed in corresponding locations). The *arrows* in (a–c) indicate incipient fluorescein diffusion into the tissues (green)

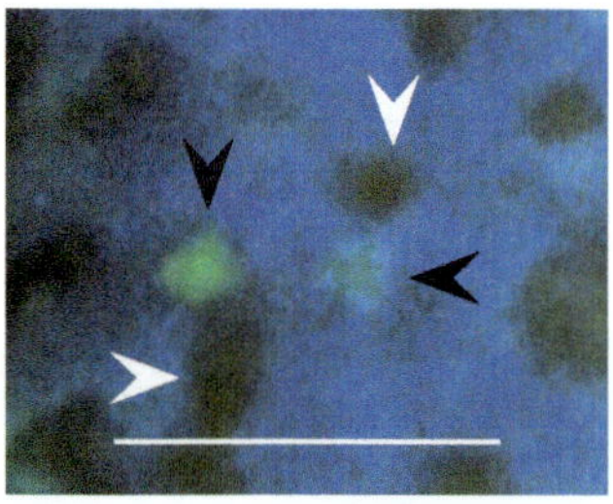

Fig. 2.4 The brownish hue of non-fluorescent staining of diseased surface cells (*white arrowheads*) contrasts with the green fluorescent one (*black arrowheads*) indicating cystic spaces

Dynamics of Punctate Fluorescein Staining (1)

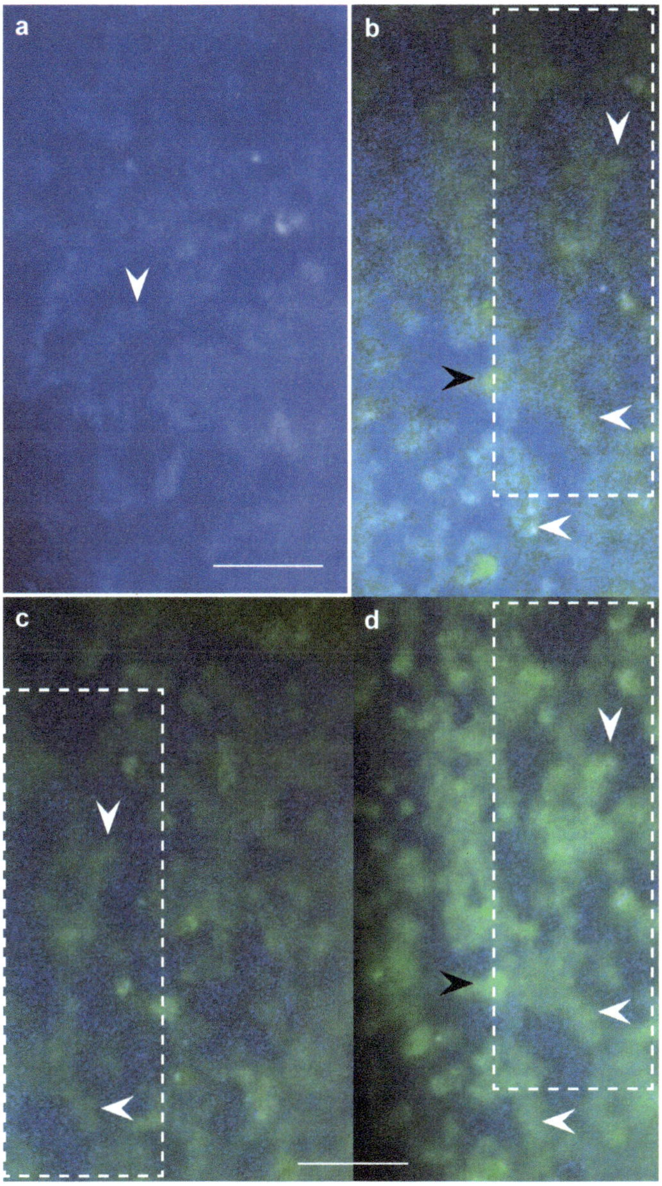

Fig. 2.5 (a) Greyish surface cells (*arrowhead*) visible before staining. (b) A different area of the same cornea. After the application of fluorescein is visible a mixture of fading non-fluorescent (yellow-brown) and incipient fluorescent (green) staining of surface cells (*white arrowheads*). Some of the more brilliantly green dots (*black arrowheads*) probably represent small cystic spaces (cf. Fig. 2.7). (c–d) The intensity of the green fluorescence increases with time; in this series, the staining seems limited to surface cells (*white arrowheads*) and cystic spaces (*black arrowheads*); so far, there is no diffusion into the stroma (cf. also Figs. 4.28, 4.29 and 4.31). (The *frames* in b–d indicate the same area; the arrowheads are placed in corresponding locations)

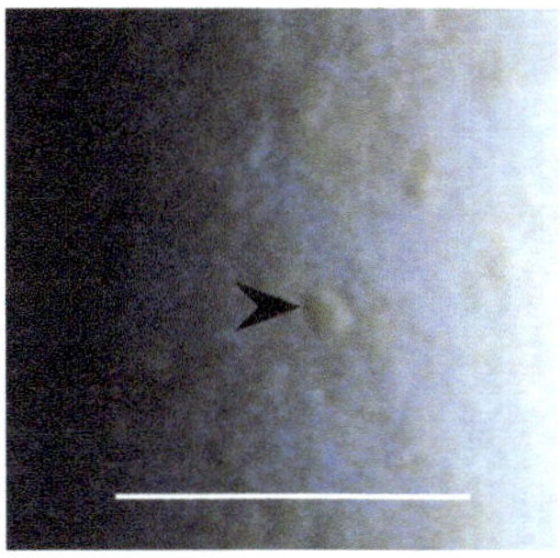

Fig. 2.6 A small cystic space (*arrowhead*) captured in the cornea shown in Fig. 2.5. The green fluorescence was not elicited in this illumination

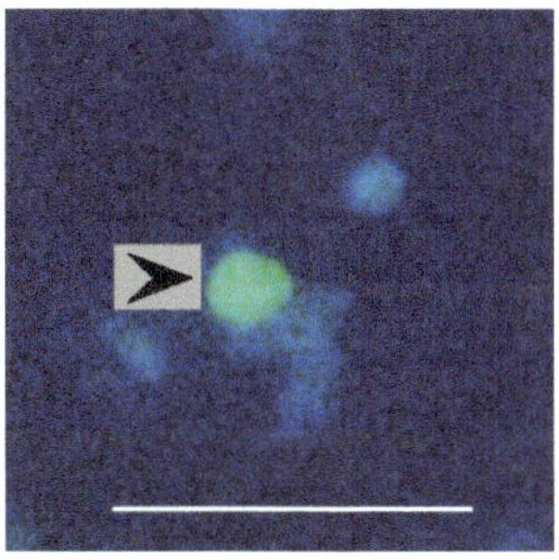

Fig. 2.7 A rounded cystic space (*arrowhead*) staining brilliantly green with fluorescein

Punctate Fluorescent Staining: Surface Cells Versus Cystic Spaces

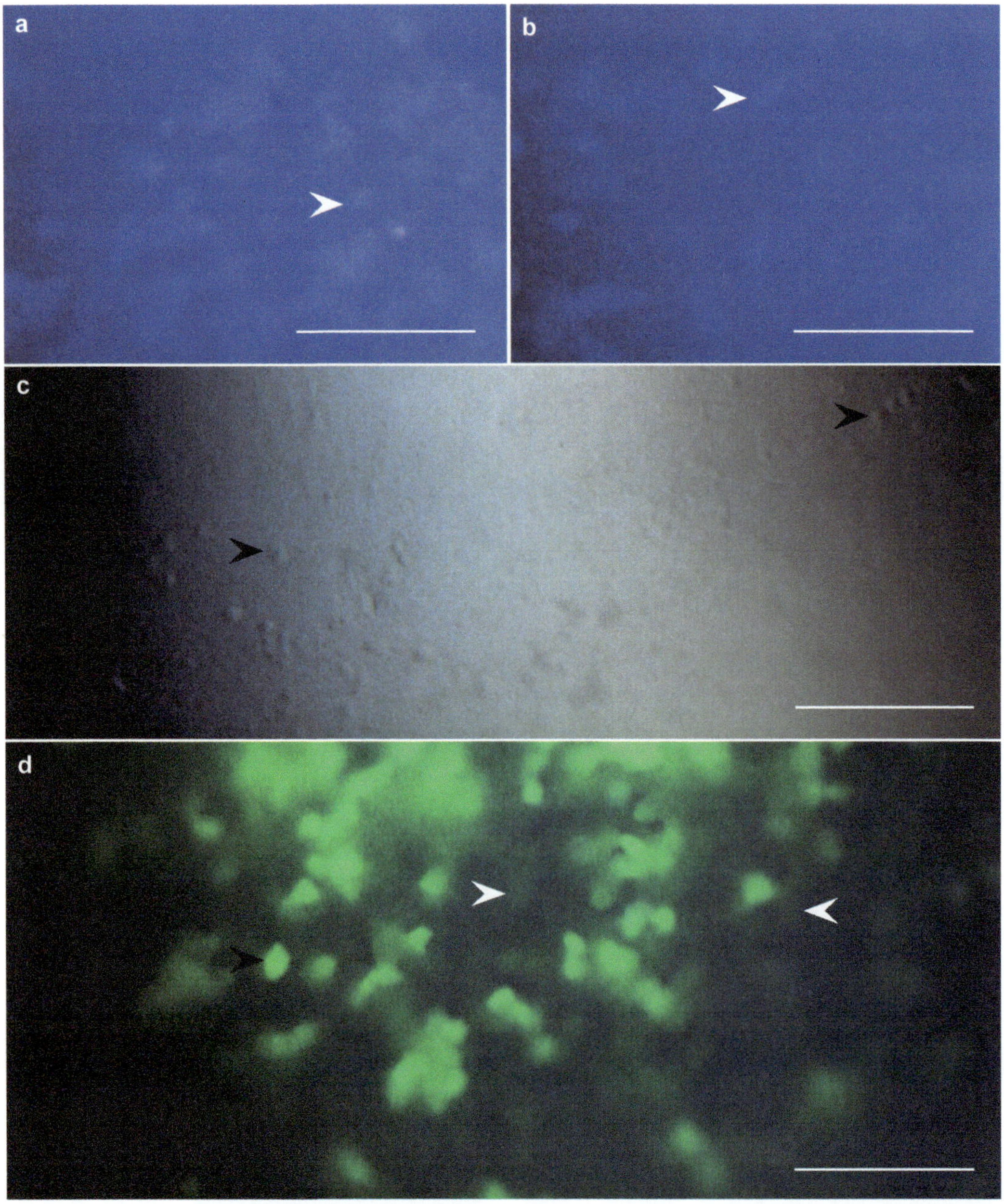

Fig. 2.8 This cornea shows (a, b) greyish surface cells (*arrowheads*) and (c) many cystic spaces (*arrowheads*). (d) After the application of fluorescein appeared many green dots; the hue varies between a brilliantly green visualising cystic spaces (*black arrowhead*) and darker one visualising surface cells (*white arrowheads*)

Dynamics of Punctate Fluorescein Staining (2)

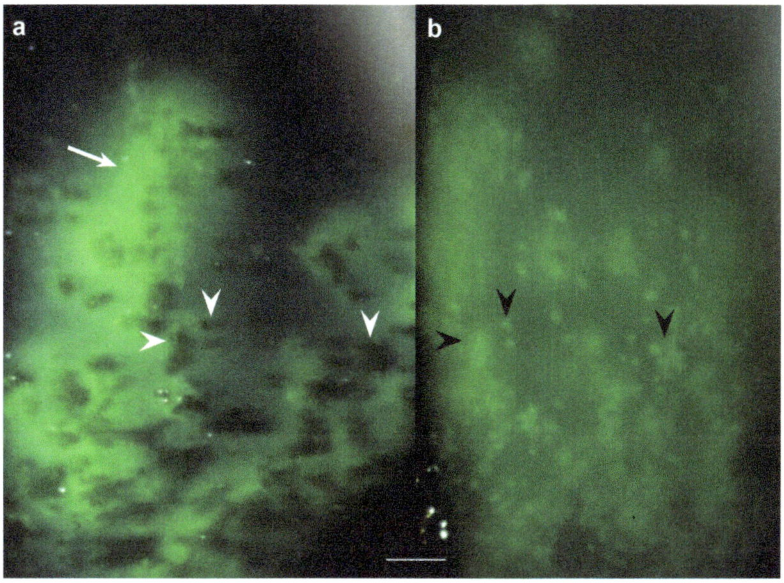

Fig. 2.9 (a) Non-fluorescent fluorescein staining of surface cells, individual or grouped (*arrowheads*) visible against green background caused by fluorescein diffusion into the tissues (*arrow*). (b) After a few minutes, the whole area appears as a green fleck; the non-fluorescent staining has transformed into a fluorescent one (green dots, *arrowheads*). (The arrowheads are placed in locations implying patterns similar to (a) but their correspondence is uncertain)

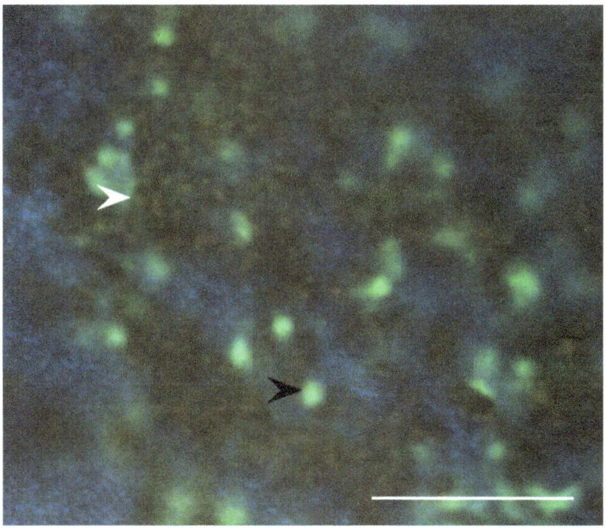

Fig. 2.10 A heavy and partly confluent non-fluorescent fluorescein staining showing many brighter dots (*white arrowhead*) surrounded by a thin darker rim. The circumscript brightly green staining indicates cystic spaces (*black arrowhead*)

Comment

An interpretation of this phenomenon captured only in two patients with impaired corneal sensitivity (cf. Figs. 4.32, 4.33, 5.2, 5.4 and 5.5) is left open.

Fluorescent (Green) Flecks in White Light

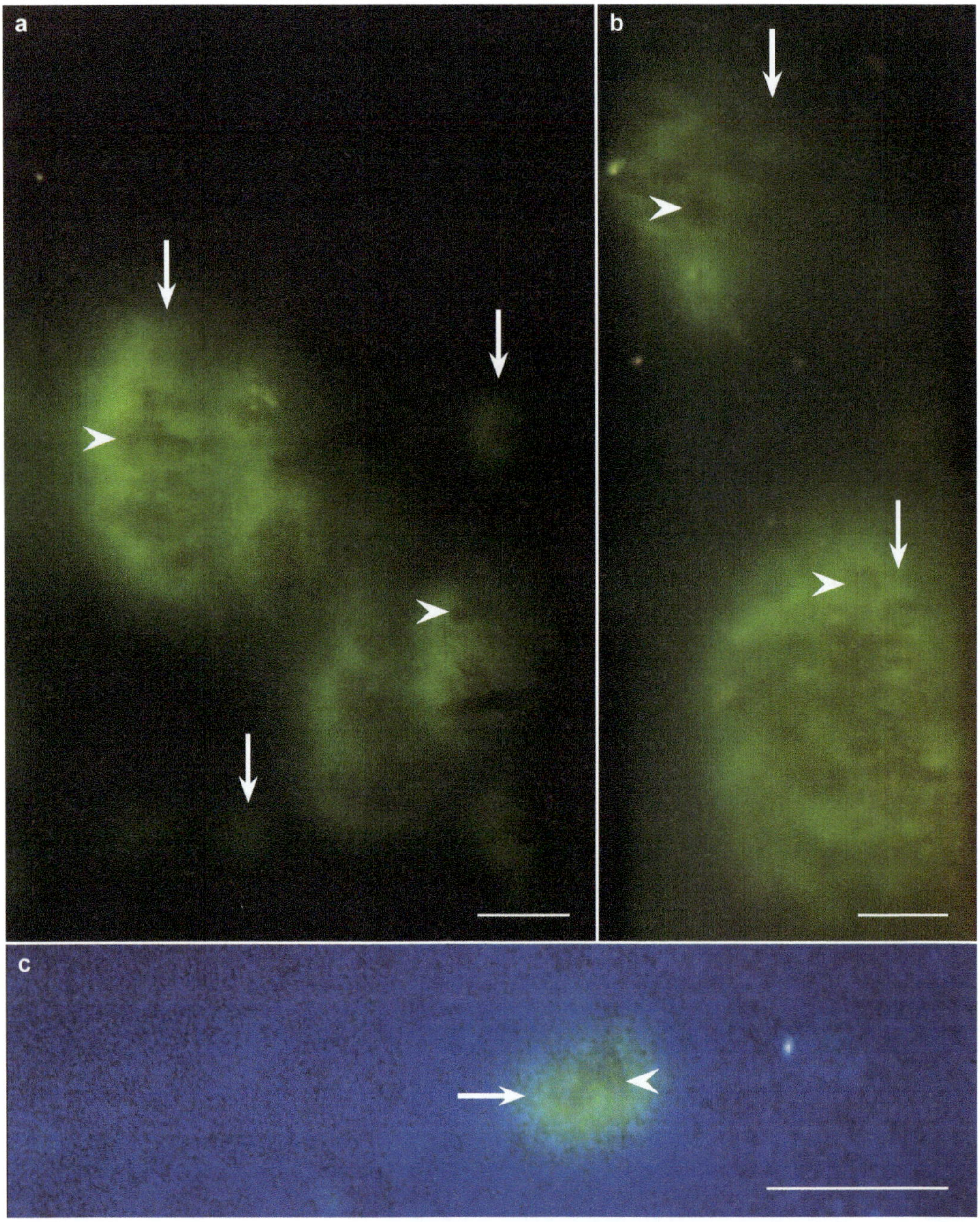

Fig. 2.11 (a–c) Fluorescent (green) flecks (*arrows*) are the result of diffusion of the dye into the tissues. Surface cells stained with non-fluorescent fluorescein (*arrowheads*) appear yellow-brown. In (a) is visible a confluence of several small flecks, (b) shows two larger flecks (*arrows*) and (c) a small solitary one

Fluorescent Flecks and Colour Filters (1)

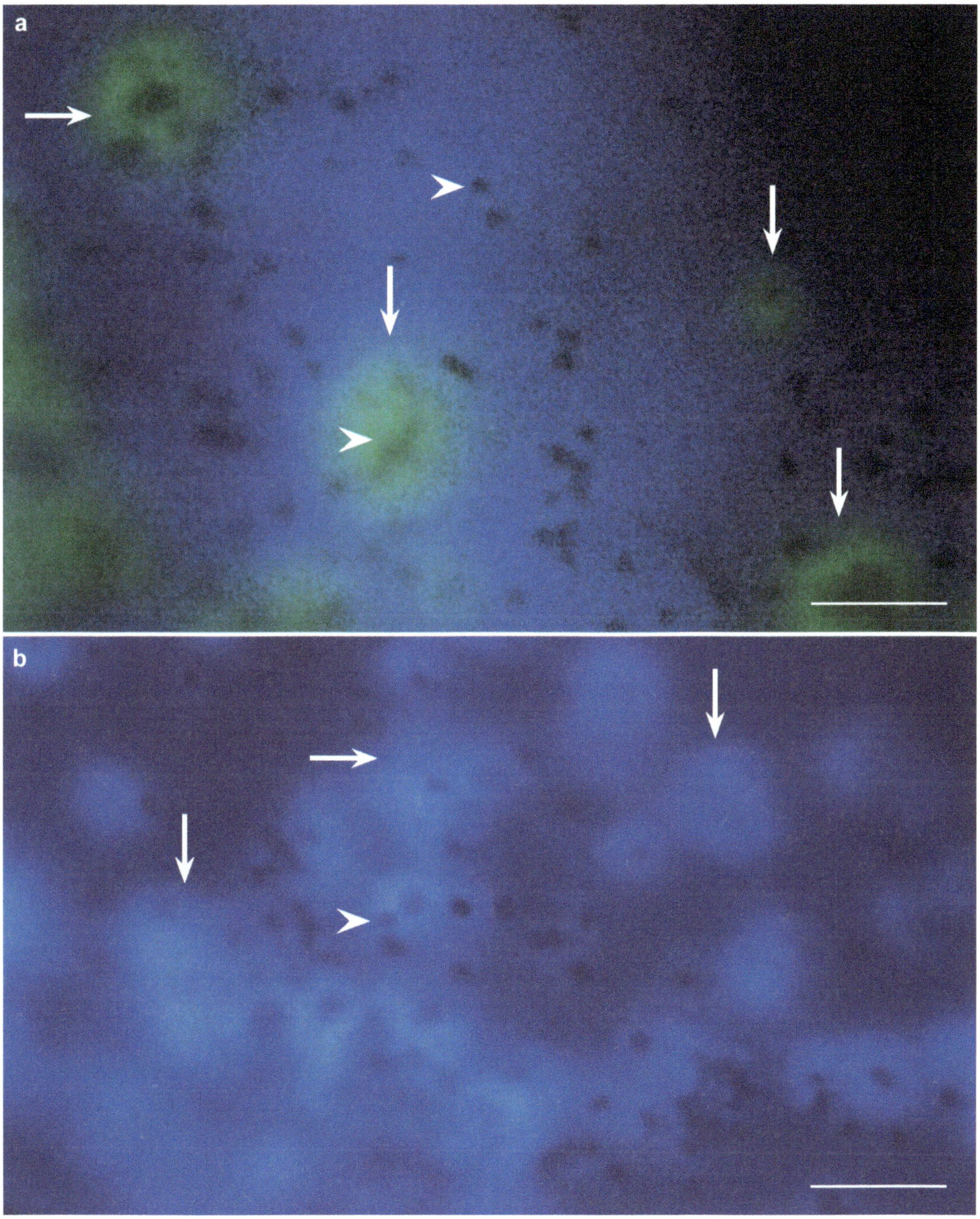

Fig. 2.12 (a, b) Fluorescent flecks (*arrows*) and non-fluorescent stained surface cells (*arrowheads*). (a) With the *green filter*, the cells are visible both within the flecks and outside them. (b) With the *blue filter*, the cells are well visible against the bright background created by the flecks but difficult to discern outside them. Also in these photographs is visible the propensity to confluence of the flecks. Cf. also Figs. 2.13 and 2.14

Fluorescent Flecks and Colour Filters (2)

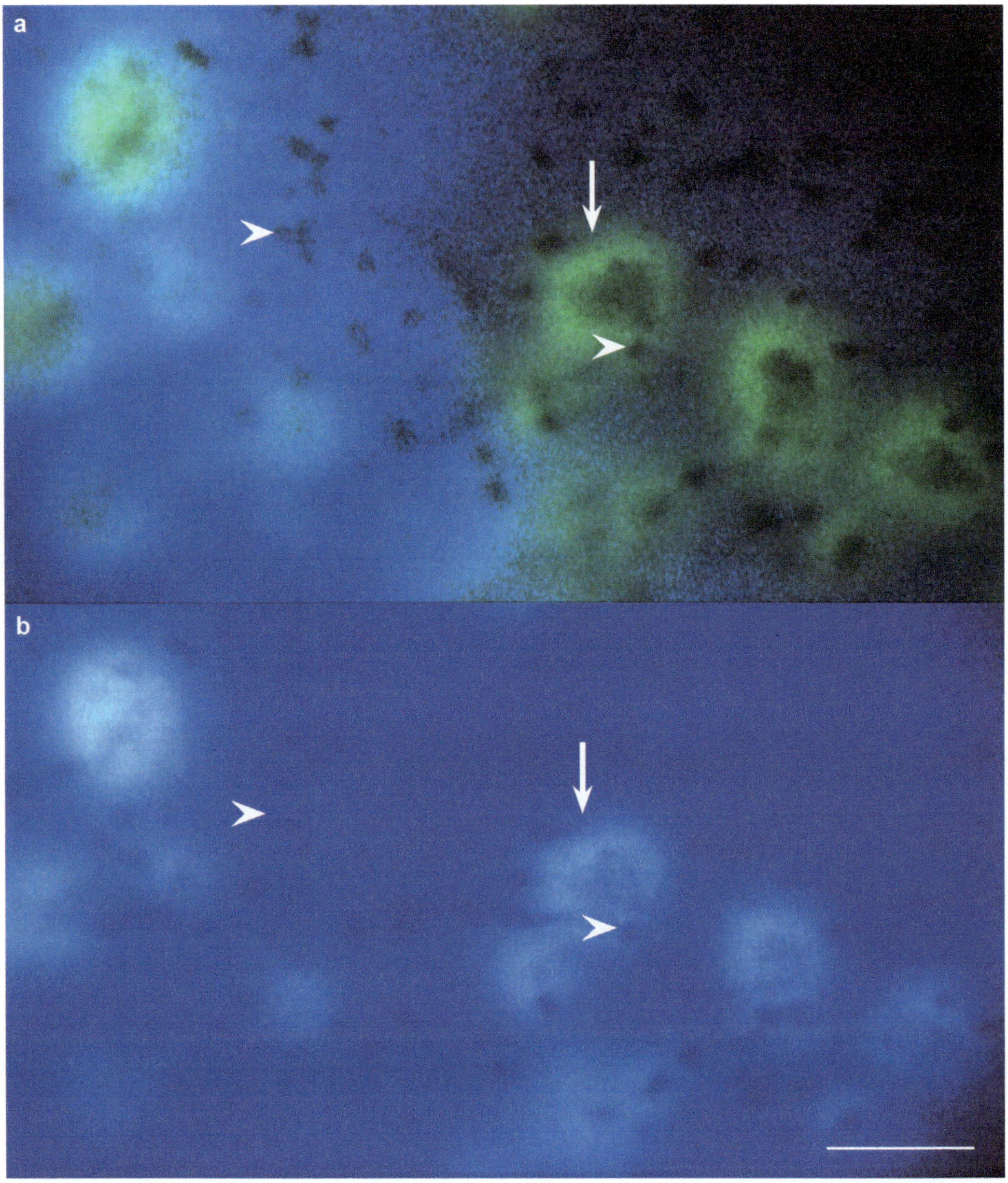

Fig. 2.13 (**a**, **b**) The same area showing fluorescent flecks (*arrows*) and non-fluorescent stained surface cells (*arrowheads*) captured with (**a**) the *green* and (**b**) the *blue filter*. The cells outside the flecks are better visible with the green filter. (The markers are placed in corresponding locations)

The Dynamics of Fluorescent Flecks; Stromal Diffusion

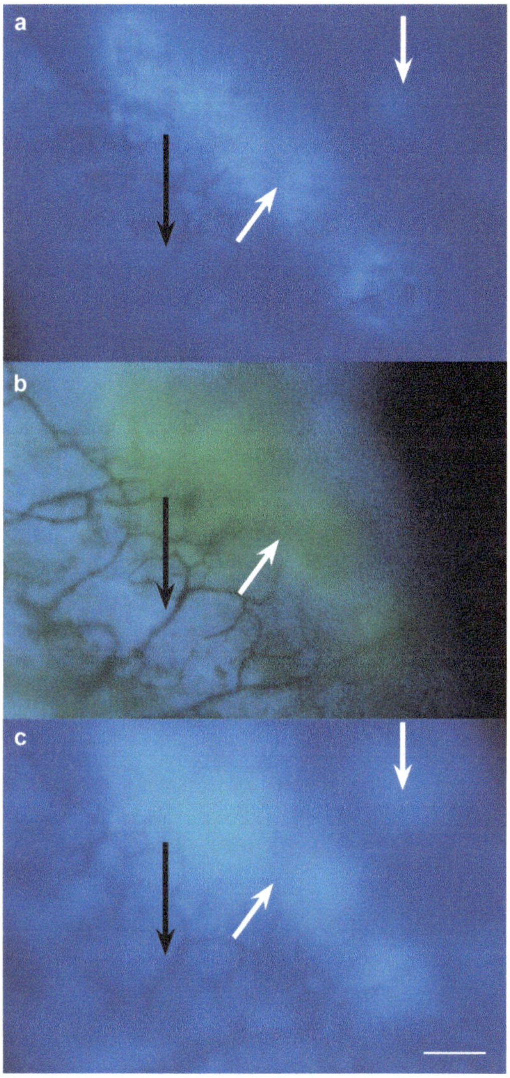

Fig. 2.14 In the strongly light-reflecting limbal area, fluorescent flecks (*arrows*) are better visible with either the blue (a and c) or the green (b) filter than in white light. The flecks enlarge with time and show propensity to confluence. The depth of fluorescein diffusion into the tissues cannot be estimated except for corneal areas in which an optical section can be created (cf. Fig. 2.15). The *black arrows* indicate limbal vessels. (The arrows are placed in corresponding locations)

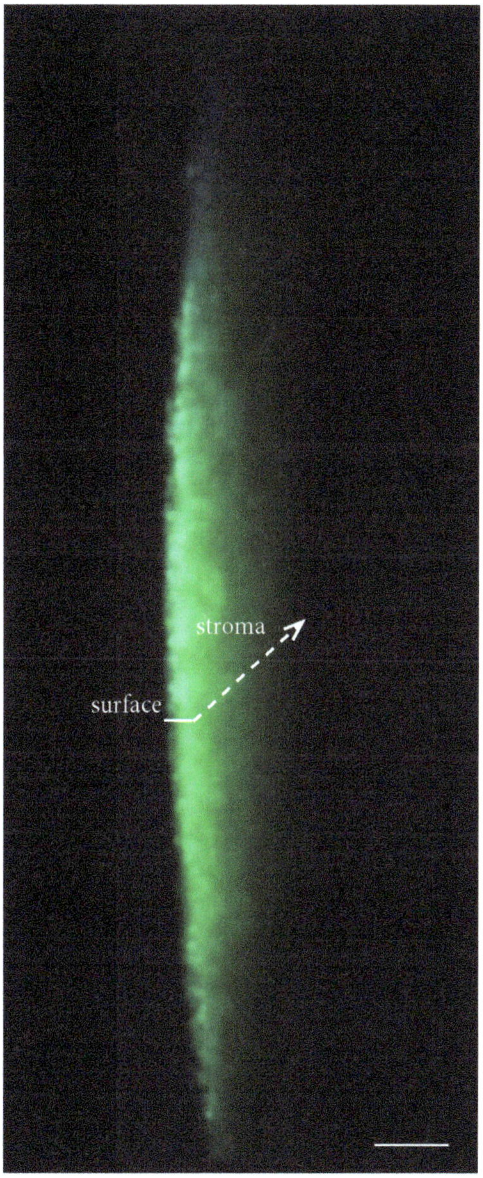

Fig. 2.15 Optical section of a cornea in which fluorescein has penetrated deeply into the stroma

Rose Bengal Staining of Surface Cells

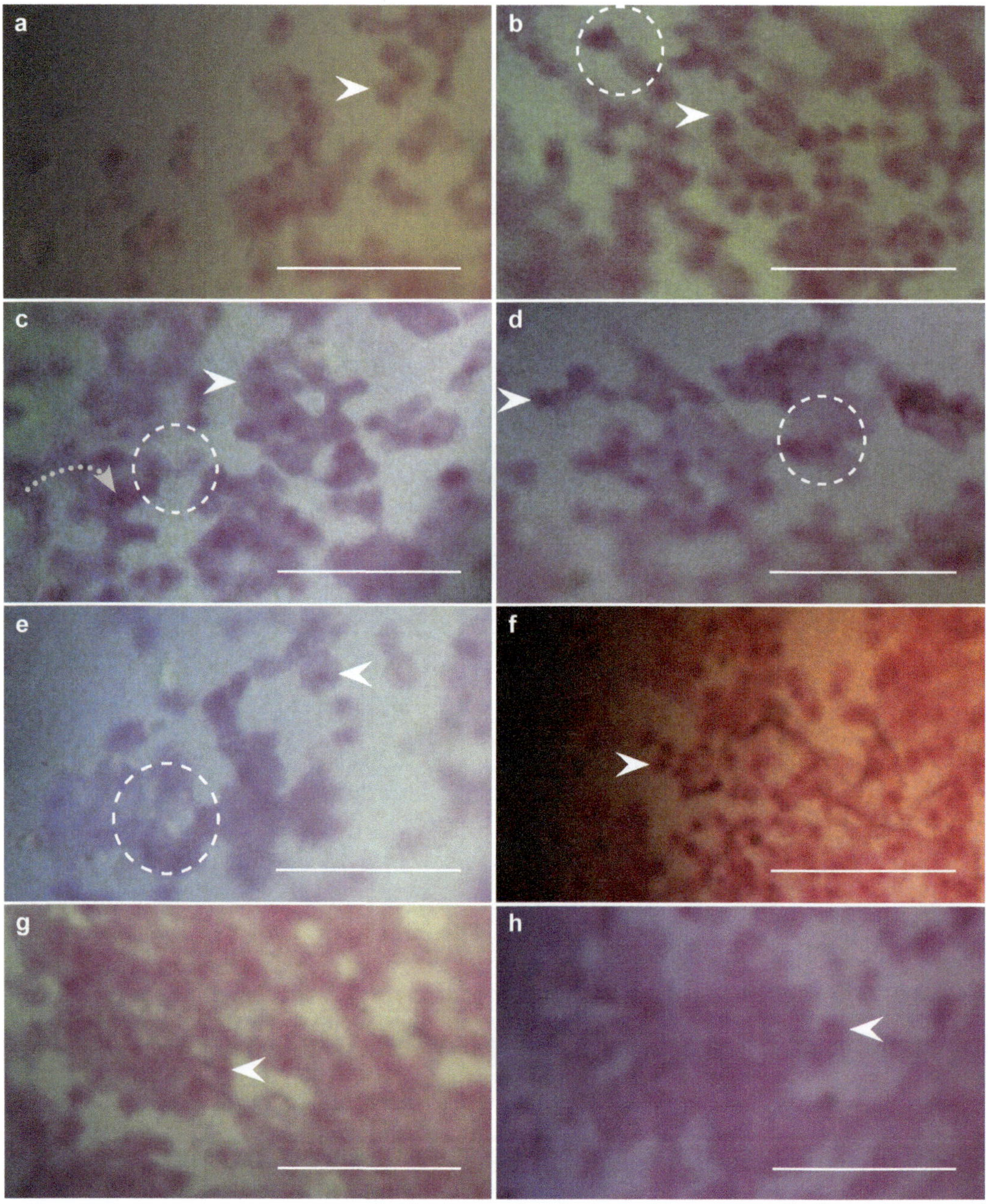

Fig. 2.16 (a–h) Variously large rose bengal stained surface cells (*arrowheads*), individual, in rows and groups. The staining densities and hues vary not only with illumination but also in cells in apposition, i.e. under approximately same illuminating conditions (b–e, *frames*). Some cells show darkly stained dots (nuclei). In places, the staining is confluent. Some of the more deeply red stained spots (c, *arrow*) are probably caused by mucus adhering to the surface (cf. Fig. 2.22)

Dynamics of Rose Bengal Stained Cells

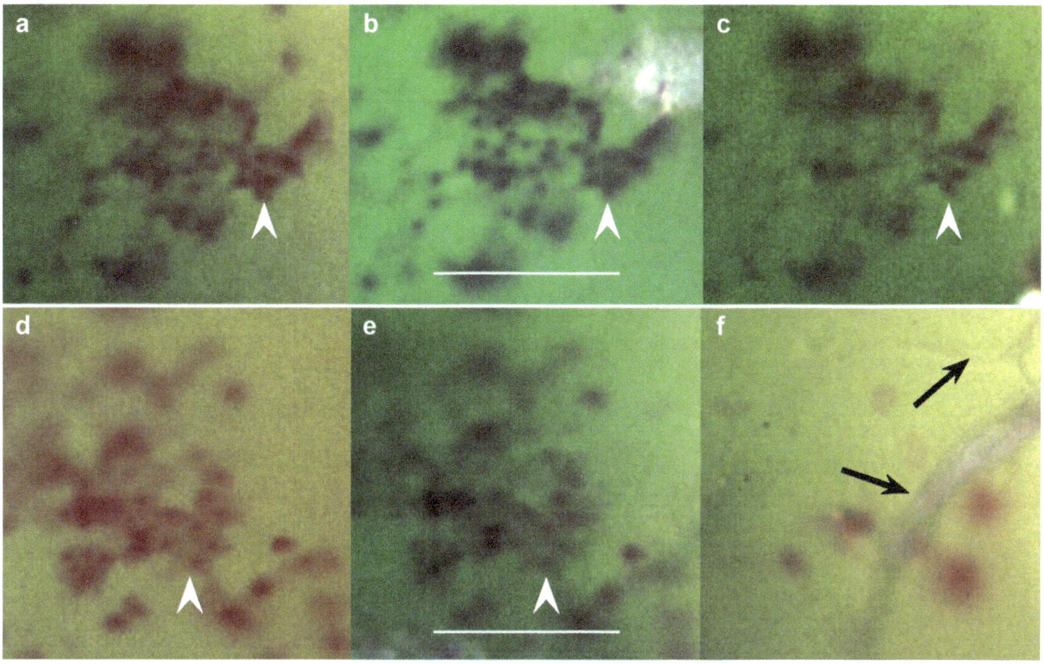

Fig. 2.17 (a–c) A group of rose bengal stained cells (*arrowheads*) in time sequence: (a) and (b) seem identical but in (c) many of the dark dots (nuclei) have disappeared. (d, e) Another area of the same cornea appears unchanged. In (f) are additionally visible mucus threads (*arrows*). (The arrowheads in a–c and in d and e are placed in corresponding locations)

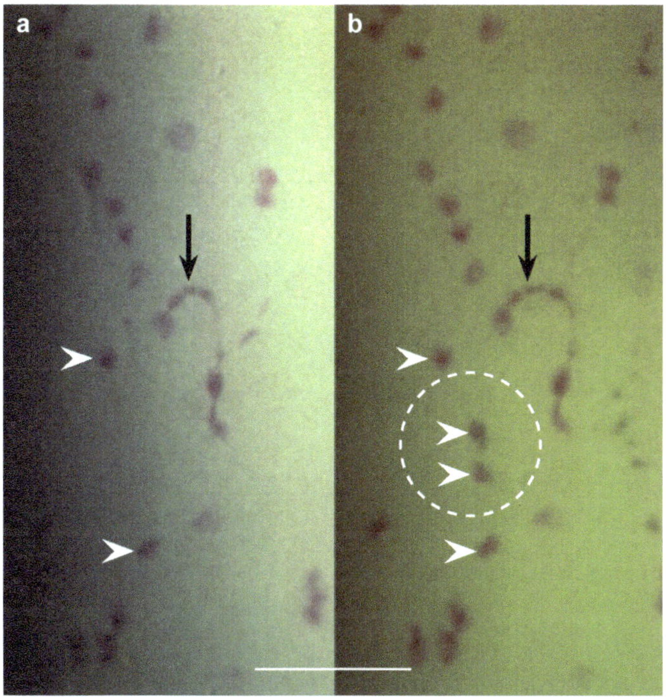

Fig. 2.18 (a, b) Two consecutive photographs of the same area. The patterns of rose bengal stained surface cells (*arrowheads*) are almost the same; in the area indicated by *frame* in (b) two new rose bengal stained cells appeared during the time elapsing between (a) and (b). The curvature of the thread (*arrows*), attached at each end to a rose bengal stained cell and forming a bow, has slightly changed. (The markers are placed in corresponding locations)

Non-fluorescent Fluorescein Versus Rose Bengal Cell Staining

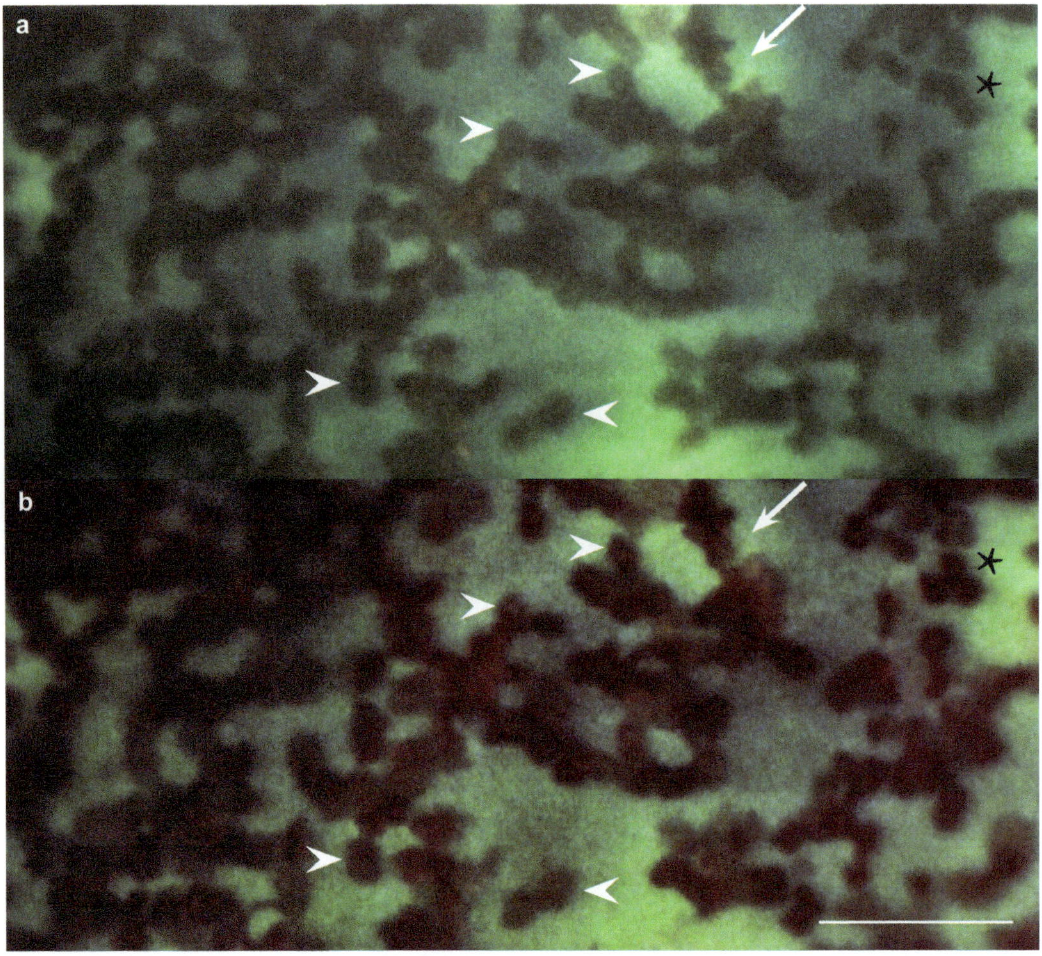

Fig. 2.19 (a) Surface cells (*arrowheads*) stained yellow/brown with non-fluorescent fluorescein. The green fluorescence (*arrow*) reveals fluorescein diffusion into the tissues. (b) The same area with rose bengal added; the red staining pattern of diseased surface cells corresponds to that in (a) with minor differences caused by displacement of some diseased surface elements (*asterisk*). (The markers are placed in corresponding locations) (Adapted from [9])

Fig. 2.21 Four consecutive photographs. (a) Fluorescent (green) stained dots (*arrowheads*); (b–d) after staining with rose bengal becomes visible that the majority of them represents diseased surface cells (*arrowheads*). In (b–d) are additionally visible mucus threads (*straight arrows*) and lumps (*bowed arrows*) moving with blinks. (The arrowheads are placed in corresponding locations)

Punctate Fluorescent Fluorescein Versus Rose Bengal Cell Staining

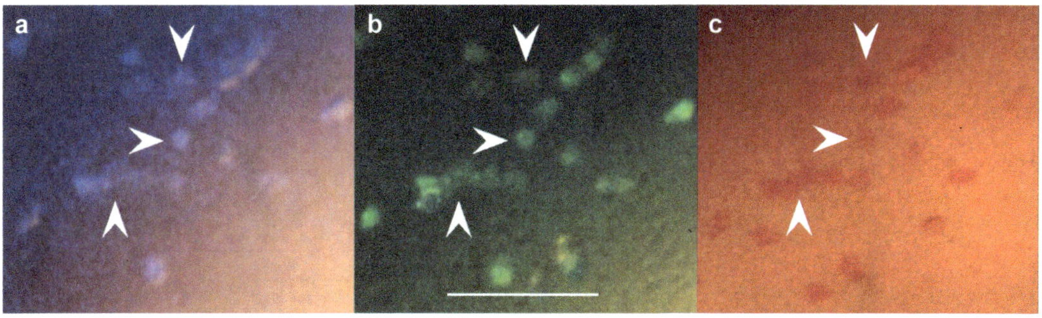

Fig. 2.20 (a) Greyish surface cells (*arrowheads*) stained (b) green with fluorescein and (c) red with rose bengal (The arrowheads are placed in corresponding locations)

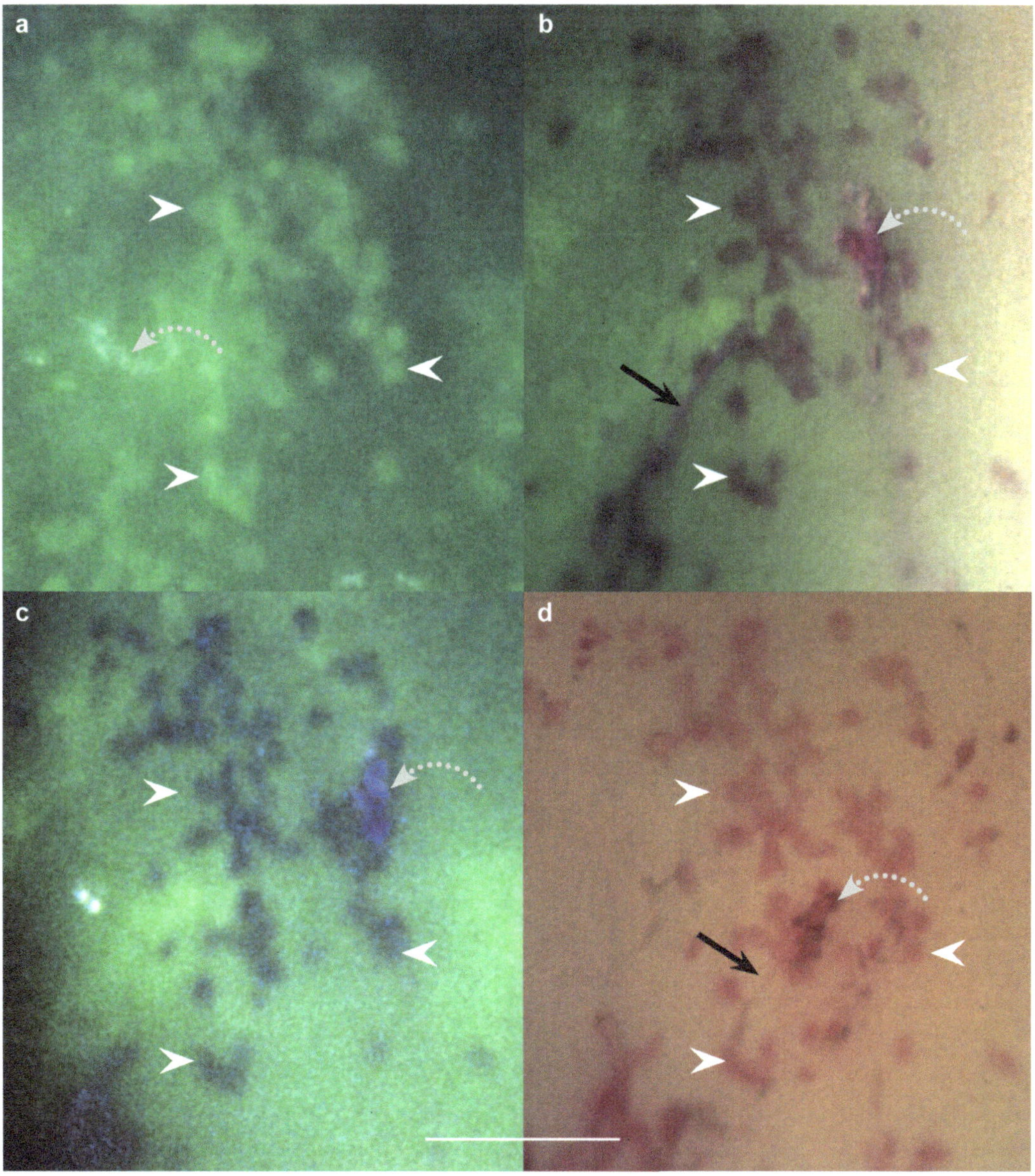

Mucus Adhering to Surface Cells

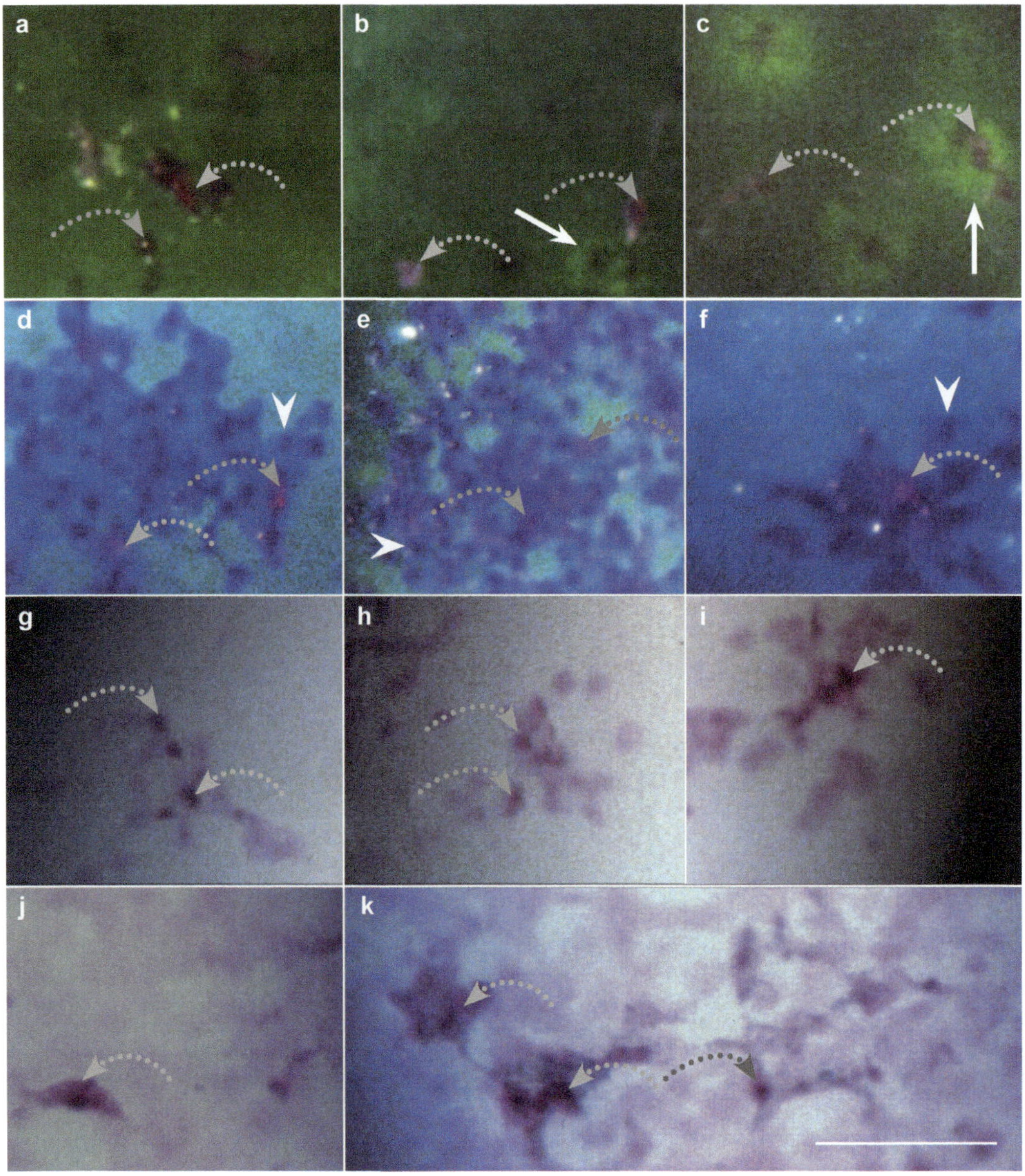

Fig. 2.22 The appearance of small rose bengal stained patches of mucus adhering to surface cells (*bowed arrows*) depends on illumination. It appears (a–f) brighter than its surroundings in focal illumination; the contrast between mucus and surface cells (*arrowheads*) staining is particularly well visible in (d–f). (g–k) The red stained mucus appears darker than its surroundings in retroillumination (cf. also Fig. 2.23). In (b, c) are additionally visible green flecks caused by fluorescein diffusion into the tissues (*straight arrows*)

Mucus Threads and Strands Adhering to the Surface

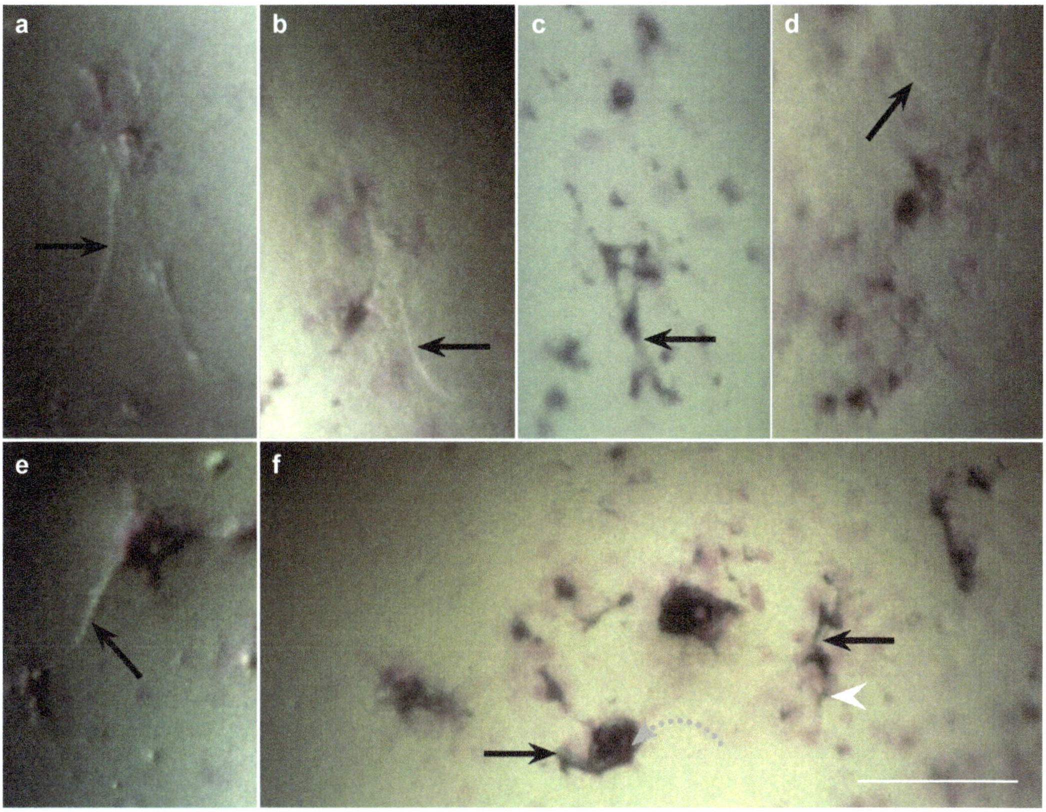

Fig. 2.23 (a–e) The curved shapes of these mucus strands (*arrows*) imply an at least partial surface attachment; in (d) the curved line (*arrow*) is suggestive of an edge of a surface-attached sheet (cf. Fig. 2.24). (f) The short threads (*straight arrows*) with attached material (*bowed arrow*) may be moving in the tear film but for the moment they seem to adhere to rose bengal stained surface cells (*arrowhead*)

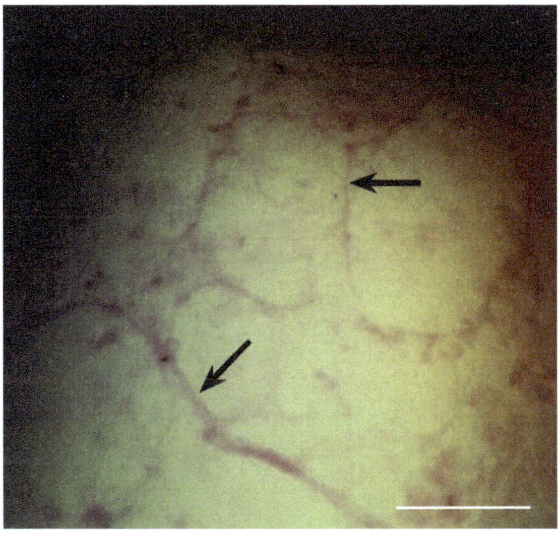

Fig. 2.24 These thicker and thinner curved rose bengal stained strands (*arrows*) seem to be rolled-up edges of a sheet adhering to the surface. (For additional examples, see Figs. 4.7–4.11)

Surface Mucus 'Plaques' and Their Dynamics (1)

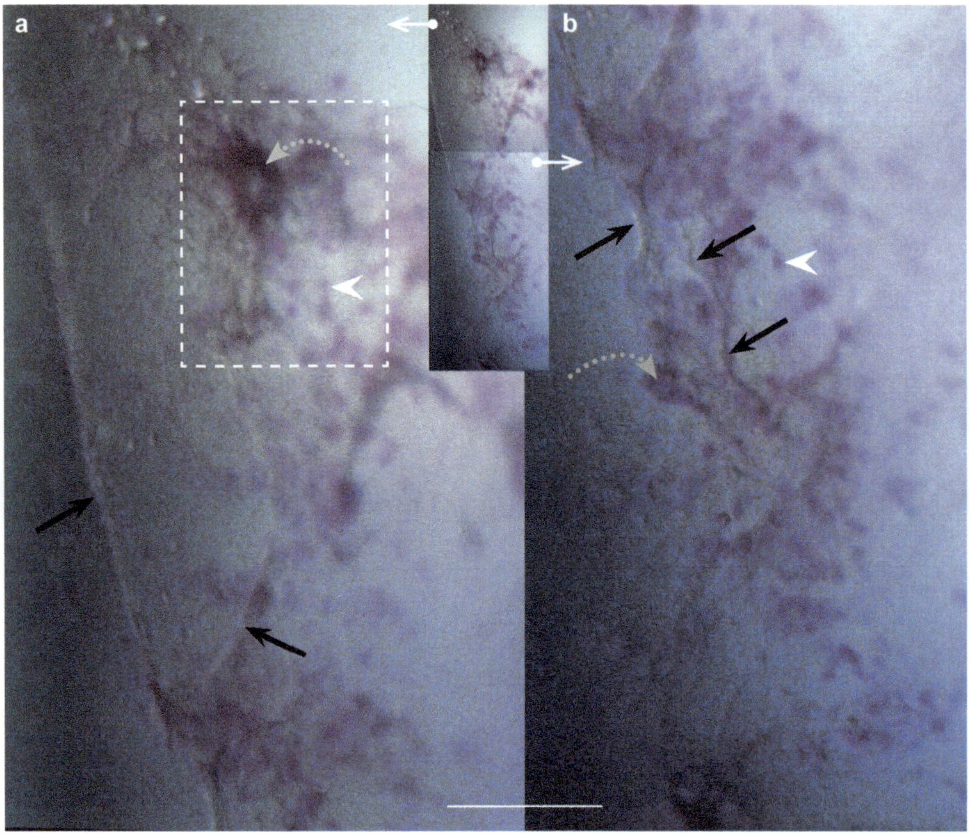

Fig. 2.25 *Inset*: survey of a larger mucus 'plaque'; (a) shows its upper and (b) its lower part at higher magnification. The mucus is visible as bowed lines *(straight arrows)* and small densely rose bengal stained areas (*bowed arrows*); the *arrowheads* indicate rose bengal stained cells. The dynamics of the area in *frame* is shown in Fig. 2.27 (opposite page)

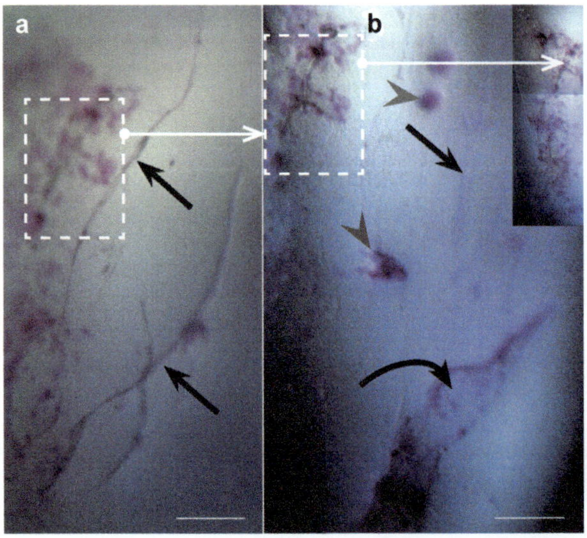

Fig. 2.26 *Inset* in (b): the same mucus 'plaque' as in Fig. 2.25. In (a, b) are visible mucus strands and threads (*straight arrows*), a crumpled mucus sheet with adhering material (b, *bowed arrow*) and lumps of material (b, *arrowheads*), all appearing and disappearing during the examination. The *frames* in (a, b) indicate the same area, shown at higher magnification in Fig. 2.28

Surface Mucus 'Plaques' and Their Dynamics (1) (cont.)

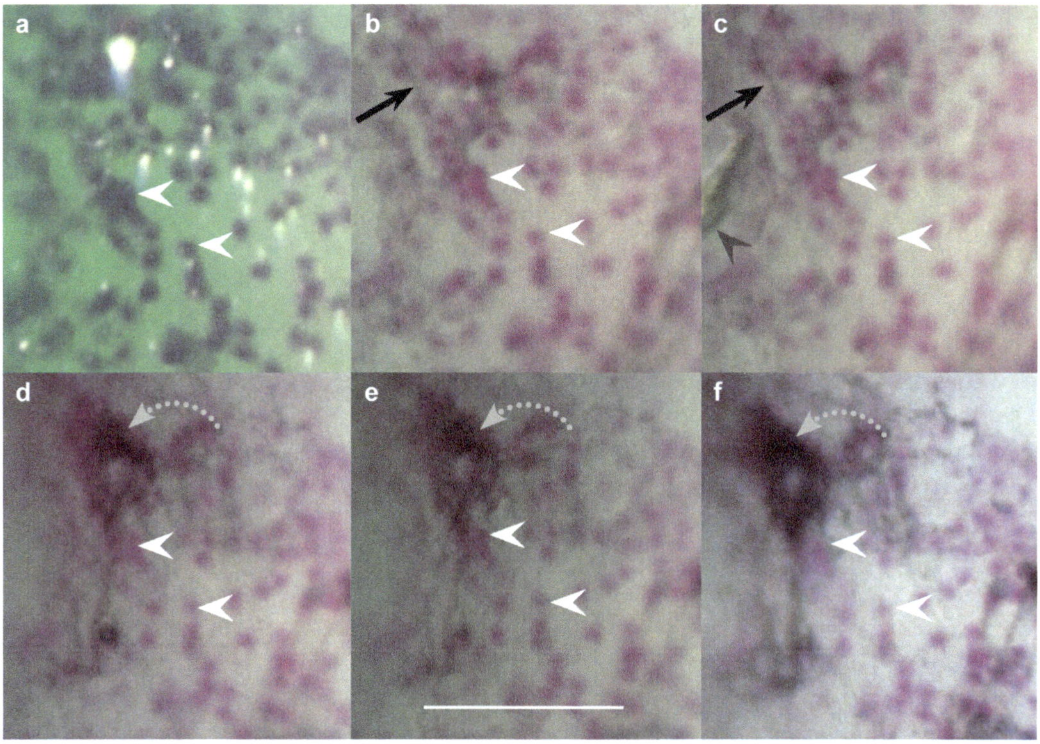

Fig. 2.27 Sequence of events occurring in the area indicated by frame in Fig. 2.25. (a–c) The *white arrowheads* indicate rose bengal stained surface cells and the *straight arrows* in (b, c) a thin mucus thread. The cell patterns appear identical in all three photographs. In (c) has appeared a lump of material (*grey arrowhead*). (d–f) show a newly attached piece of mucous material (*bowed arrows*) that remains in place. (The markers are placed in corresponding locations, the white arrowheads throughout the series)

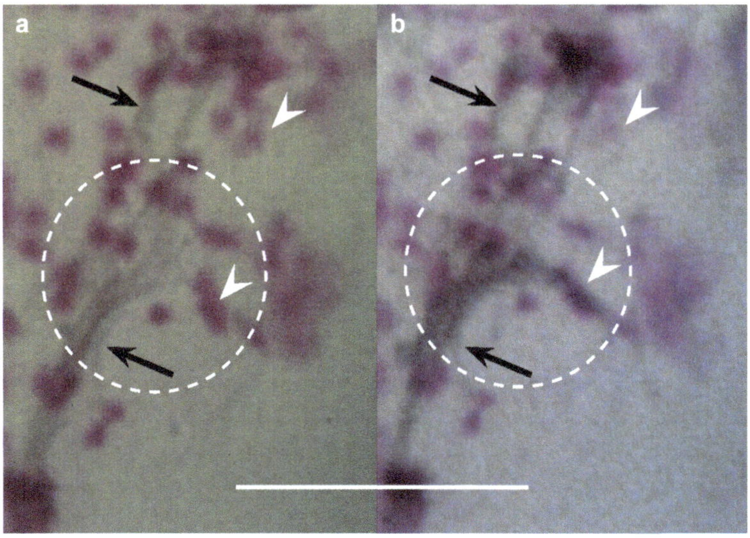

Fig. 2.28 The area indicated by frames in Fig. 2.26. (a, b) The *arrows* point to mucus threads and the *arrowheads* to rose bengal stained cells. Only minor changes (in *frame*) have occurred during the time elapsing between the two photographs. (The markers are placed in corresponding locations)

Surface Mucus 'Plaques' and Their Dynamics (2)

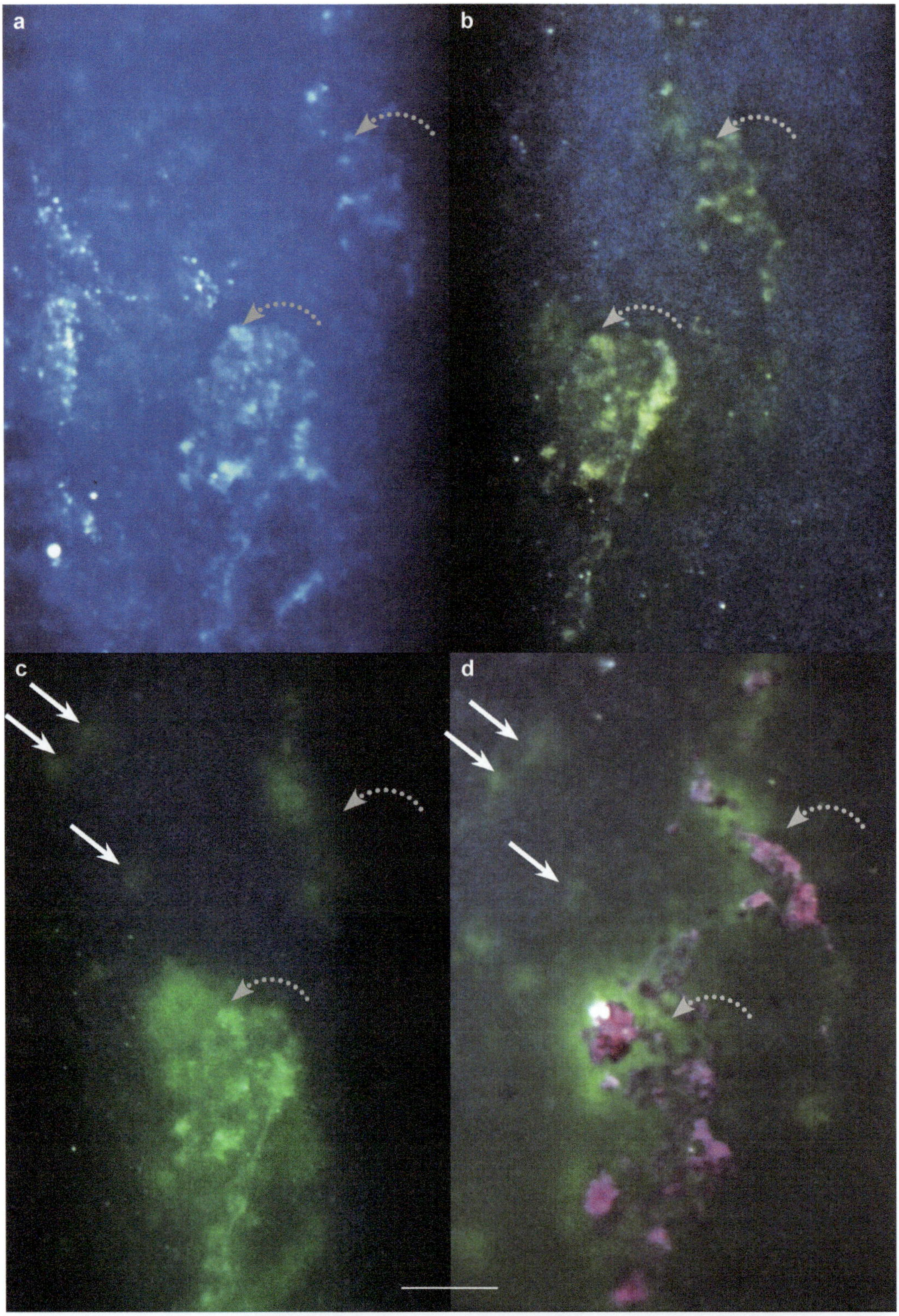

Surface Mucus 'Plaques' and Their Dynamics (2) (cont.)

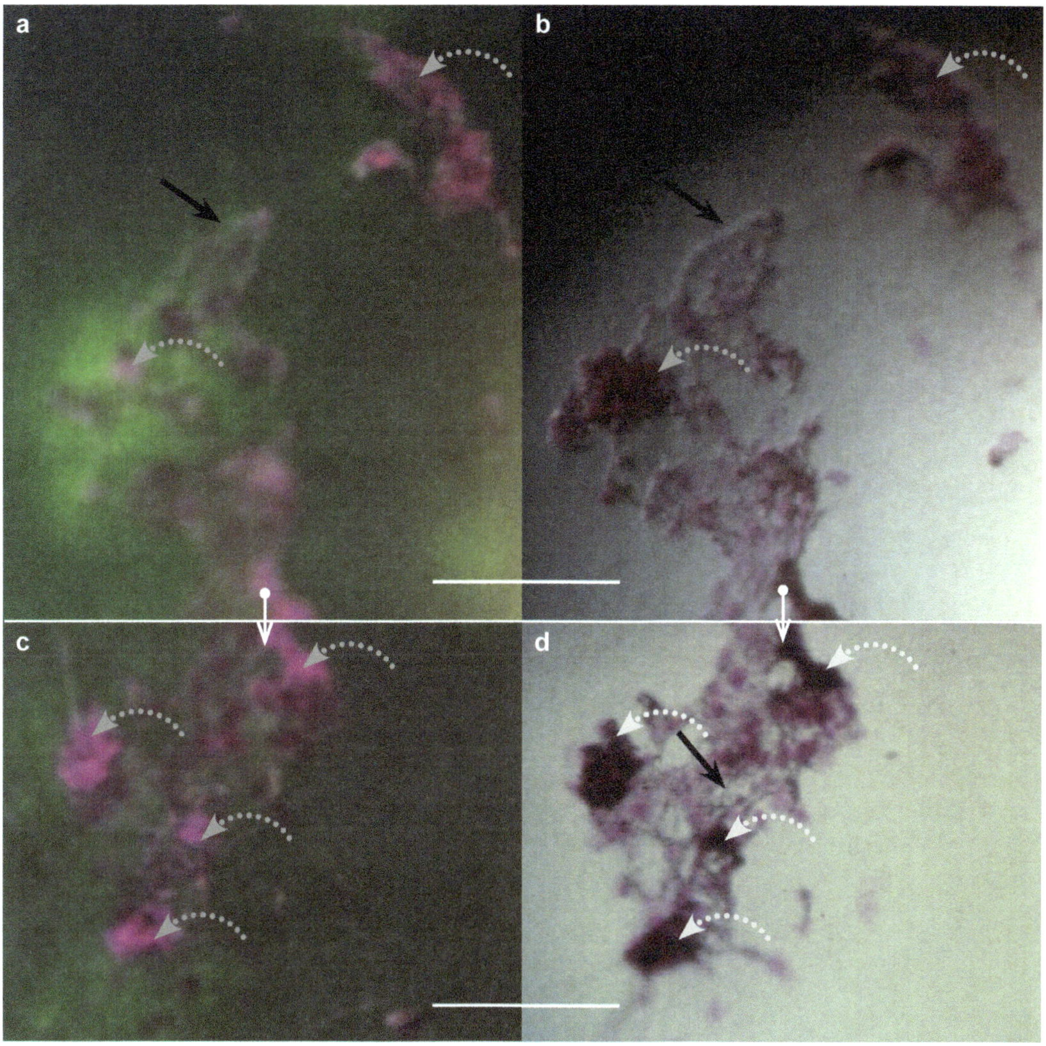

Fig. 2.30 (a, b) The upper and (c, d) the lower part of Fig. 2.29d. The *bowed arrows* indicate pieces of surface-adherent mucus, brightly red/pink in focal (a and c) and dark (b and d) in retroillumination. The *straight arrows* indicate mucus strands and threads. The patterns are similar but not identical because of changes occurring with blinks. (The markers are placed in corresponding locations in each pair of the photographs)

Fig. 2.29 (a) Before staining are visible areas (*bowed arrows*) containing strongly light-reflecting patches, lines and dots. (b) Early after the application of fluorescein appears green staining caused by fluorescein diffusion into the tissues in these areas (*bowed arrows*). Later on (c) the green staining appears more brilliant; the *straight arrows* indicate small fluorescent (green) flecks. (d) After the application of rose bengal, there is a new pattern showing brightly red/pink stained mucus adhering to green flecks (*bowed arrows*), in (a–c) placed in corresponding locations and in (d) placed with the small green flecks serving as (very approximate) reference points; some details are shown in Fig. 2.30; cf. also Fig. 5.24

Fluorescent Fluorescein and Rose Bengal Staining in Combination. Example 1

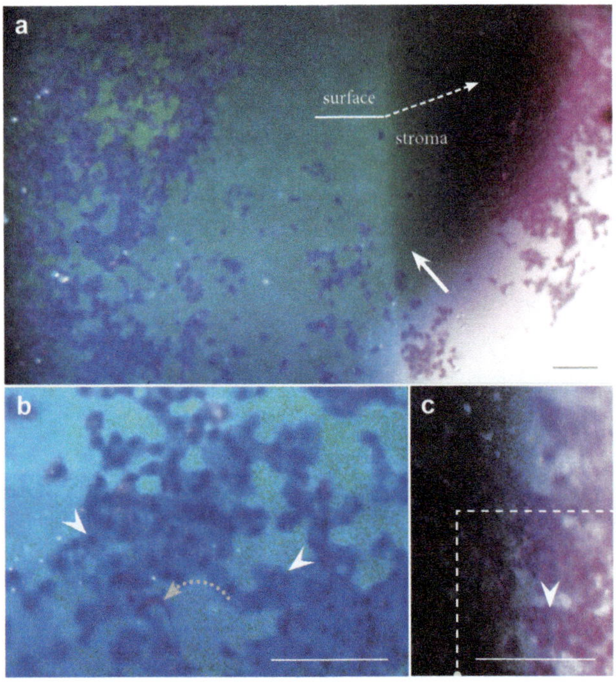

Fig. 2.31 (a) Survey. Heavy rose bengal staining, in the left part of the picture seen against green background caused by fluorescein diffusion (*arrow*) into the tissues, and in the right one in light reflected from the iris (cf. Fig. 4.19); the hue varies with background illumination. (b) Of the variously large cells (*arrowheads*), many show a distinct dark dot (nucleus); attached mucus (*arrow*) appears brightly red/pink. (c) In an area of heavy staining, cell nuclei (*arrowhead*) are difficult to discern. The area in *frame* is shown in Fig. 2.32

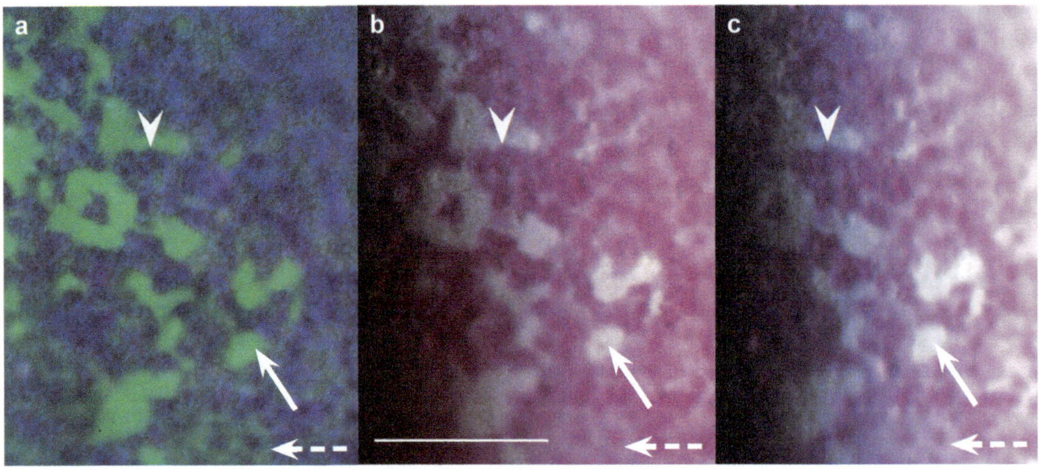

Fig. 2.32 The area in frame in Fig. 2.31. In areas showing heavy rose bengal staining, (a) darker dots (nuclei, *arrowheads*) are well discernible against green background but (b, c) more difficult so against a deeply red one. The brightly green hue of fluorescein diffusing into the tissues (a, *plain arrow*) indicates an absence of (discernible) rose bengal staining (cf. b, c) and its dirty hue (a, *dashed arrow*) a week one (cf. b, c). (The markers are placed in corresponding locations)

Fluorescent Fluorescein and Rose Bengal Staining in Combination. Example 2

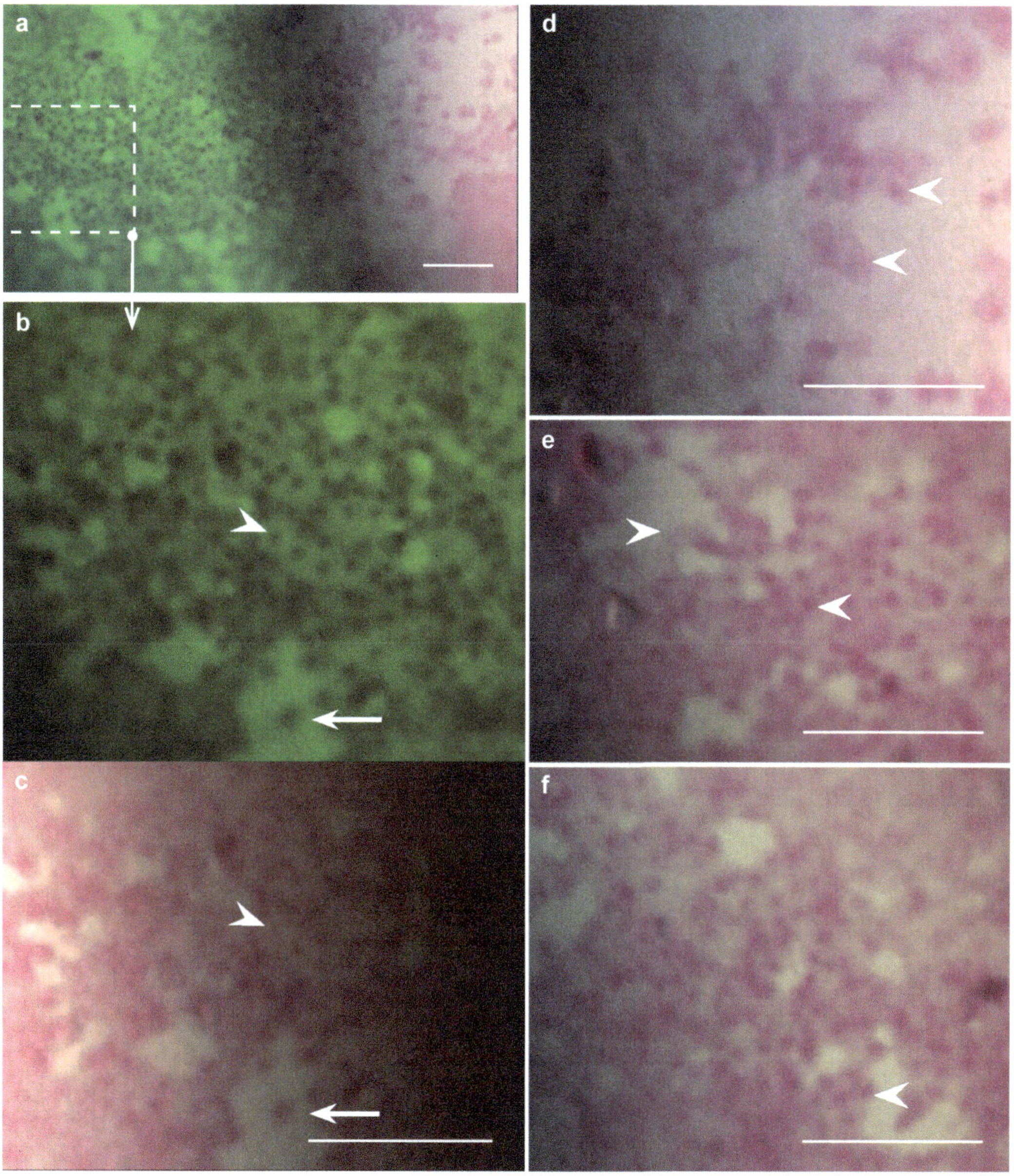

Fig. 2.33 (a) Survey of an area showing fluorescein diffusion (green) into the tissues and many rose bengal stained surface cells. (b) The area in *frame* in (a) shows rows of smaller and larger rose bengal stained surface cells *(arrowhead)* in apposition and green stained in-between areas *(arrows)*. (c) The same area as in (b); the green staining is not visible in retroillumination. (The markers are placed in corresponding locations.) (d–f) Different areas of the same cornea showing smaller and larger rose bengal stained surface cells *(arrowheads)*, some with and others without a deeply red stained dot (nucleus)

Surface Changes Captured in the Same Cornea at the Same Occasion

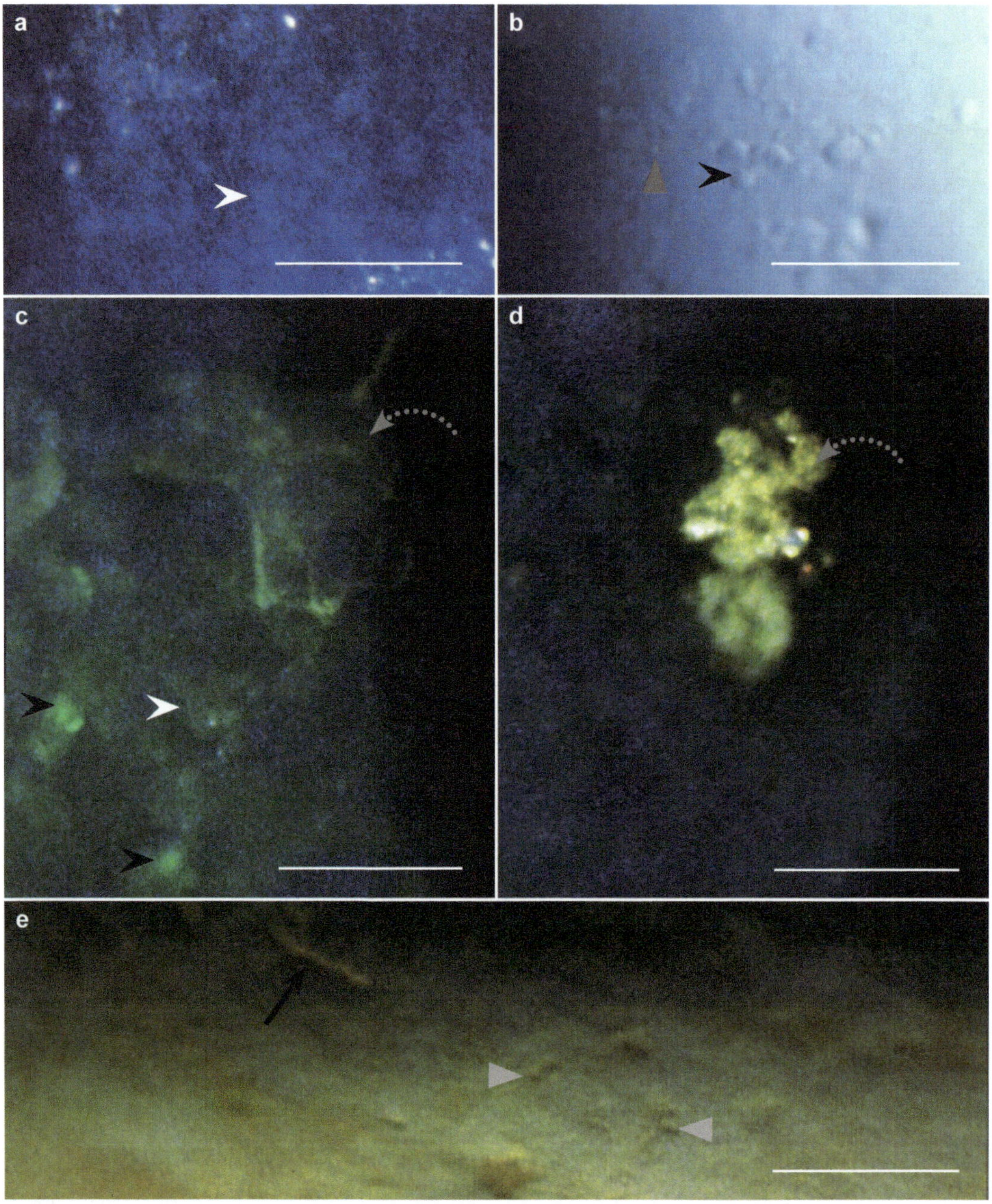

Fig. 2.34 Before staining, the cornea shows (a) greyish surface cells *(arrowhead)* and bright light-reflecting dots and (b) cystic spaces *(black arrowhead)* and rounded bodies (*grey arrowhead*). Shortly after the application of fluorescein is visible (c) a weak green staining revealing surface cells (*white arrowhead*) and a brilliantly green one indicating cystic spaces (*black arrowheads*); the *arrows* indicate (c) a flat mucus sheet and (d) a crumpled one. In (e), the *arrow* indicates a mucus strand and the *arrowheads* rounded bodies; in this illumination, fluorescein staining appears yellow

Surface Changes Captured in the Same Cornea at the Same Occasion (cont.)

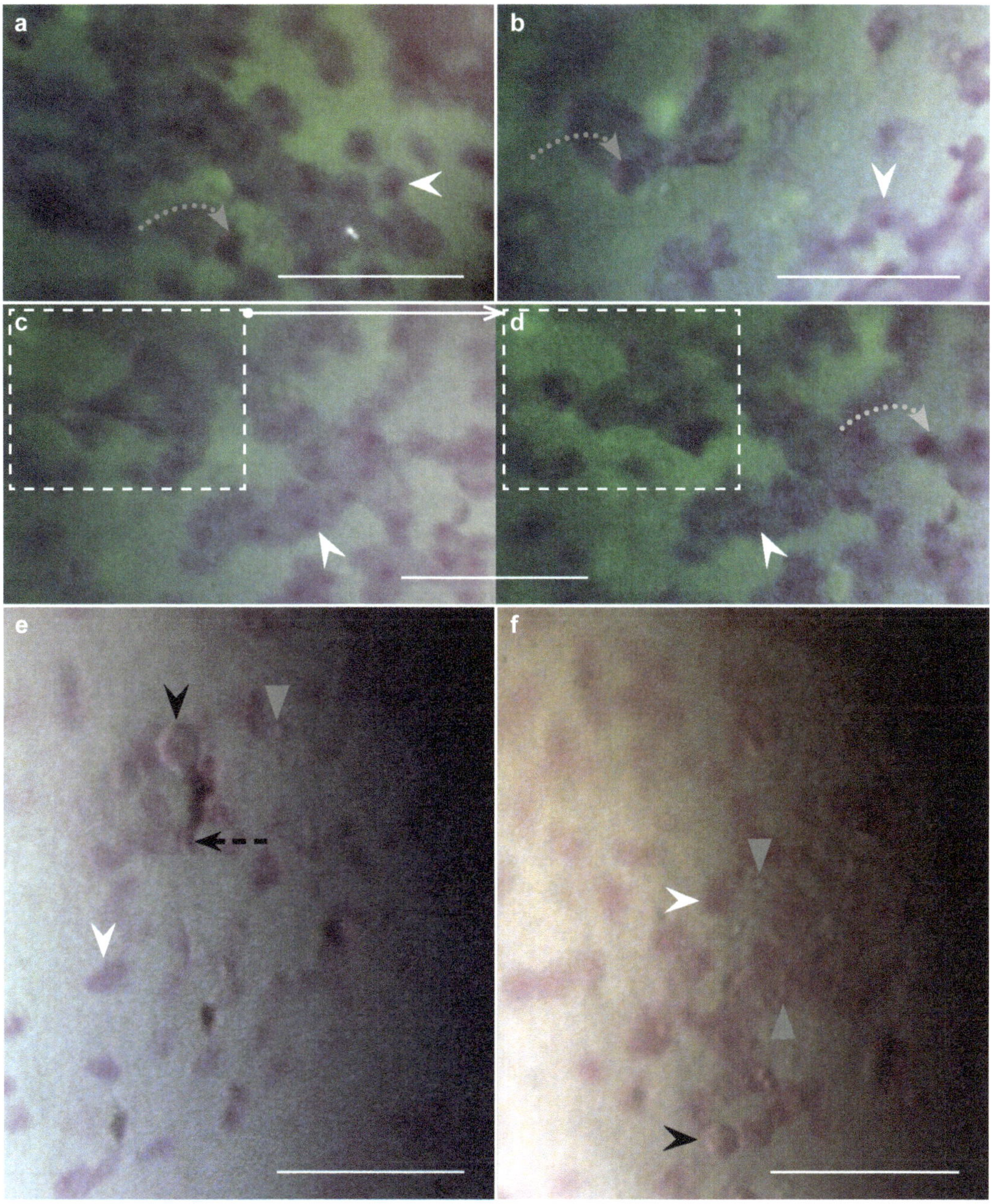

Fig. 2.35 (a–d) Rose bengal stained surface cells (*arrowheads*), with or without deeply red stained dots (nuclei), and mucus adhering to some of the cells (*arrows*). (c, d) show the same area; the arrow in (d) indicates surface mucus not visible in (c) and the *frames* highlight some other changes occurring during the examination. (The arrowheads in c and d are placed in corresponding locations.) (e, f) In these areas are visible rose bengal stained cells (*white arrowheads*) lacking deeply stained dots (nuclei), cystic spaces (*black arrowheads*), rounded bodies (*grey arrowheads*), and a small filament (*arrow*)

Epithelial Infiltrates (?)

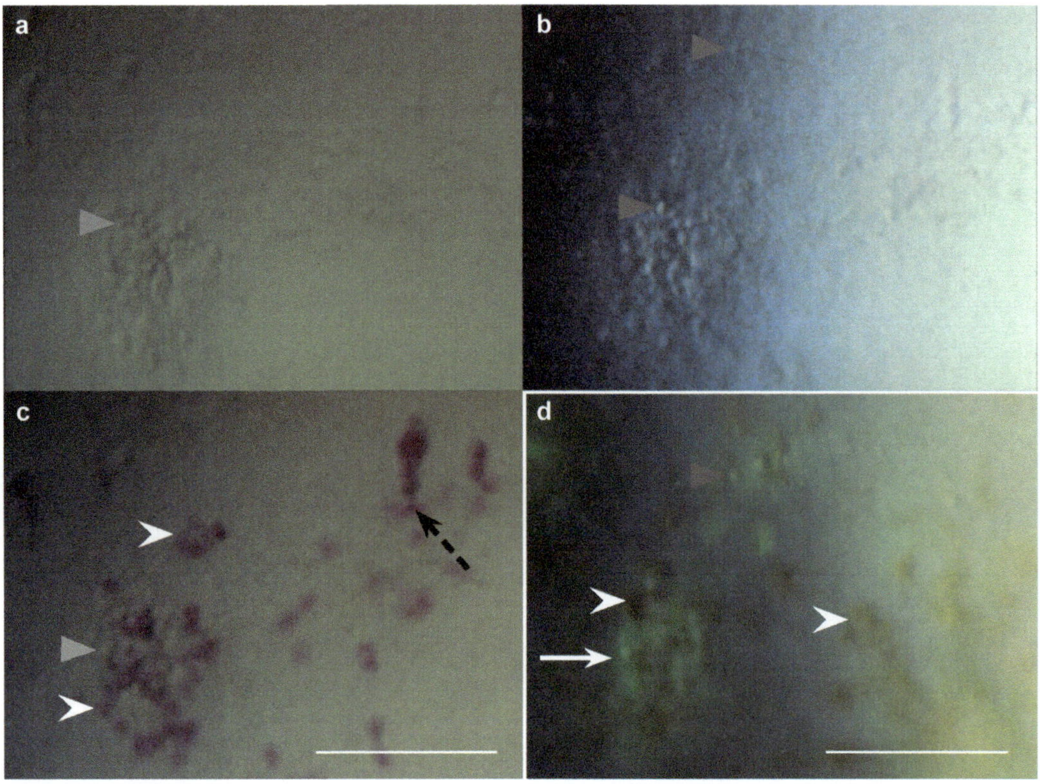

Fig. 2.36 (a–c) The same area. Rounded bodies (*grey arrowheads*) and rose bengal stained surface cells (*white arrowheads*), individual or grouped; the *dashed arrow* in (c) indicates attachment point of a small filament. (d) A small fleck, showing fluorescein diffusion into the tissues (green, *white arrow*); yellow-brown (non-fluorescent) stained surface cells (*white arrowheads)* are present within the fleck and outside it, rounded bodies (*grey arrowhead*) are visible outside it (cf. Fig. 4.1)

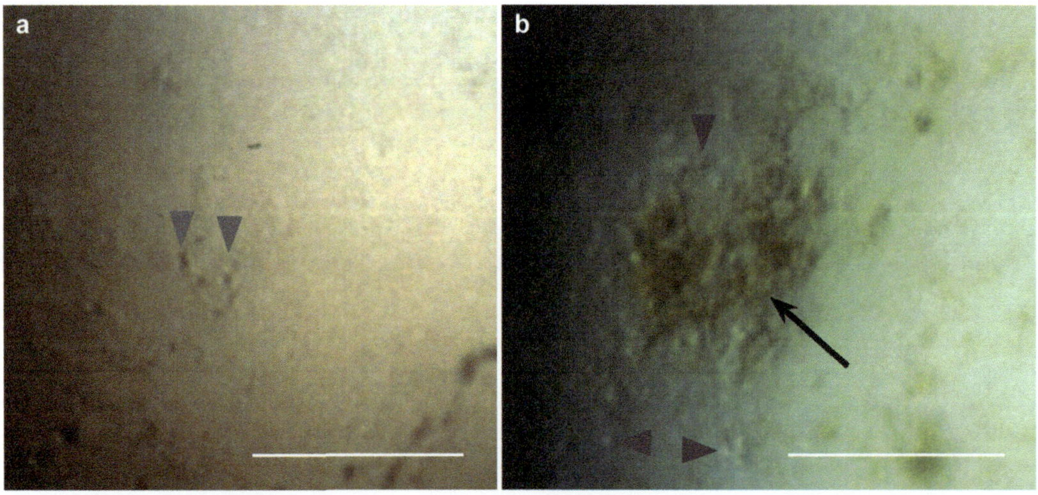

Fig. 2.37 (a) Rounded bodies (*arrowheads*), spread on the surface and (b) concentrated in a small area (*arrow*); the latter reminds of epithelial infiltrates (such as occurring in the acute stage of adenovirus infection and in Thygeson's superficial punctate keratitis)

Fluorescent Flecks (2, Additional Features)

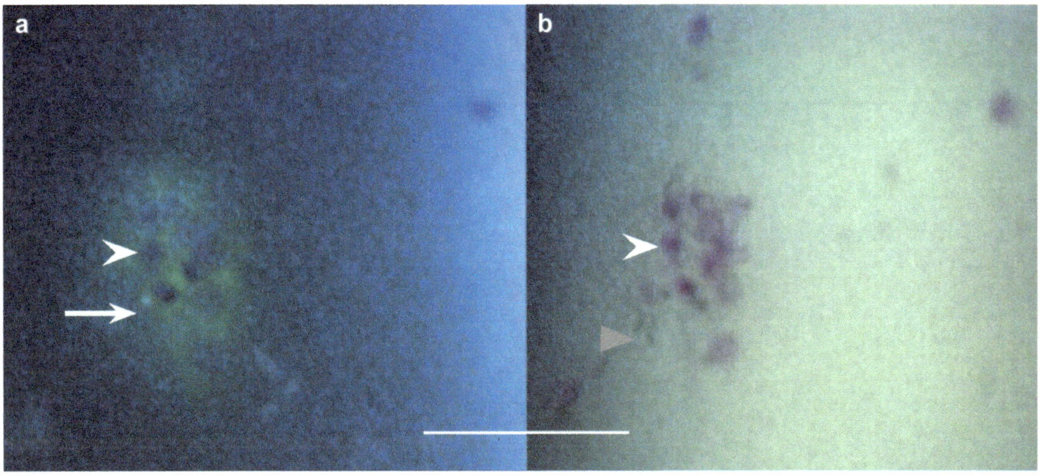

Fig. 2.38 (a, b) A small fleck showing fluorescein diffusion into the tissues (*arrow*) and rose bengal stained surface cells (*white arrowhead*). In (b) are visible rounded bodies (*grey arrowhead*). (The white arrowheads are placed in corresponding locations)

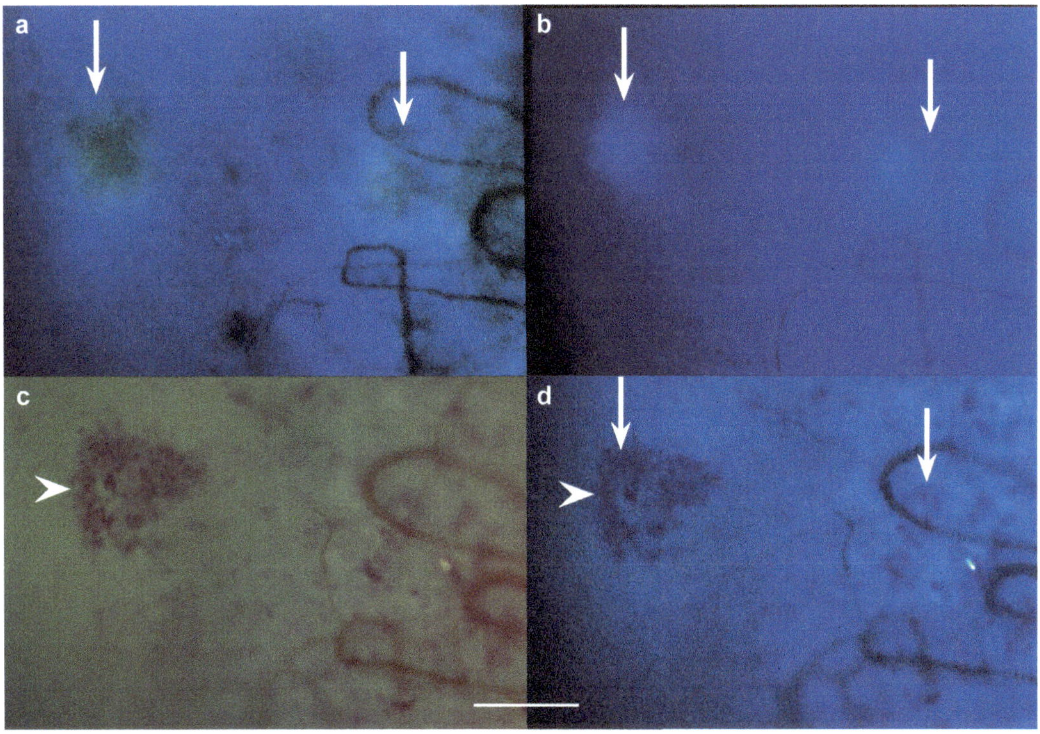

Fig. 2.39 Small corneal flecks (*arrows*) close to the limbus visualised with (a) fluorescein and green filter, (b) fluorescein and blue filter, (c) rose bengal in white light and (d) rose bengal and green filter. Where non-fluorescent (dark, yellow) fluorescein staining (a) is present, rose bengal staining (c, d) can be expected. (The markers are placed in corresponding locations)

Fluorescent Flecks (2, Additional Features) (cont.)

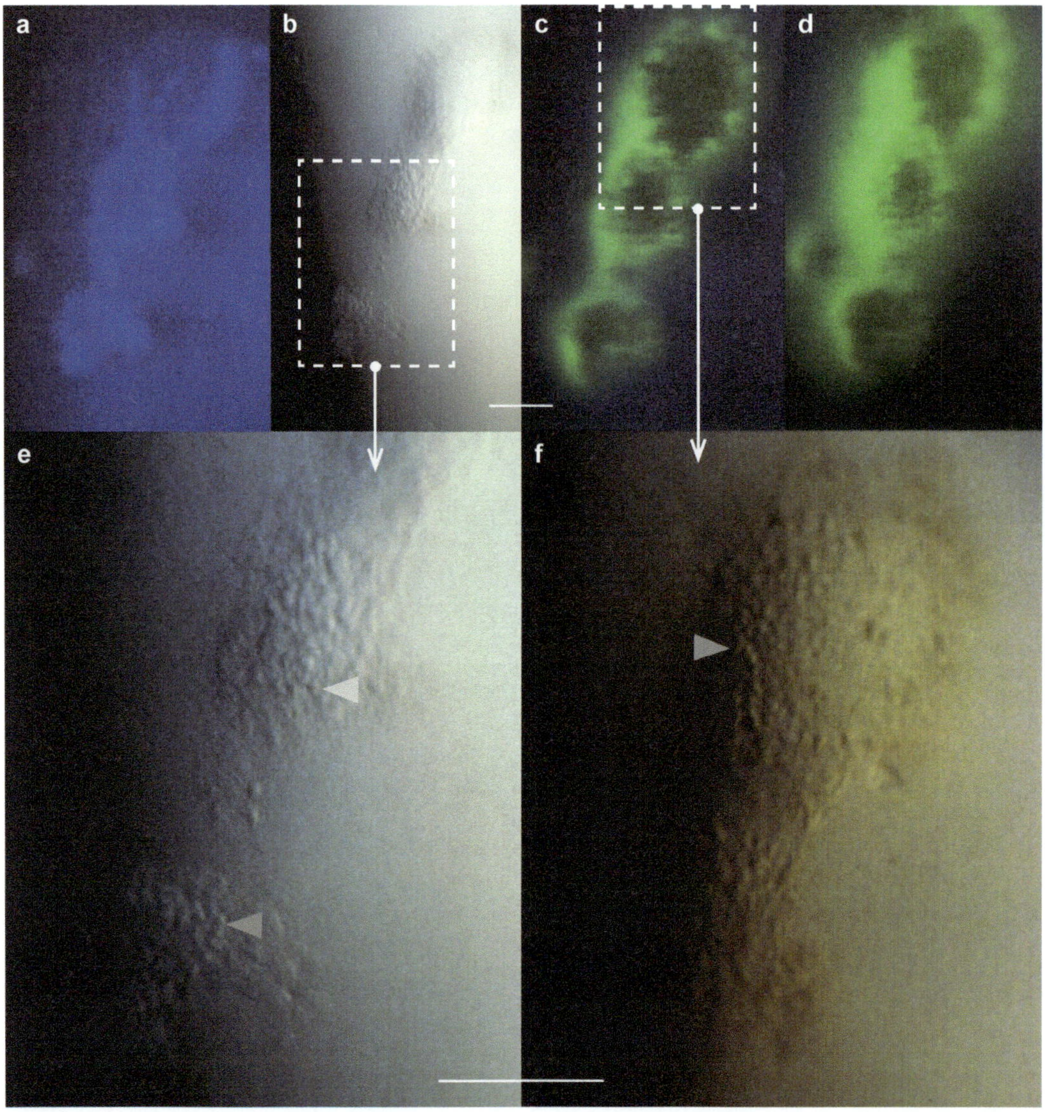

Fig. 2.40 (a–d) This figure with undulating borders is (a) partly light-reflecting, (b) appears granular, (c) shows a non-fluorescent (dark) and a fluorescent (green) staining, caused by fluorescein diffusion into the tissues, which (d) enlarges with time. In all photographs is visible that the shape of the fleck is a result of confluence of smaller lesions. The areas in *frames* are shown at higher magnification in (e, f); in both are visible rounded bodies (*arrowheads*) (cf. Figs. 2.48, 4.12, 4.15, and 4.17)

Fluorescent Flecks (2, Additional Features) (cont.)

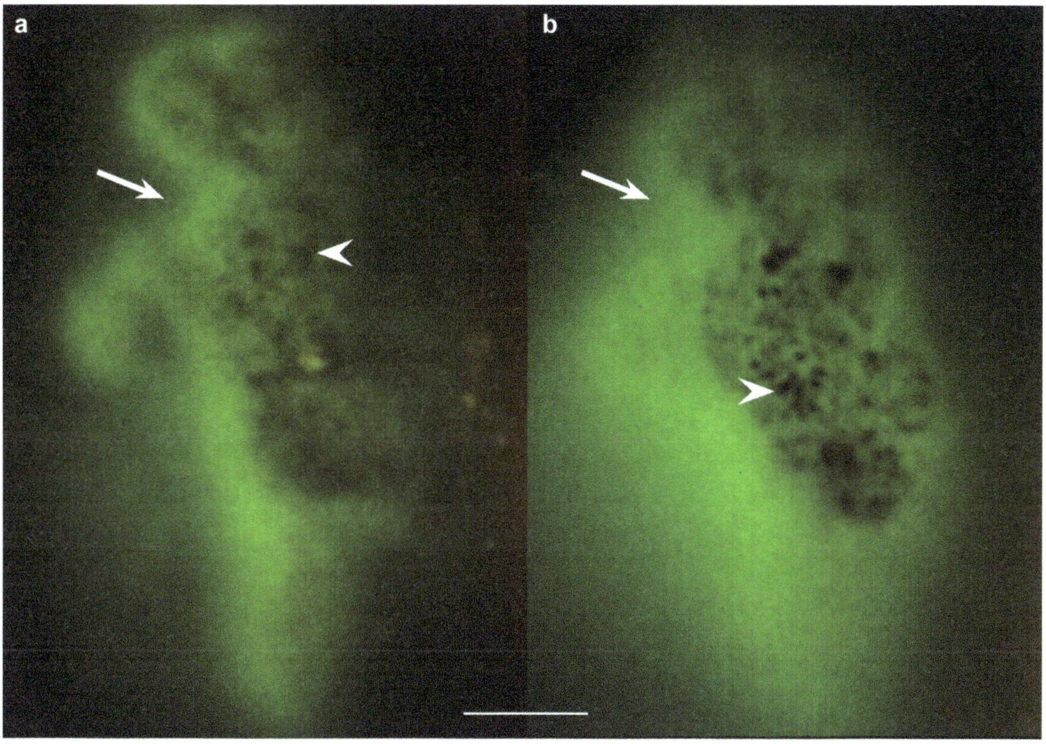

Fig. 2.41 A fleck showing (a) non-fluorescent stained surface cells (*arrowhead*) and (b) rose bengal stained ones (*arrowhead*). The undulating borders in (a) imply a result of confluence of several flecks (cf. Fig. 2.40). The area of green staining (*arrows*) caused by fluorescein diffusion into the tissues enlarges with time

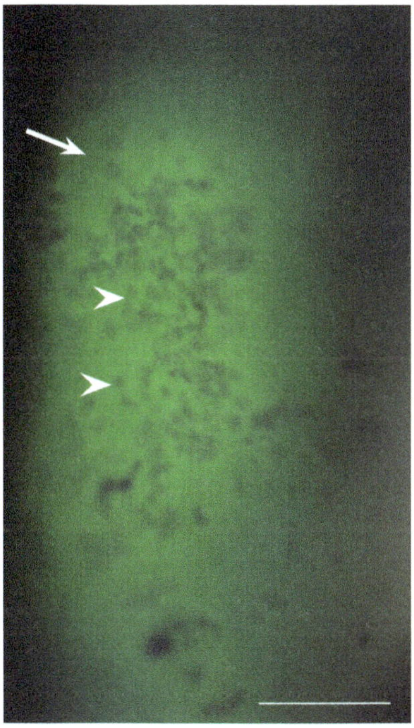

Fig. 2.42 The extensive fluorescein diffusion into the tissues (green, *arrow*) implies that this fleck was captured some time after the application of the dye. The *arrowheads* indicate rose bengal stained surface cells

Fluorescent Flecks (2, Additional Features) (cont.)

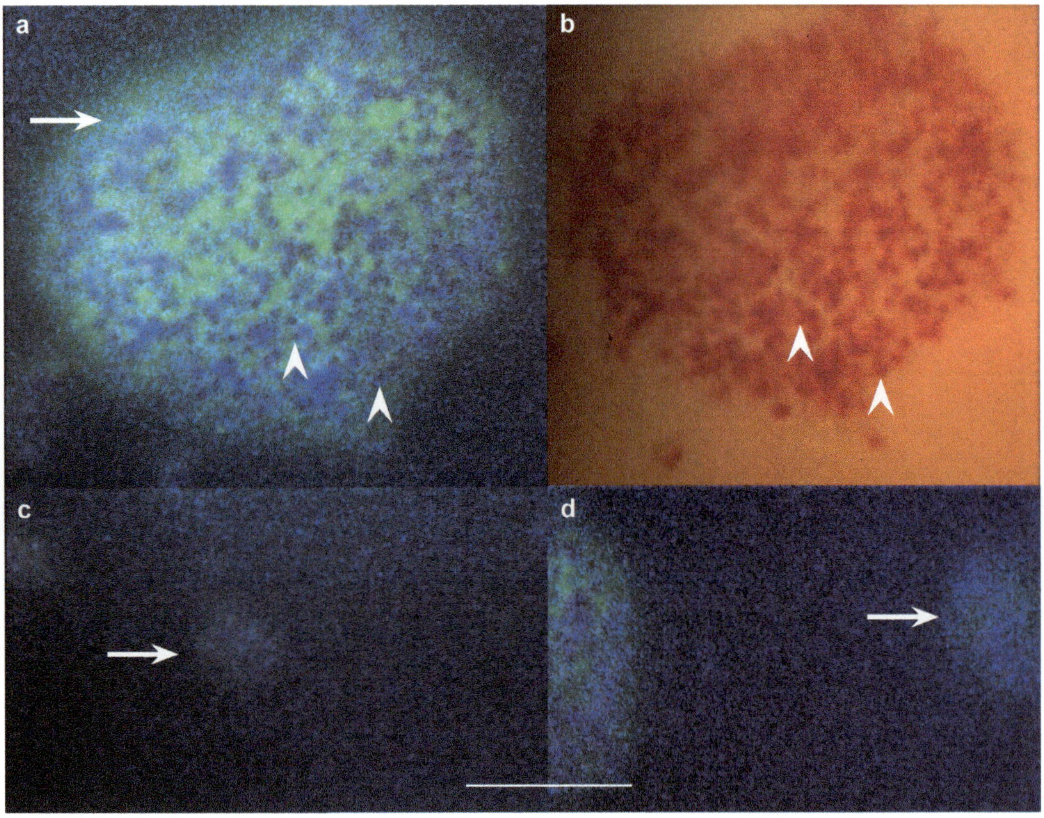

Fig. 2.43 A large rounded fleck showing (a) green fluorescein staining (*arrow*) and (a, b) many small rose bengal stained cells (*arrowheads*). (c, d) Small flecks are present in the surroundings (*arrows*). (The arrowheads are placed in corresponding locations)

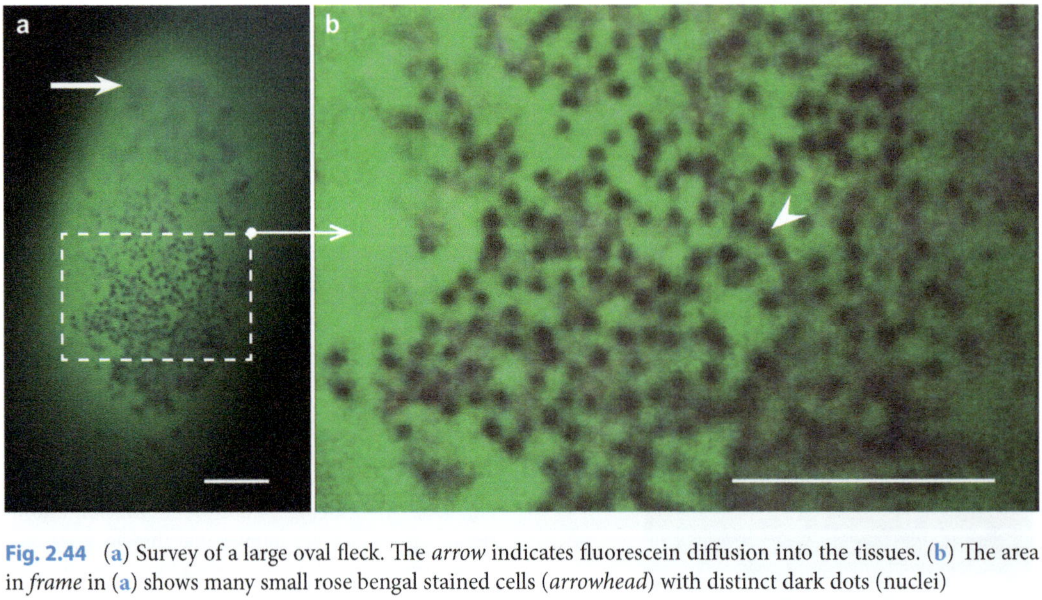

Fig. 2.44 (a) Survey of a large oval fleck. The *arrow* indicates fluorescein diffusion into the tissues. (b) The area in *frame* in (a) shows many small rose bengal stained cells (*arrowhead*) with distinct dark dots (nuclei)

Fluorescent Flecks (2, Additional Features) (cont.)

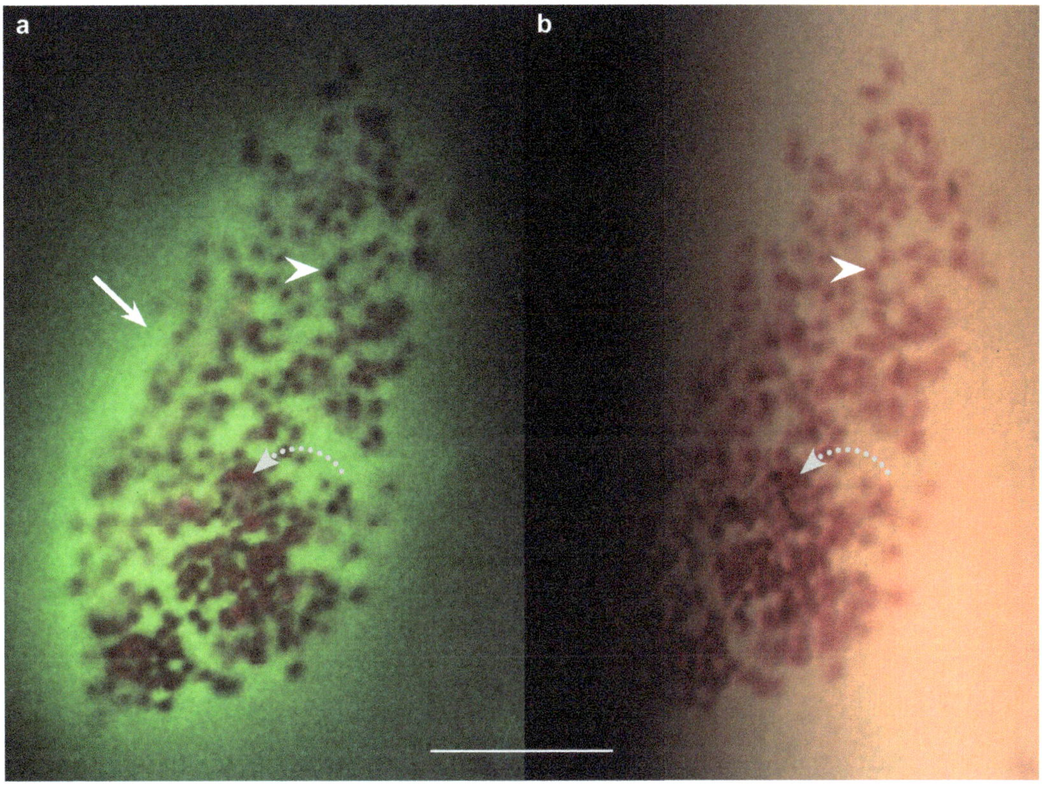

Fig. 2.45 An oval fleck showing (a) fluorescein diffusion into the tissues (green, *straight arrow*) and (a, b) small rose bengal stained nucleated cells (*arrowheads*) with mucus adhering to some of them (*bowed arrows*). (The markers are placed in corresponding locations)

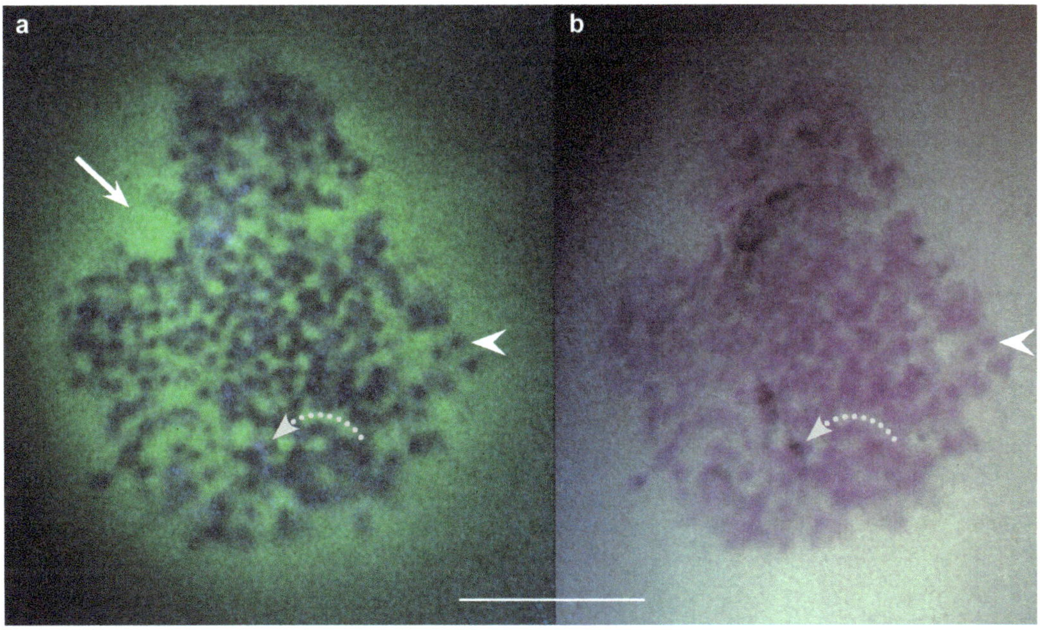

Fig. 2.46 A fleck showing (a) fluorescein diffusion into the tissues (green, *straight arrow*) and (a, b) small rose bengal stained nucleated cells (*arrowheads*) with mucus adhering to some of them (*bowed arrows*). (The markers are placed in corresponding locations) (Adapted from [3])

Fluorescent Flecks (2, Additional Features) (cont.)

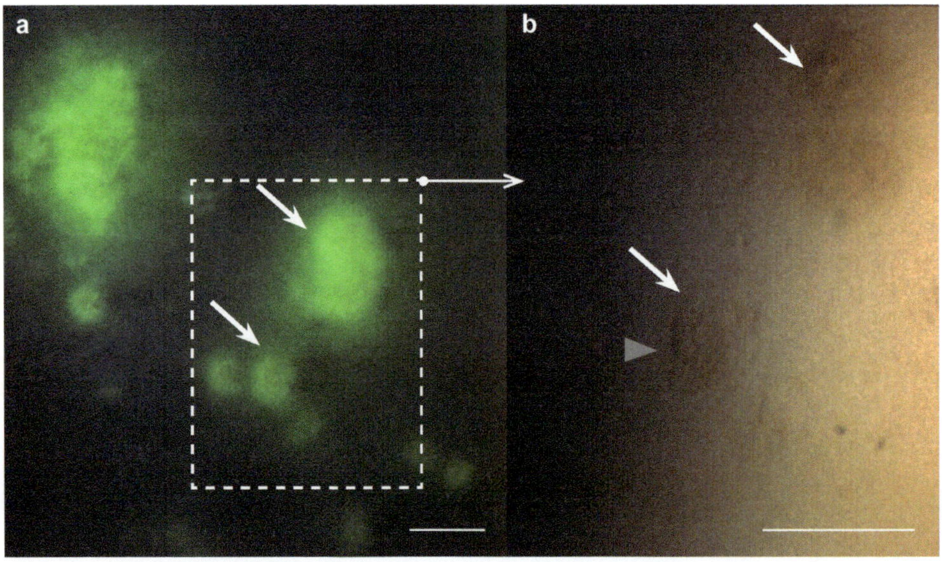

Fig. 2.47 (a) Survey capturing several larger and smaller green flecks (*arrows*) close to each other. The area in *frame* is shown in (b): the flecks appear darker than their surroundings; the arrowhead indicates a spot in which is visible a fine granularity. (The arrows in a and b are placed in corresponding locations)

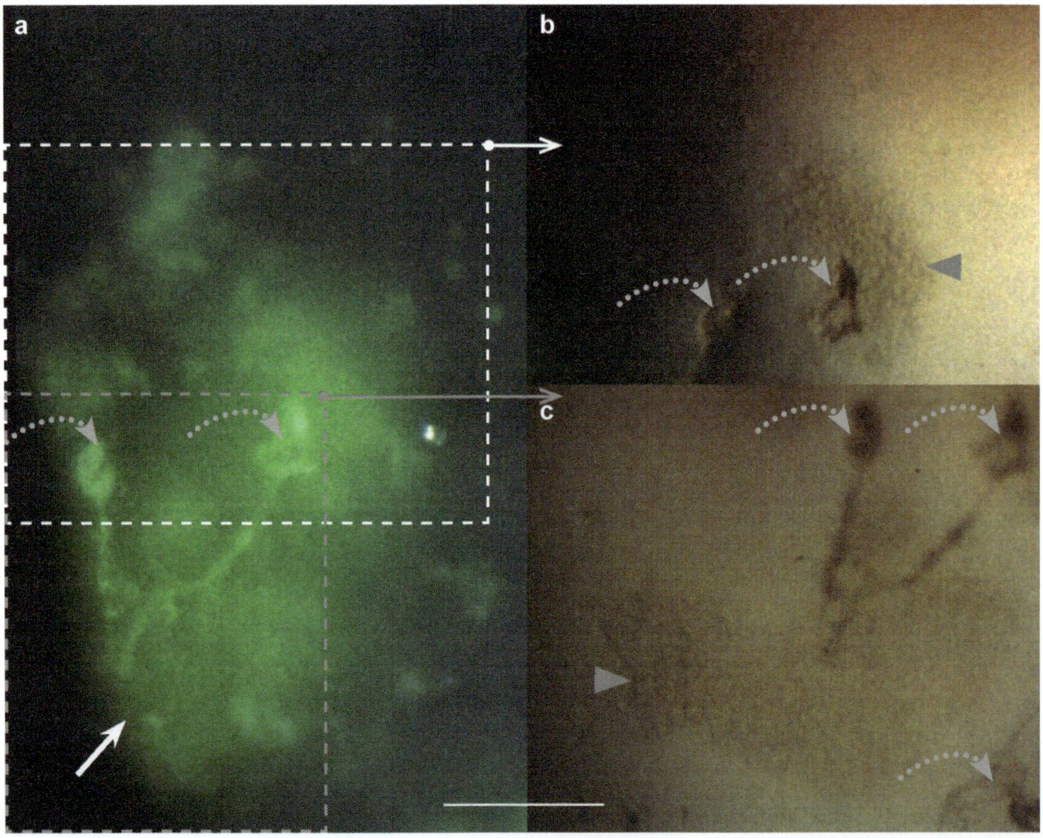

Fluorescent Flecks (2, Additional Features) (cont.)

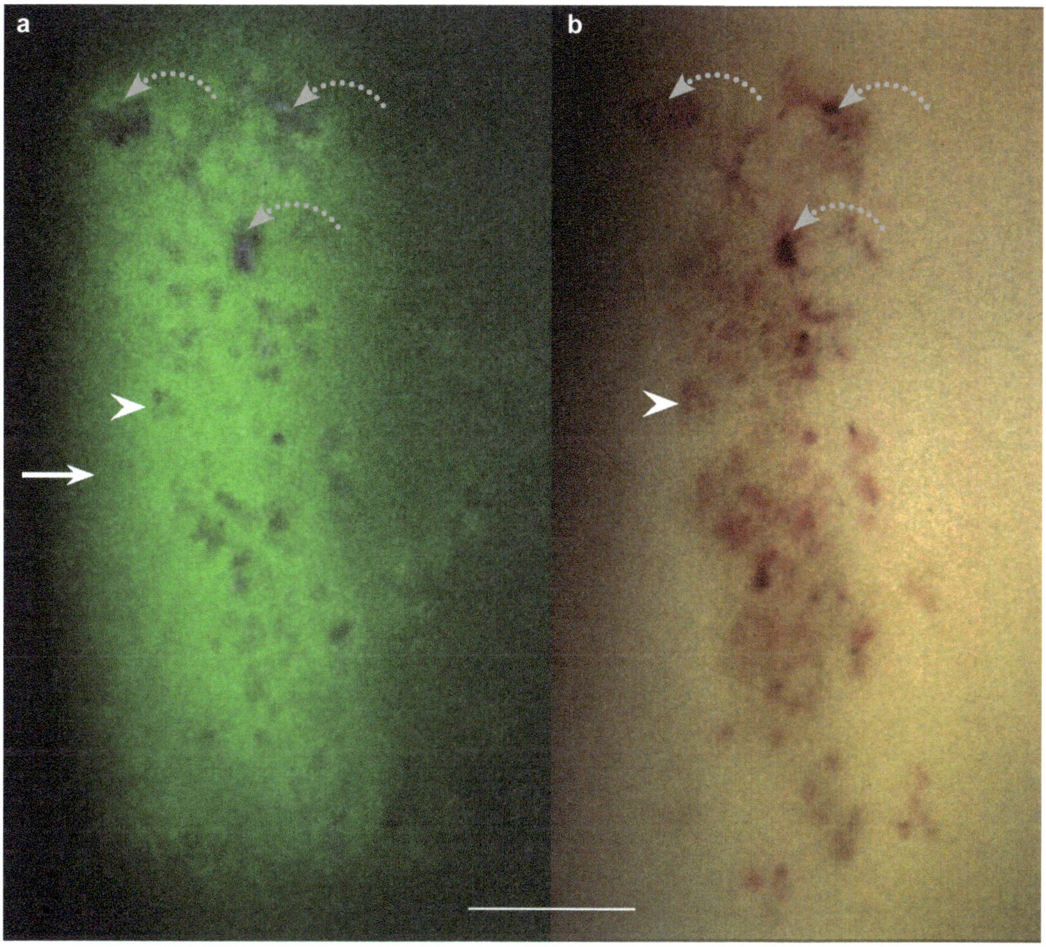

Fig. 2.49 The same cornea as in Fig. 2.47. A fleck showing surface-adherent mucus (*bowed arrows*), fluorescein diffusion into the tissues (green, *straight arrow* in a) and rose bengal stained surface cells/cell fragments *(arrowheads*). (The markers are placed in corresponding locations)

Fig. 2.48 The same cornea as in Fig. 2.47. (a) A larger green fleck (*white arrow*) resulting from confluence of smaller ones. In the areas in *frames* is visible in (b) and (c) a fine granularity (*arrowheads*). The mucus (*bowed arrows*) within the area of the fleck changes position but seems partly attached to the surface. An additional piece of mucus is visible in (c) (right lower corner, *bowed arrow*)

Adverse Effect of Rose Bengal (1)

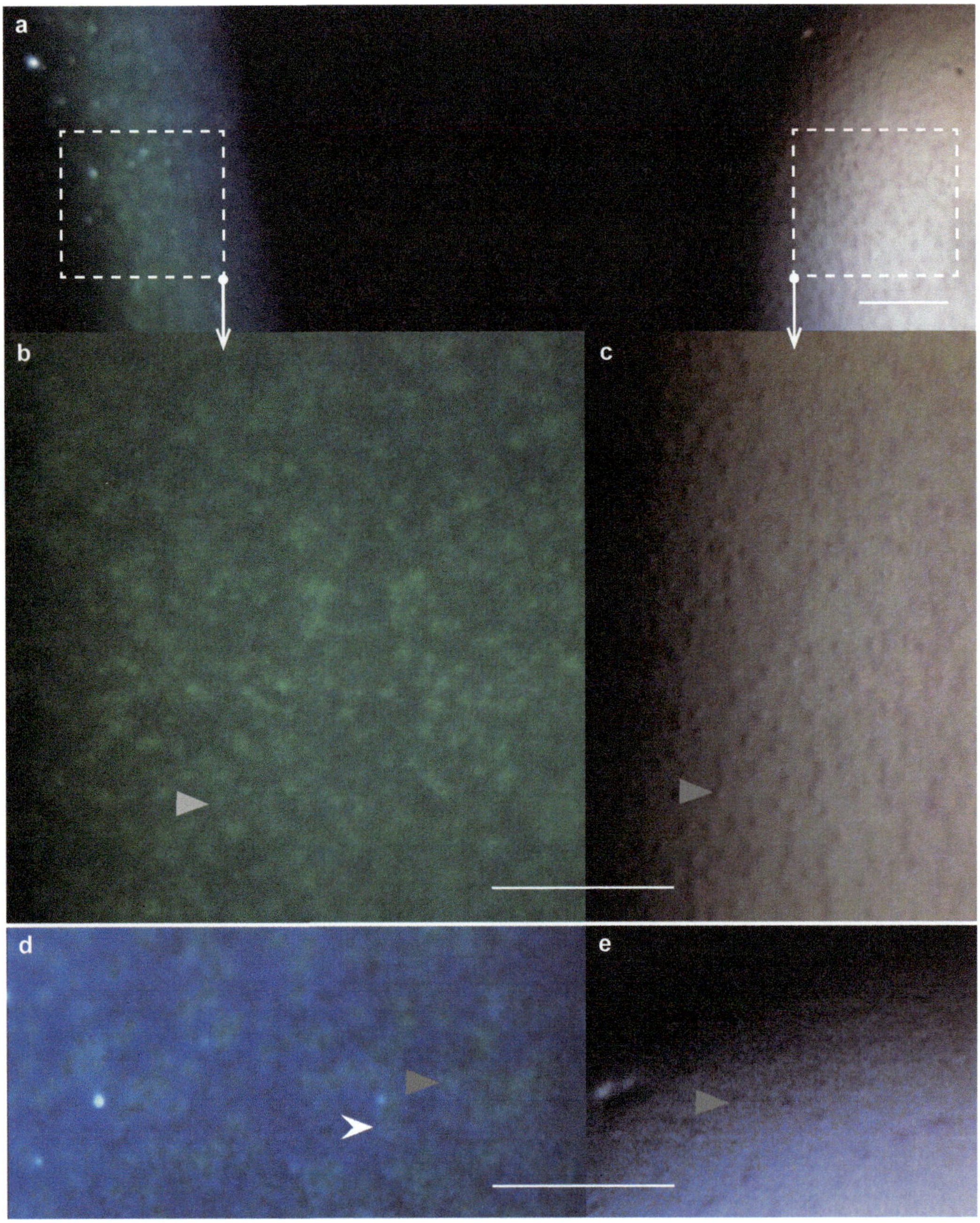

Fig. 2.50 Green corneal stipple in two corneae after the application of rose bengal in eyes preinstalled with fluorescein. Both corneae appeared normal before staining. (a) Survey. The areas in frames are shown at higher magnification in (b, c). (b) In the left part, many brightly green dots (*arrowhead*) are visible through the still green stained tear film. (c) In the right part are visible many rounded bodies (*arrowhead*). (d, e) show another cornea. (d) Fluorescein has disappeared from the tear film; visible are bright dots (*grey arrowhead*) and larger green dots (*white arrowhead*) that probably represent surface cells (cf. Fig. 2.51). (e) Also here are visible many rounded bodies (*arrowhead*)

Adverse Effect of Rose Bengal (2)

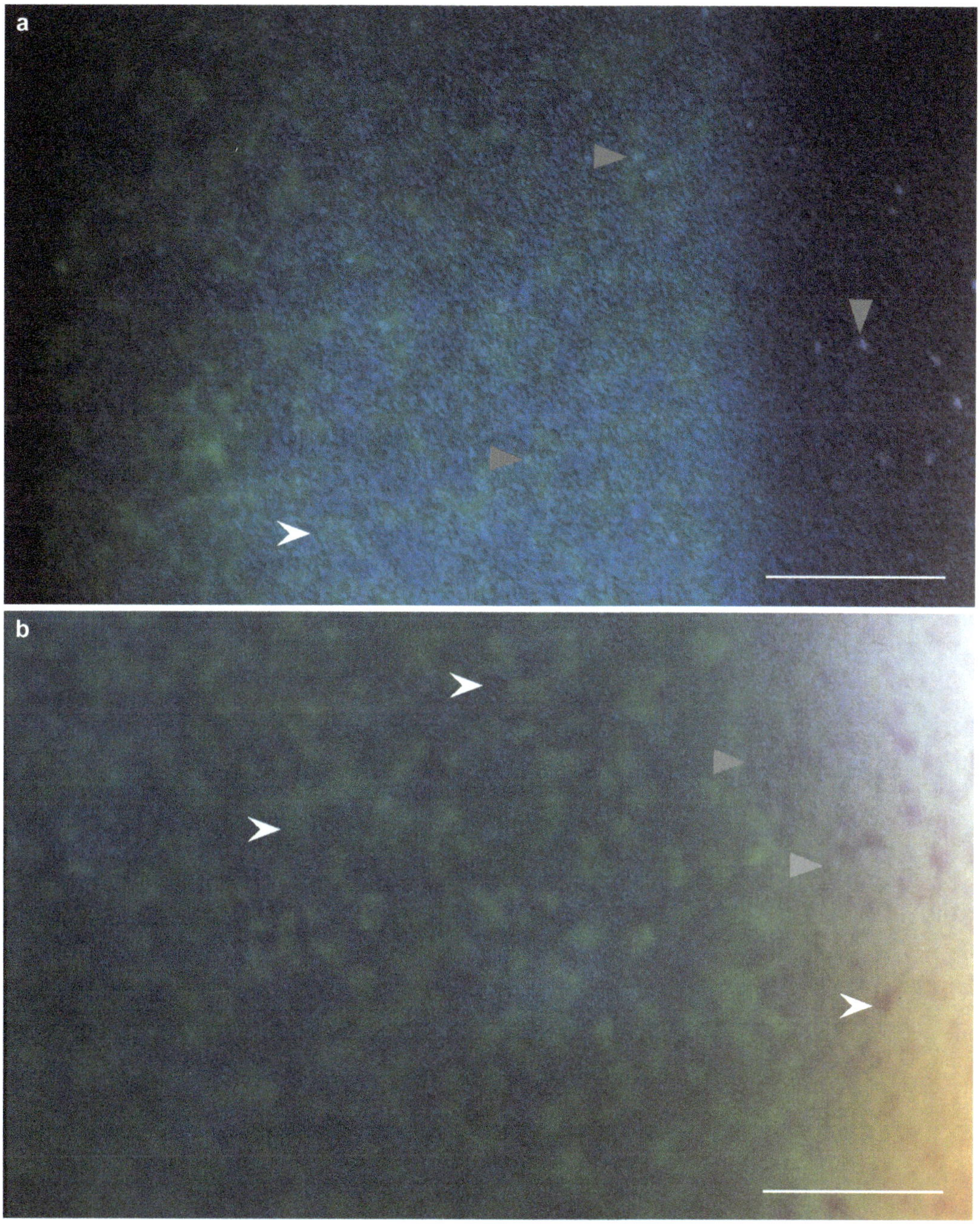

Fig. 2.51 Green corneal stipple in two corneae after the application of rose bengal in eyes preinstalled with fluorescein. Before staining both corneae appeared normal. (a) In the left part of the picture are visible myriads of bright dots, some small and rounded (*grey arrowheads*), others as larger green dots (*white arrowhead*) probably representing surface cells. In the right part are visible rounded bodies (*grey arrowhead*). (b) Also in this cornea appeared myriads of green dots after the application of rose bengal. The *white arrowheads* indicate green (left) and red (right) stained dots compatible with surface cells. Rounded bodies are only faintly visible (*grey arrowheads*) (If observed after the fluorescein had disappeared from the tear film, this cornea might have shown a fine punctate fluorescein staining before the application of rose bengal)

Mechanical Surface Damage

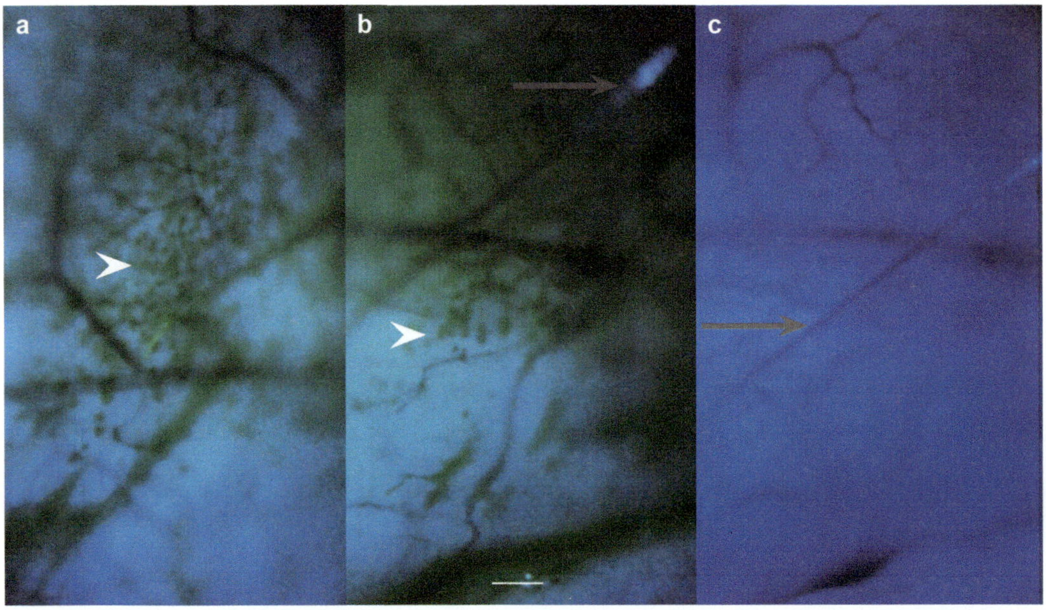

Fig. 2.52 (a–c) Damaged surface cells staining with non-fluorescent fluorescein (*arrowheads*) in trichiasis. An offending eyelash is indicated by *arrow*. (Conjunctival surface; a, b green filter, c blue filter)

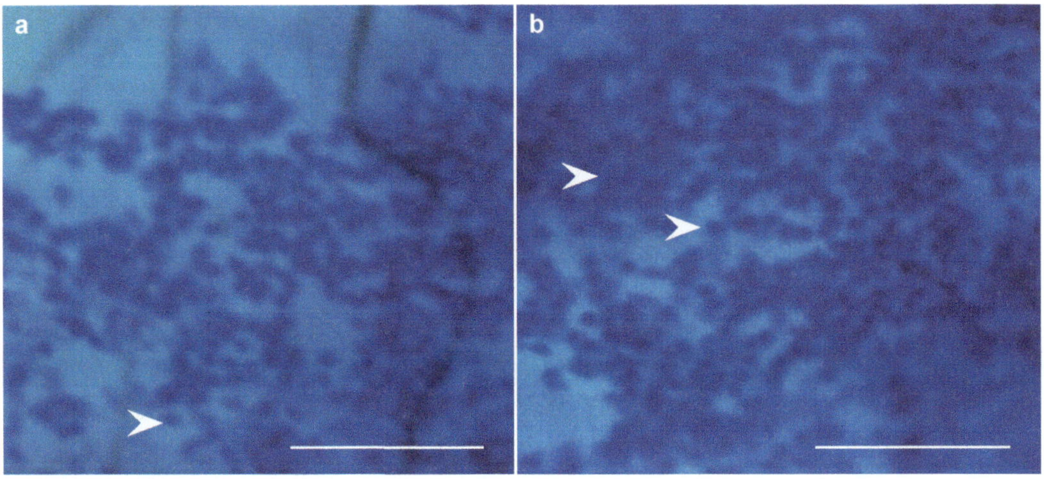

Fig. 2.53 (a, b) Surface damage caused by contact with paper strip used in Schirmer test; visible are many small rose bengal stained cells (*arrowheads*). (Conjunctival surface, green filter)

Addendum

An additional example of mechanical surface damage is shown in Fig. 4.31.

Fluorescent Flecks Versus HSV. Surface-Adherent Mucus Versus HZO Mucus Plaques

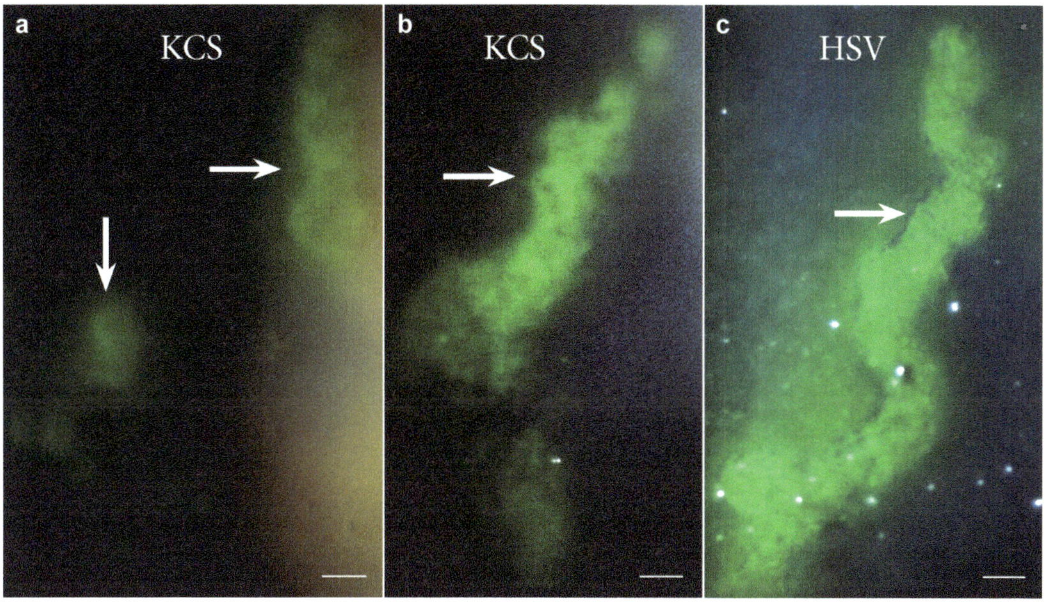

Fig. 2.54 (a, b) Green flecks *(arrows)* in KCS, individual and confluent; the figures with undulating borders remind of (c) herpes simplex virus lesions (HSV) (a Adapted from [3]; c Adapted from [11])

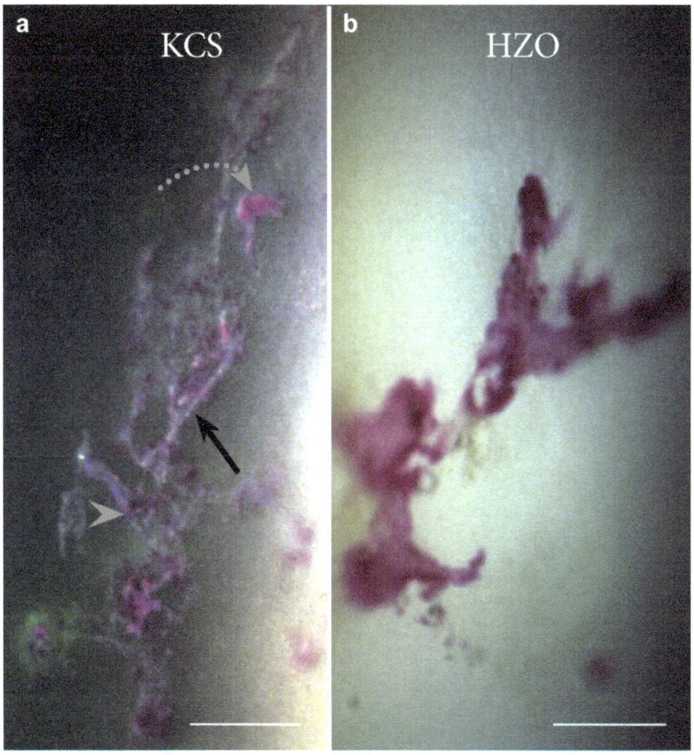

Fig. 2.55 (a) In KCS, mucus adhering to the surface shows threads (*straight arrow*) and patches (*bowed arrow*); the figure contains also cell debris (*arrowhead*). (b) For comparison, a typical red stained mucus plaque in herpes zoster ophthalmicus (HZO) (Adapted from [5, 12])

The Conjunctival Surface 3

In comparison with the cornea, observations of the conjunctival surface meet with two obstacles: one is the conjunctival pliability and the other the light originating in the underlying strongly light-reflecting sclera.

Conjunctival movements with eye movements and blinks result both in lateral displacements and in level differences. This does not disturb slit-lamp examinations but at a higher magnification level it is difficult to obtain comparable images capturing the same area.

The *scleral light reflection* not only effectively defies attempts to identify surface changes without the aid of diagnostic dyes but also renders fluorescein staining invisible. With *fluorescein sodium*, some staining can be visualised by manipulating the primary light source but the resulting area of visibility is rather small for practical purposes. *Colour filters*, such as present in a standard slit lamp, solve the problem. Fluorescein staining is visualised by either of them: the *green* filter better highlights its non-fluorescent (adherent) property and the *blue* filter the fluorescent one; it is easy to use them interchangeably. With *rose bengal*, the use of filters is optional; the staining is visible better with the green than with the blue one but neither of them reveals additional information.

Fluorescein sodium visualises, by its *non-fluorescent* staining property, diseased surface cells as dark dots (dark punctate staining). By its *fluorescent* property, it visualises: (1) *cystic spaces* (bright punctate staining) and (2) *surface disruptions* visible as bright *flecks*. The *dynamics* of fluorescein staining shows two phenomena: (1) the non-fluorescent staining is relatively short-lived and sooner or later transforms into a fluorescent (bright) one, and (2) the bright flecks may appear after some delay or rapidly and enlarge slowly or rapidly; in severe cases, large areas may appear bright within short.

Rose bengal visualises diseased surface cells.

With the two dyes, *diseased surface cells* are visualised as *dark dots* (non-fluorescent fluorescein), *bright dots* (fluorescent fluorescein) and *red dots* (rose bengal). There is a correspondence between the three but with the bright dots it is difficult to decide which of them visualises surface cells and which visualises other cystic spaces; as a detection of cystic spaces before staining is not possible, their existence in the conjunctival epithelium can neither be confirmed nor verified by the present method. Cells stained with non-fluorescent fluorescein stain also with rose bengal; they are present individually, in rows or groups, sometimes in apposition and other times with unstained slits between them, and the staining may be confluent with no discernible details. The cells show a variety of shapes and sizes (about 15–50 μm), and variously large cells may be present close to each other. The density of staining varies, also in cells close to each other and thus captured under approximately same illuminating conditions. In some cells, rose bengal (but not fluorescein) additionally reveals deeply stained dots interpreted as cell nuclei; nuclei are also visualised with *lissamine green*, sometimes used as an alternative to rose bengal.

Hence, with the dyes, the conjunctival epithelium shows phenomena comparable to the corneal ones save for one – the mucus. Larger structures similar to those adhering to the cornea have not been captured, but it may be that small amounts of mucus adhering to rose bengal stained cells (cf. cornea) could not be visualised because of the illuminating conditions.

Similarly to the cornea, conjunctival surface changes may concern the whole surface but usually are most pronounced in the interpalpebral area. The above examples (with the exception of Fig. 3.1) show the nasal conjunctiva. Additional examples are included in Chaps. 4 and 7.

H.M. Tabery, *Keratoconjunctivitis Sicca and Filamentary Keratopathy*,
DOI 10.1007/978-3-642-31028-7_3, © Springer-Verlag Berlin Heidelberg 2012

Punctate Non-fluorescent Fluorescein Staining

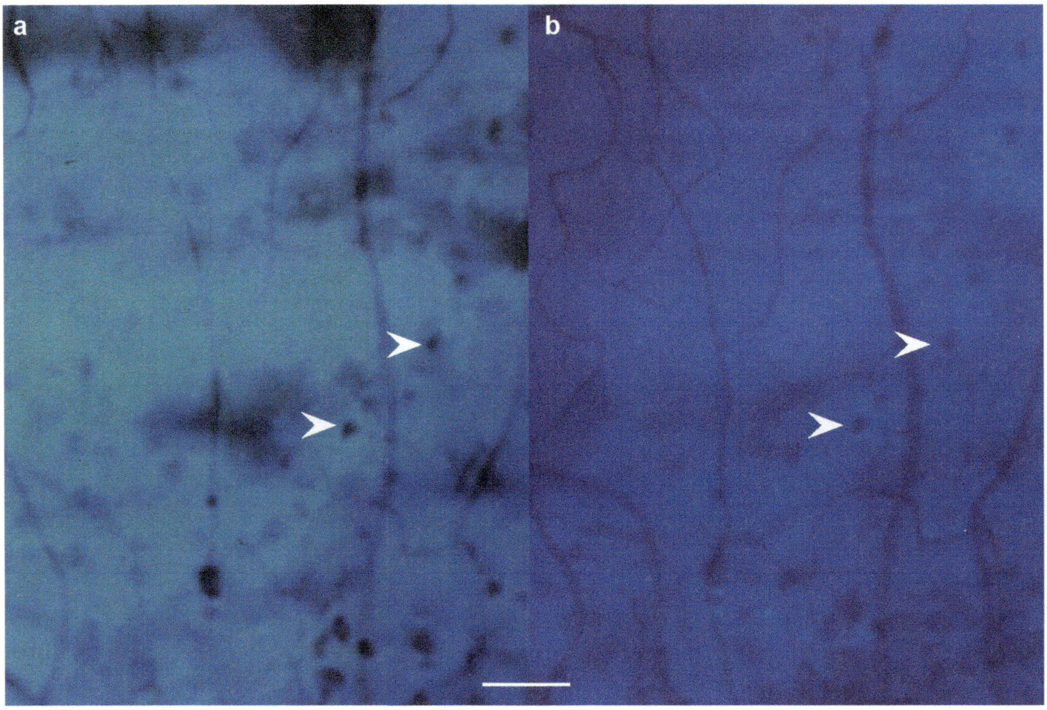

Fig. 3.1 Surface cells staining with non-fluorescent fluorescein (*arrowheads*) are visible both with (a) the green and (b) the blue filter but easier discernible with the green one. (The arrowheads are placed in corresponding locations; superior conjunctiva)

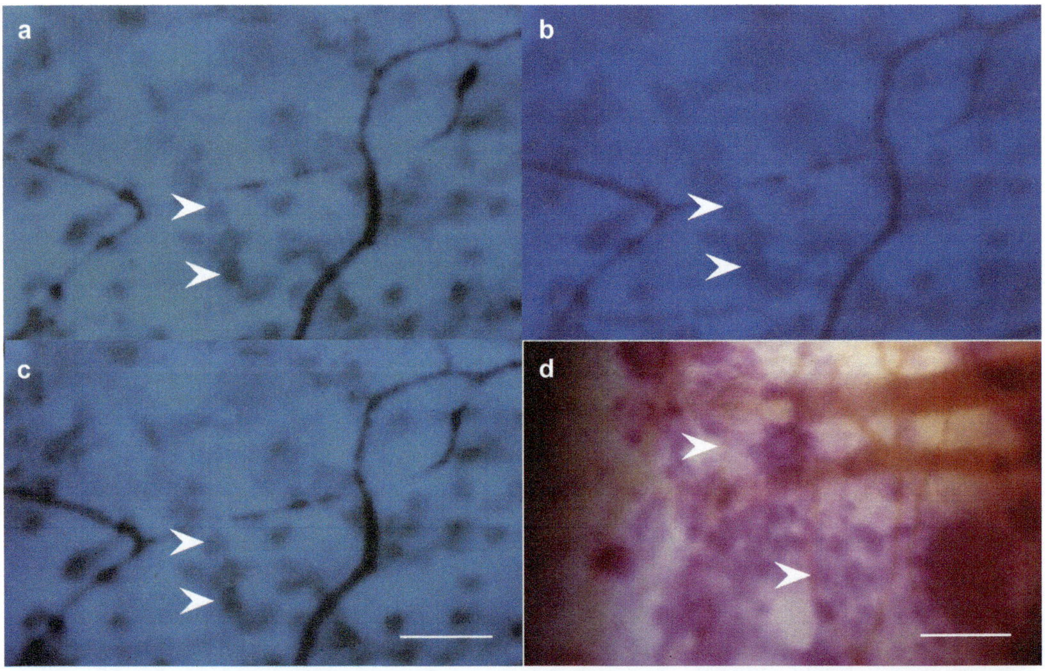

Fig. 3.2 The varying density of non-fluorescent fluorescein cell staining (*arrowheads*) is visible in consecutive photographs taken with (a and c) the green filter but not in that with (b) the blue one. (The arrowheads are placed in corresponding locations.) (d) shows a similarly varying density of rose bengal cell staining (*arrowheads*) in a different area of the same conjunctiva

Punctate Fluorescent Fluorescein Staining

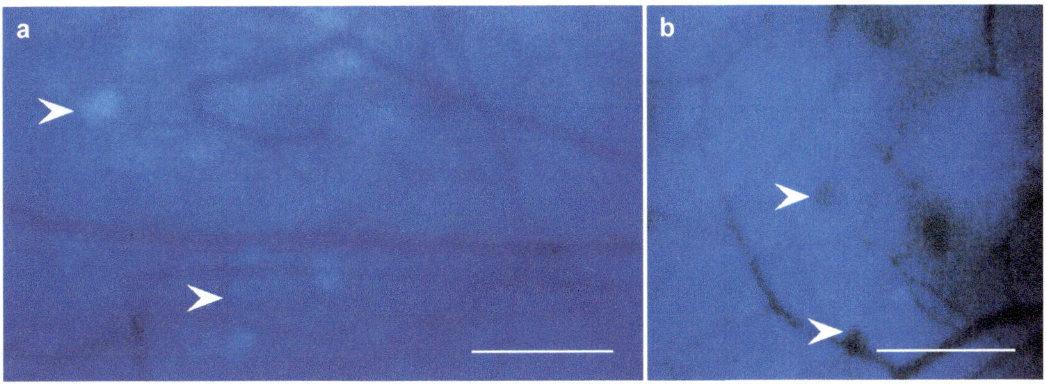

Fig. 3.3 (a) Punctate fluorescent (bright) fluorescein staining (*arrowheads*) visualised with the blue filter. (b) Punctate non-fluorescent (dark) fluorescein staining (*arrowheads*) visualised with the green filter

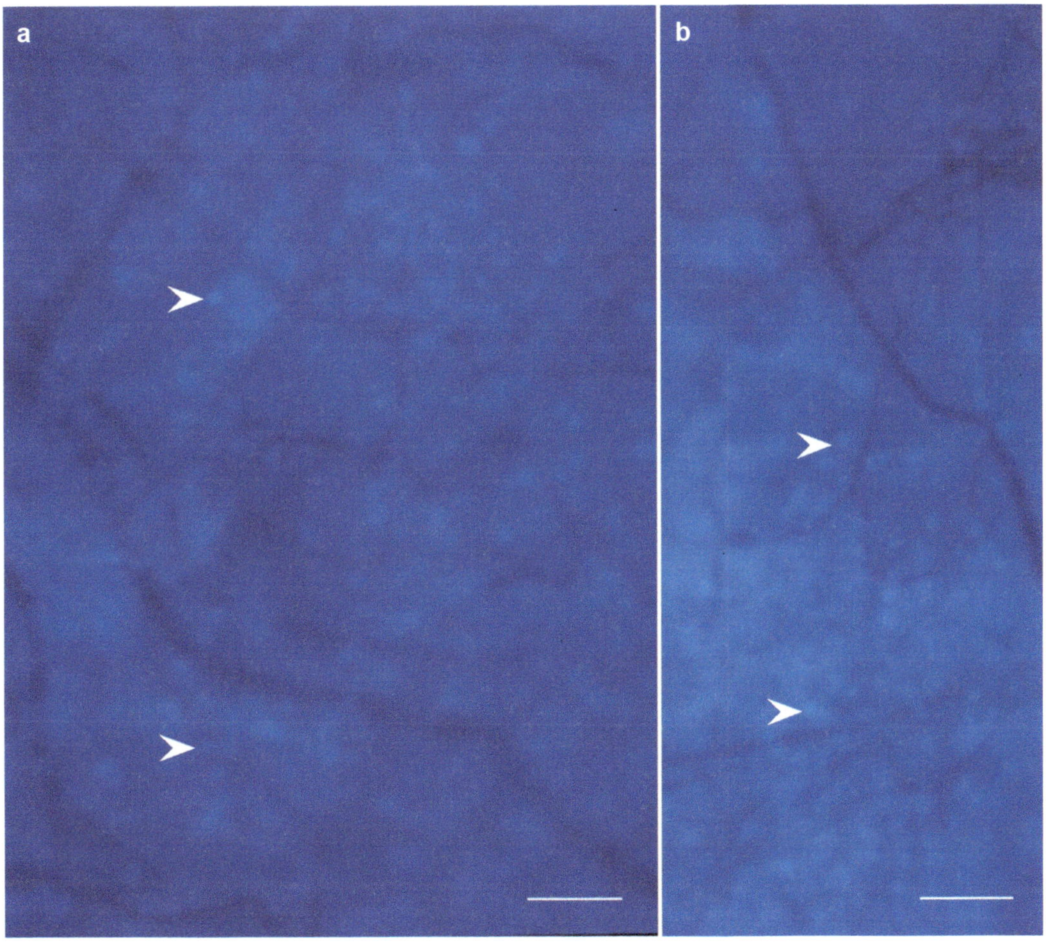

Fig. 3.4 (a, b) Survey of a punctate fluorescent fluorescein staining visualised with the blue filter. The fluorescent (bright) dots (*arrowheads*) are the result of penetration of green stained fluid below diseased cells and/or into other cystic spaces (cf. Fig. 3.7, overleaf, and Fig. 3.10)

Punctate Fluorescent Fluorescein Versus Rose Bengal Cell Staining

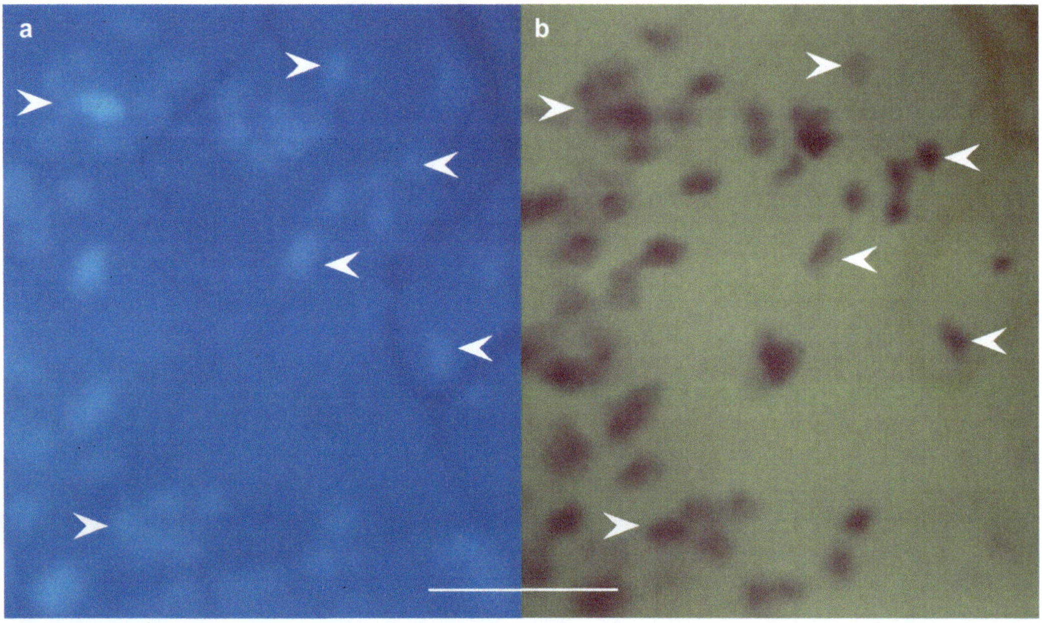

Fig. 3.5 (a) Punctate fluorescent staining and, for comparison, (b) the same area after the application of rose bengal. The *arrowheads* indicate surface cells visualised in both photographs. Cf. Fig. 3.10. (Some discrepancies are caused by cell detachments from the surface and cell movements with blinks; (a) blue filter)

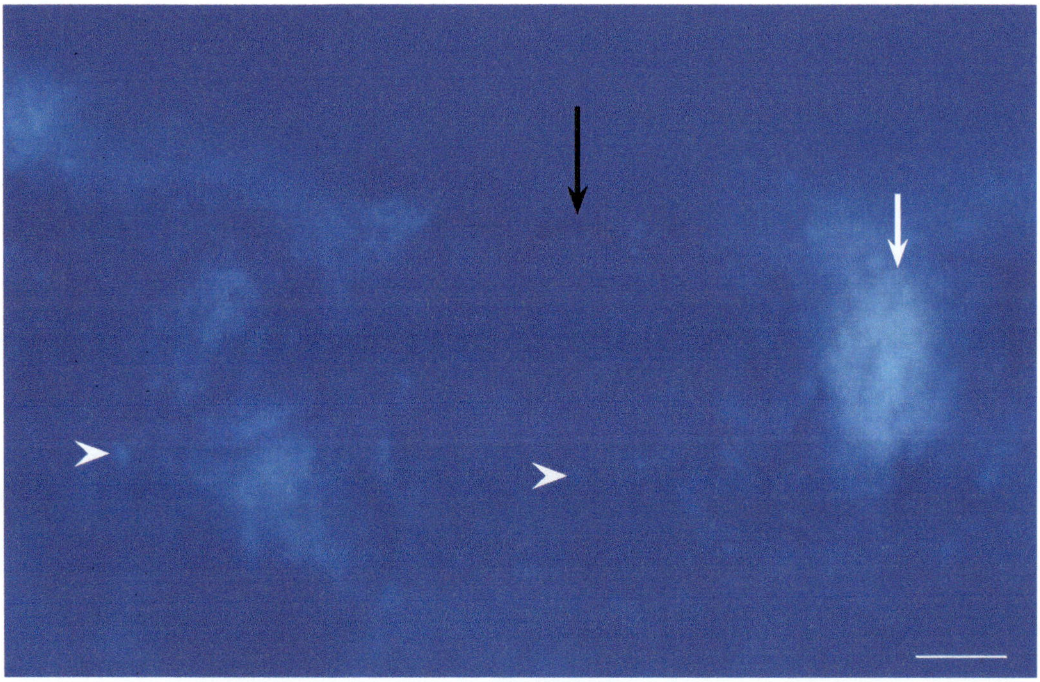

Fig. 3.6 A fluorescent fleck (*white arrow*) and punctate fluorescent staining (*arrowheads*) at the lower corneal limbus. The *black arrow* indicates a limbal vessel. (Blue filter)

Fluorescent Flecks

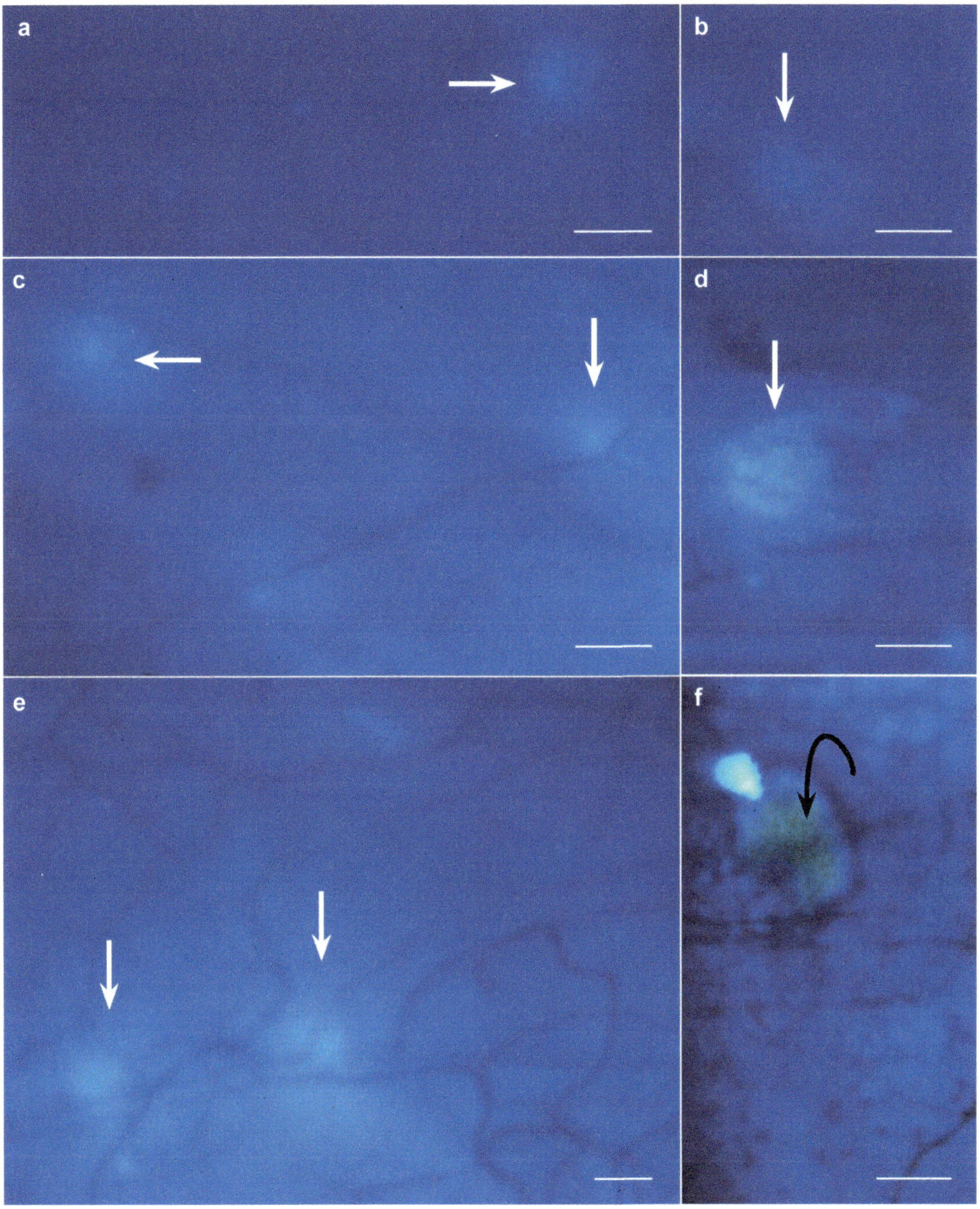

Fig. 3.7 (a–e) Low-magnification photographs showing variously large fluorescent flecks (*arrows*) caused by fluorescein diffusion into the tissues. (f) For comparison, pooling of fluorescein visible shortly after the application of the dye (*arrow*); it indicates a depressed area (epithelial erosion). (Blue filter)

Non-fluorescent Fluorescein Versus Rose Bengal Cell Staining (1)

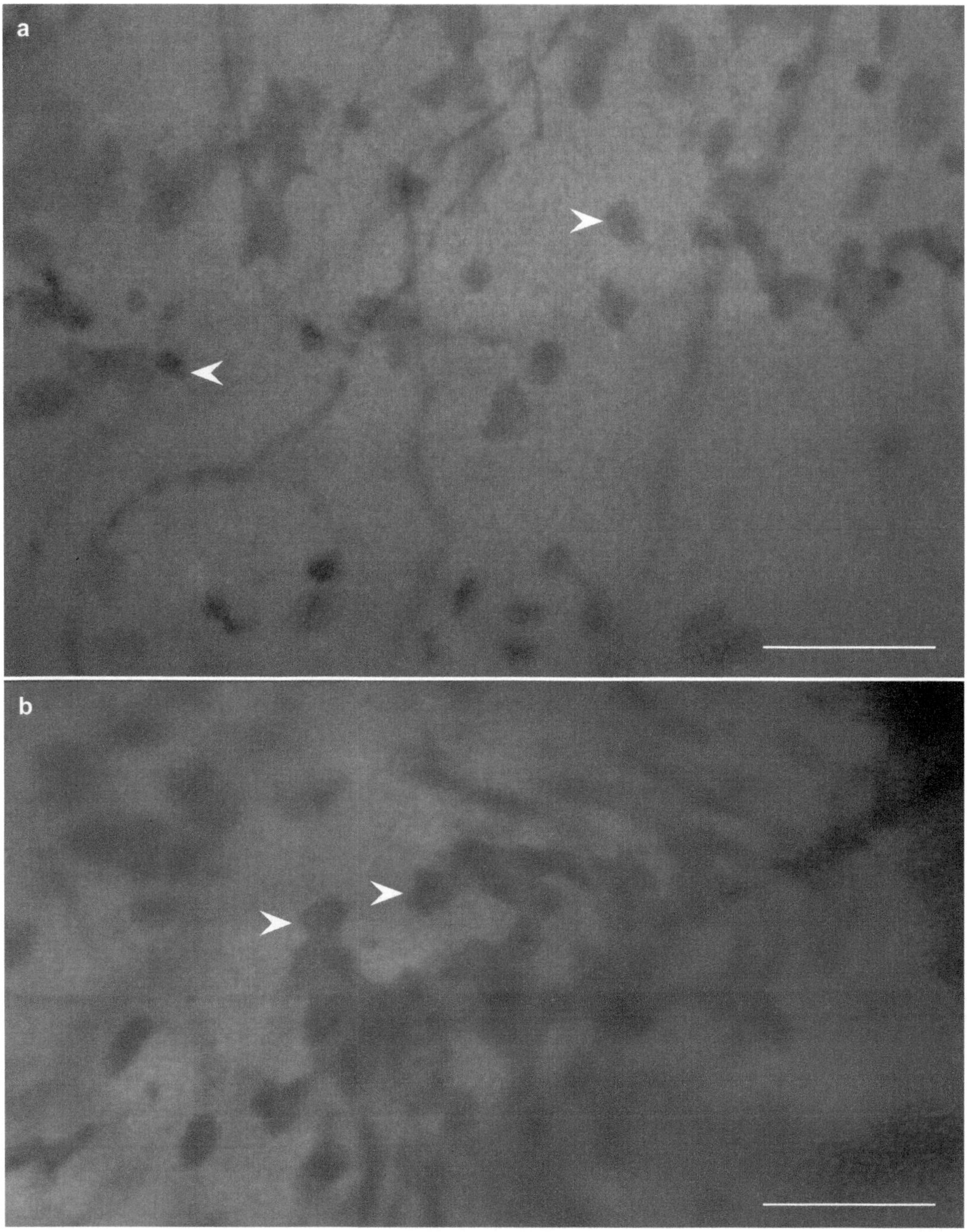

Fig. 3.8 With the green filter are visible cells (*arrowheads*) staining with (a) non-fluorescent fluorescein and (b) rose bengal; some of the rose bengal stained cells show a darkly stained dot (nucleus)

Non-fluorescent Fluorescein Versus Rose Bengal Cell Staining (2)

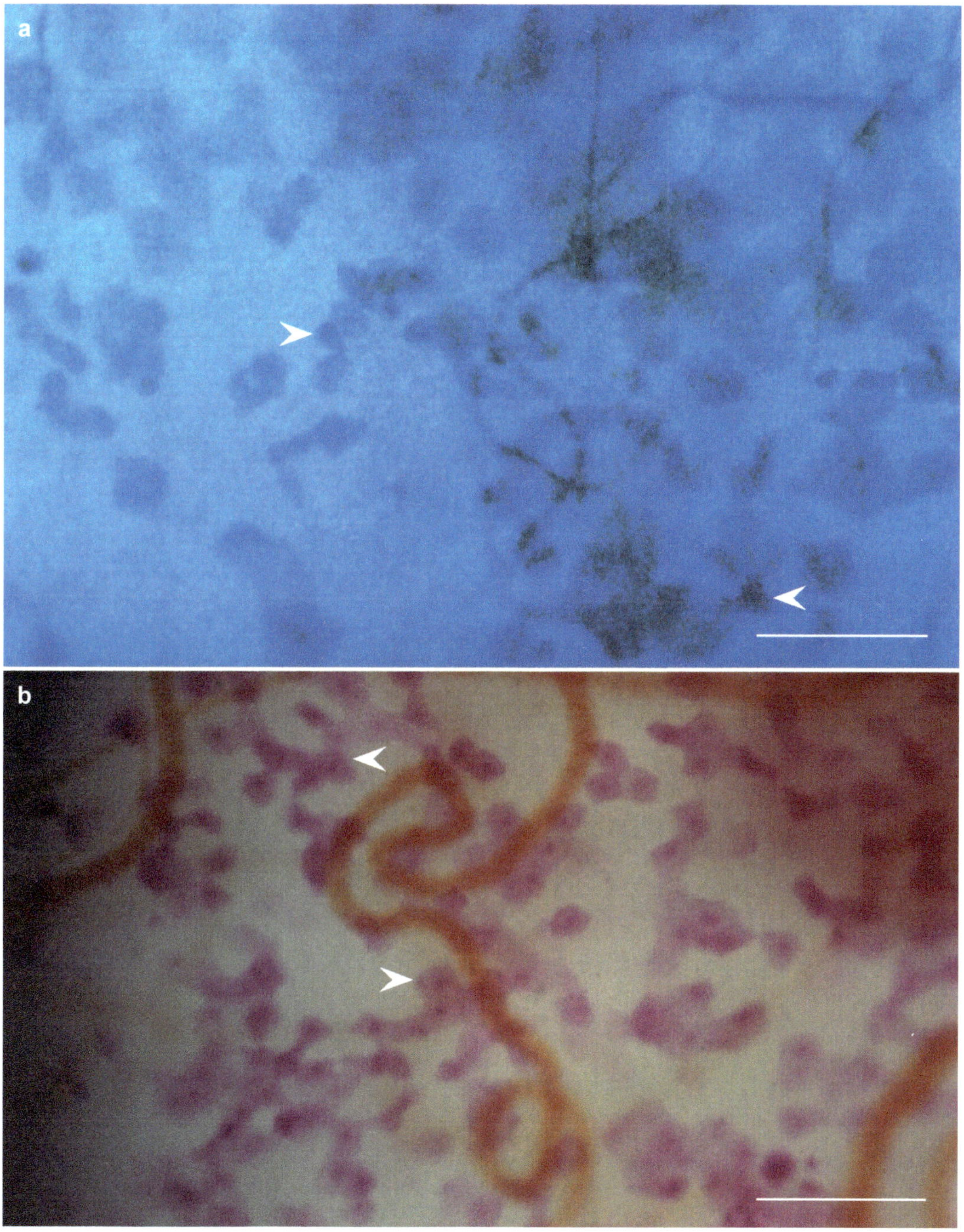

Fig. 3.9 Surface cells (*arrowheads*) visualised with (a) non-fluorescent fluorescein and green filter and (b) with rose bengal in white light. The pictures are very similar but distinct, deeply stained dots (nuclei) are clearly discernible only with rose bengal

Punctate Fluorescein Versus Rose Bengal Cell Staining

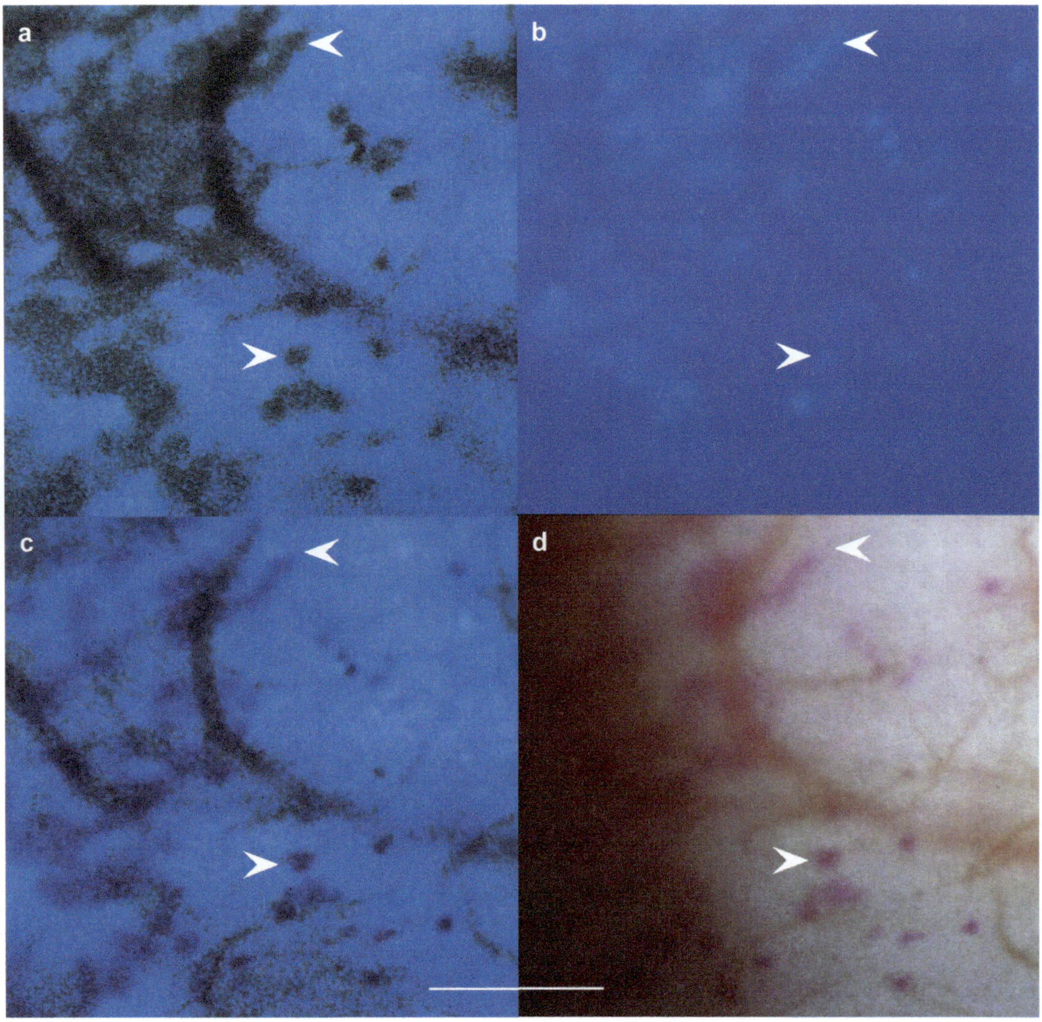

Fig. 3.10 Surface cells (*arrowheads*) visualised in the same area with (a) non-fluorescent fluorescein, (b) fluorescent fluorescein, (c) rose bengal and green filter and (d) rose bengal in white light. The patterns match. (The arrowheads are placed in corresponding locations; cf. also Fig. 6.18)

Rose Bengal Versus Lissamine Green Cell Staining

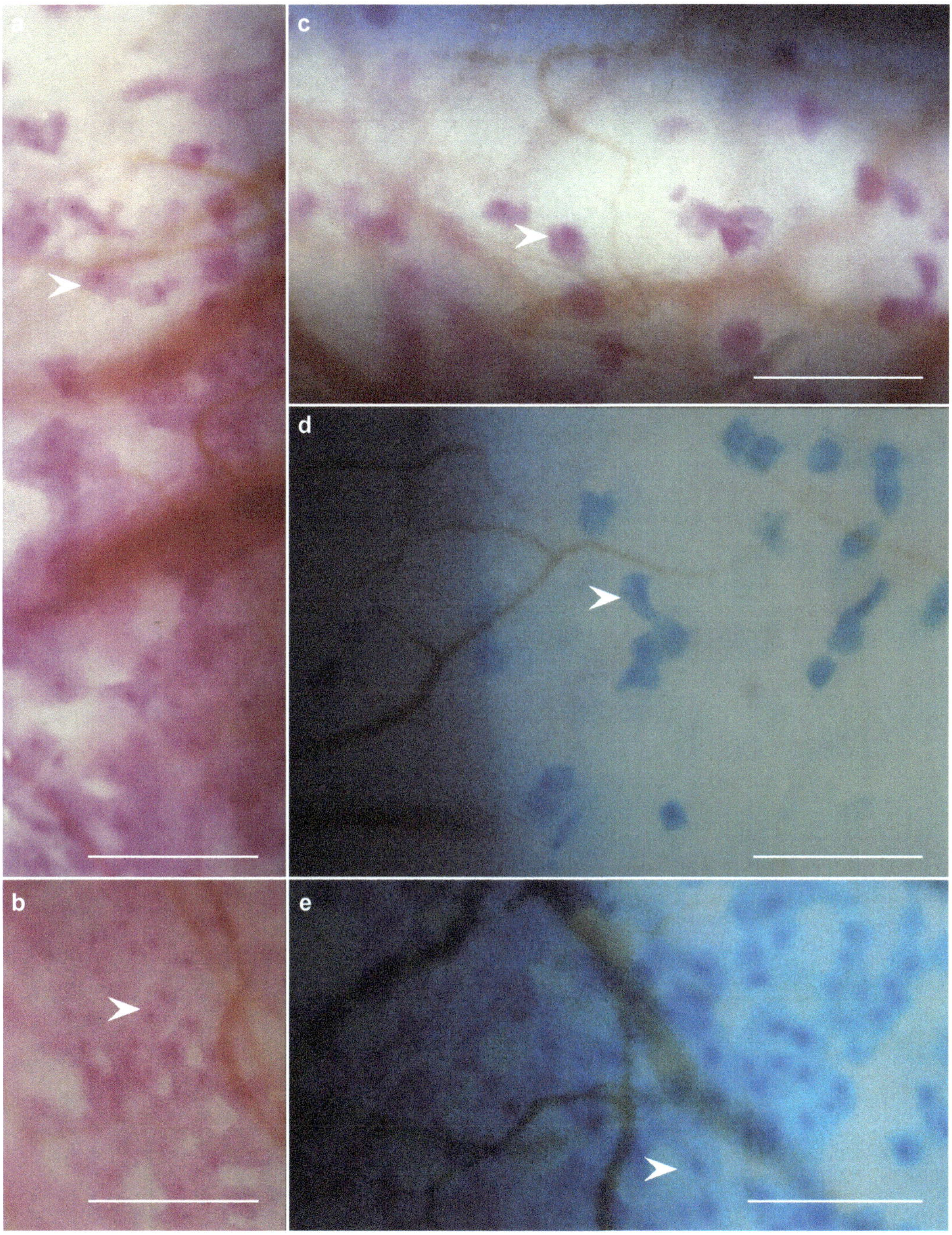

Fig. 3.11 Surface cells (*arrowheads*) visualised with (a–c) rose bengal and (d, e) lissamine green; the results are comparable

Additional Examples of Rose Bengal Cell Staining (1)

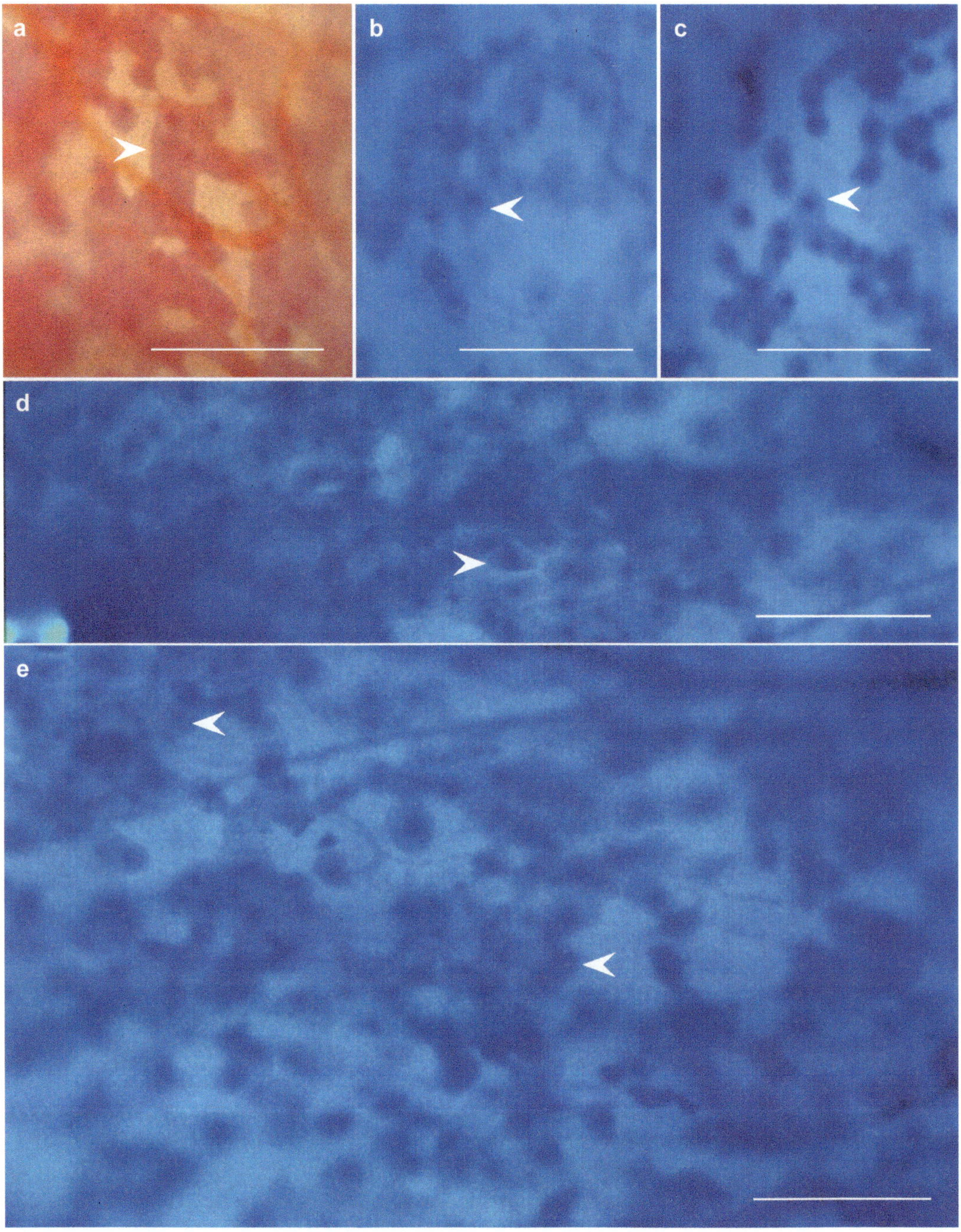

Fig. 3.12 (a–c) Rose bengal stained surface cells (*arrowheads*) captured (a) in white light and (b, c) with the green filter in different areas of the same conjunctiva. (d, e) Rose bengal stained surface cells (*arrowheads*) captured with the green filter in different areas of the same conjunctiva

Additional Examples of Rose Bengal Cell Staining (2)

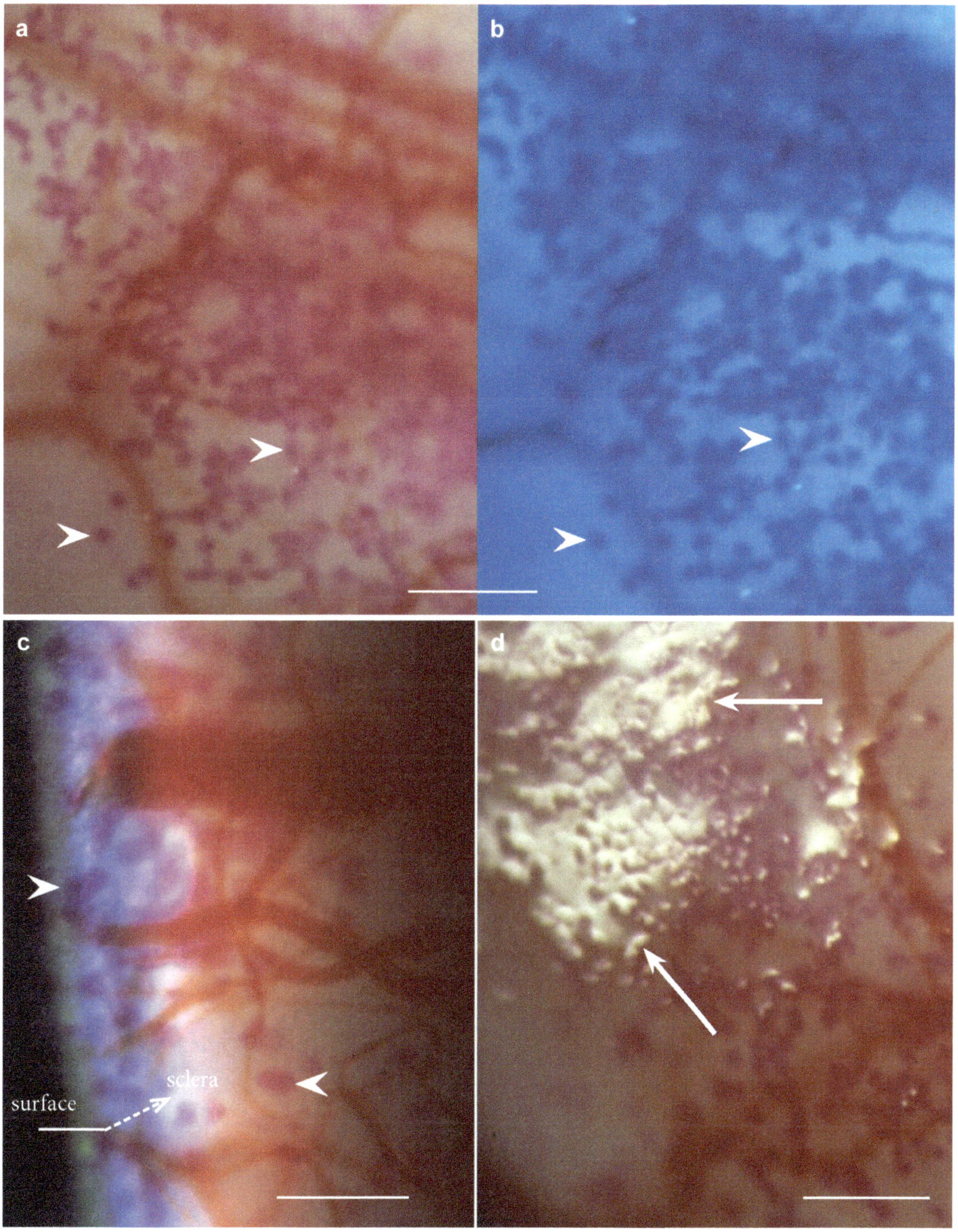

Fig. 3.13 (a, b) Rose bengal cell staining (*arrowheads*) captured in the same area (a) in white light and (b) with the green filter. (The arrowheads are placed in corresponding locations.) (c) With a narrow light beam the strong light-reflection from the sclera obliterating the visibility of the green fluorescence of fluorescein can be avoided; the hue of the red staining (*arrowheads*) varies with illumination. (d) shows conjunctival specular light reflection (*arrows*) revealing surface irregularities

Additional Examples of Rose Bengal Cell Staining (3)

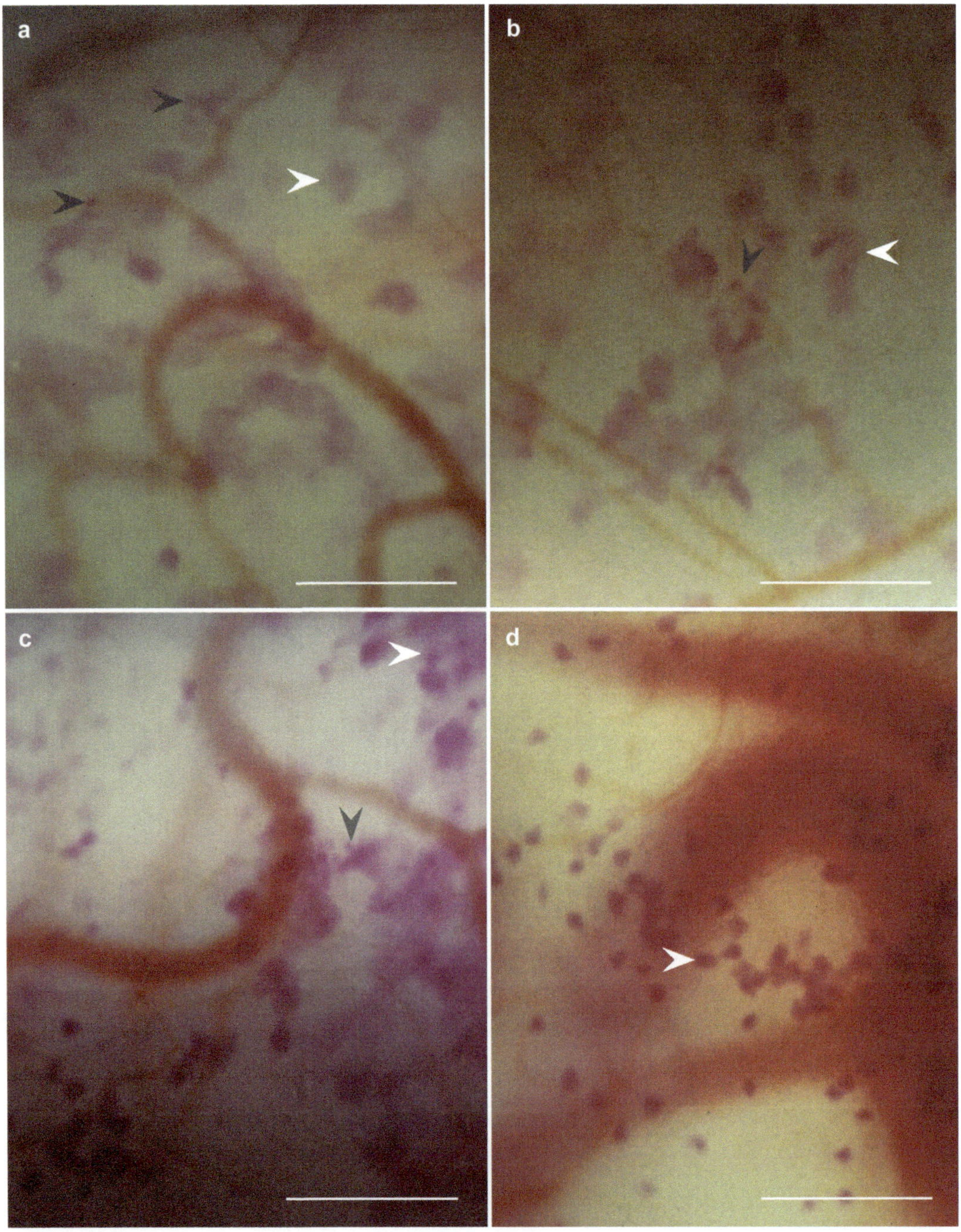

Fig. 3.14 (a, b) Areas showing more or less deeply rose bengal stained surface cells (*white arrowheads*): (a, b) without deeply stained dots (nuclei), (c) small and larger cells of which some contain a deeply stained dots (nuclei) and (d) small cells. The *grey arrowheads* in (a–c) indicate red stained dots, possibly cell fragments

Additional Examples of Rose Bengal Cell Staining (4)

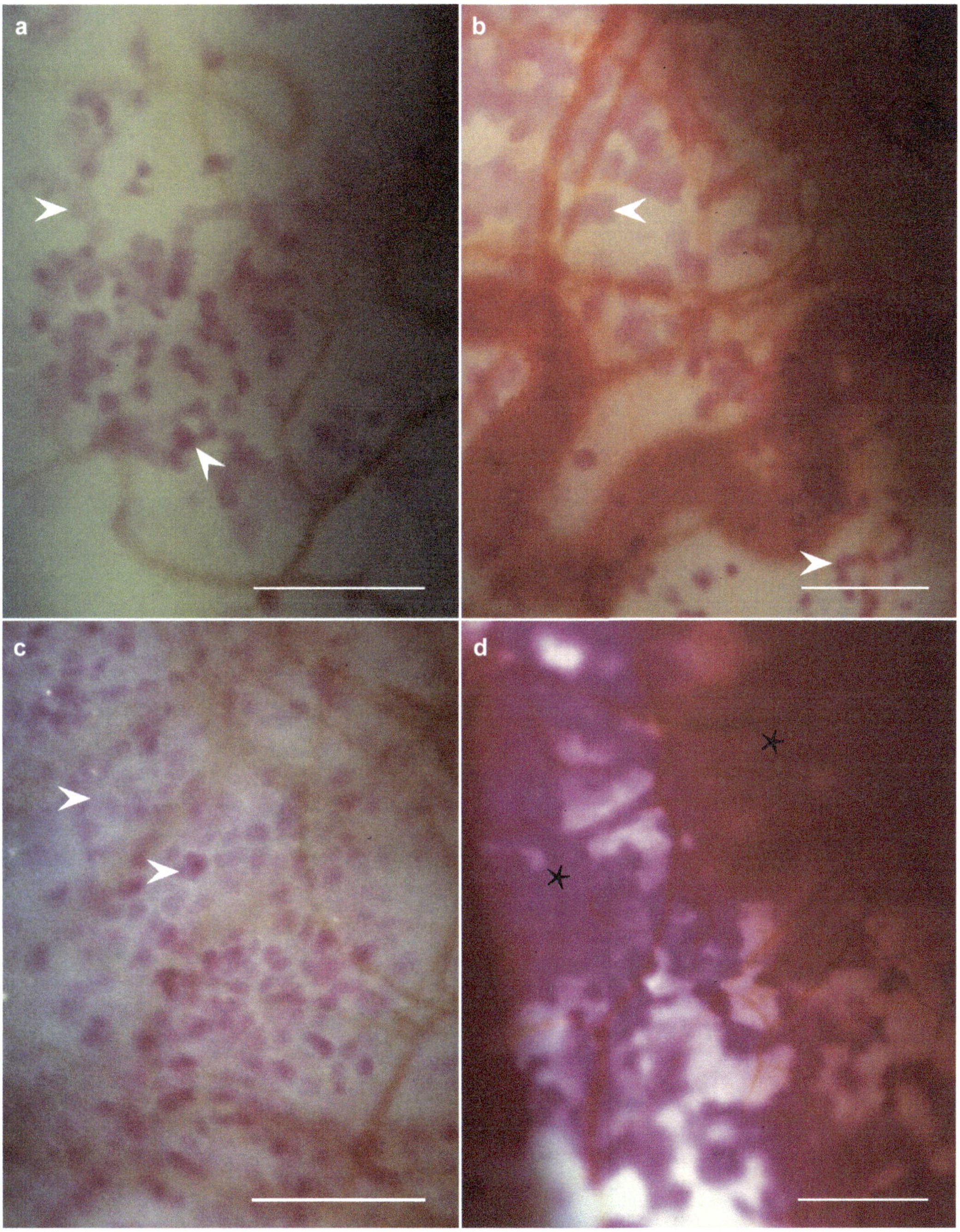

Fig. 3.15 Areas showing rose bengal stained surface cells (*arrowheads*): in (a and c) is visible varying staining density, in (b) larger and small cells and in (d) areas of confluent staining with no discernible details (*asterisks*)

Additional Examples of Rose Bengal Cell Staining (5)

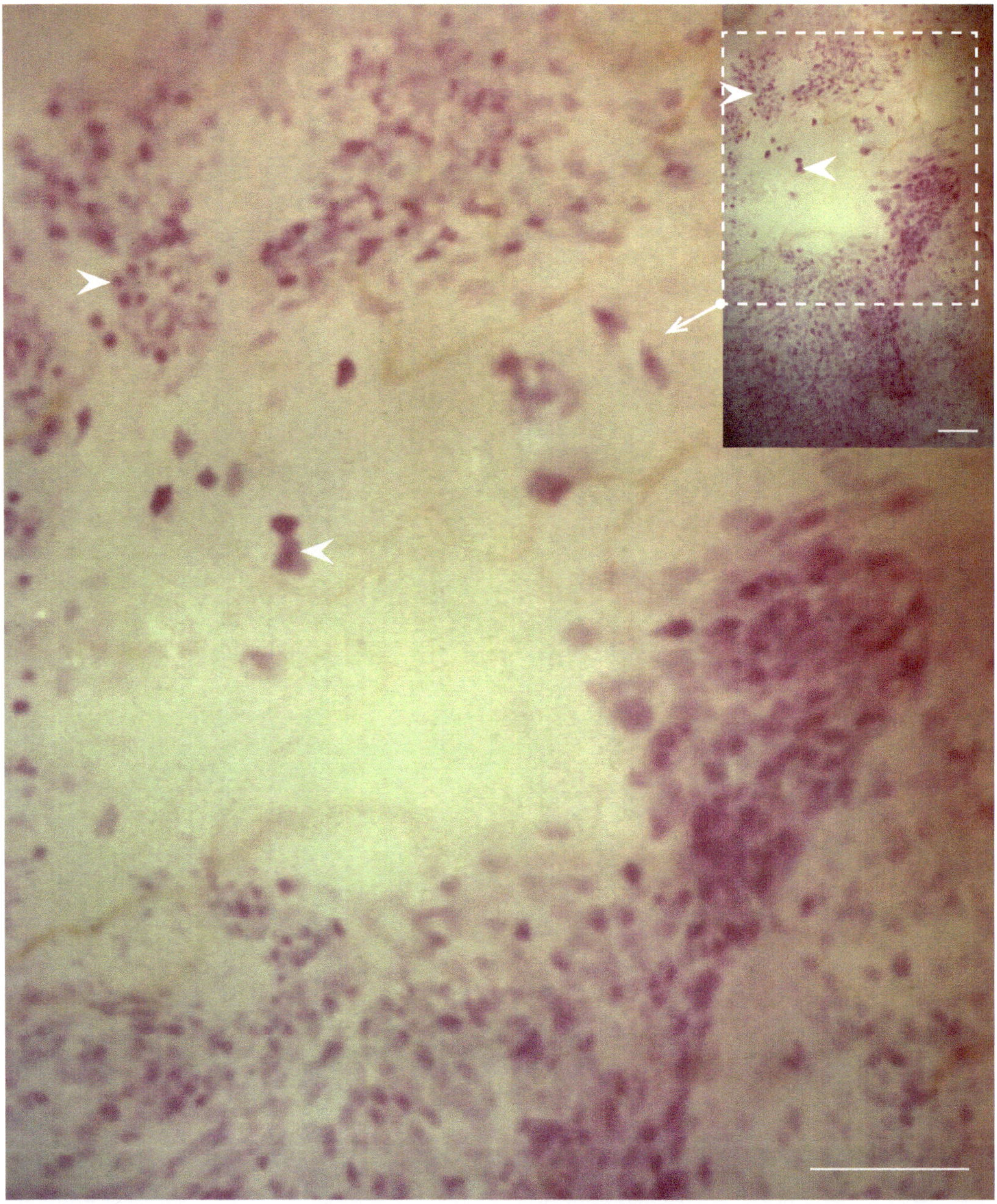

Fig. 3.16 *Inset*: Survey. The area in *frame* shows many variously shaped and more or less deeply stained surface cells (*arrowheads*); in places, deeply stained dots might represent cell nuclei. (The arrowheads are placed in corresponding locations)

Additional Examples of Rose Bengal Cell Staining (6)

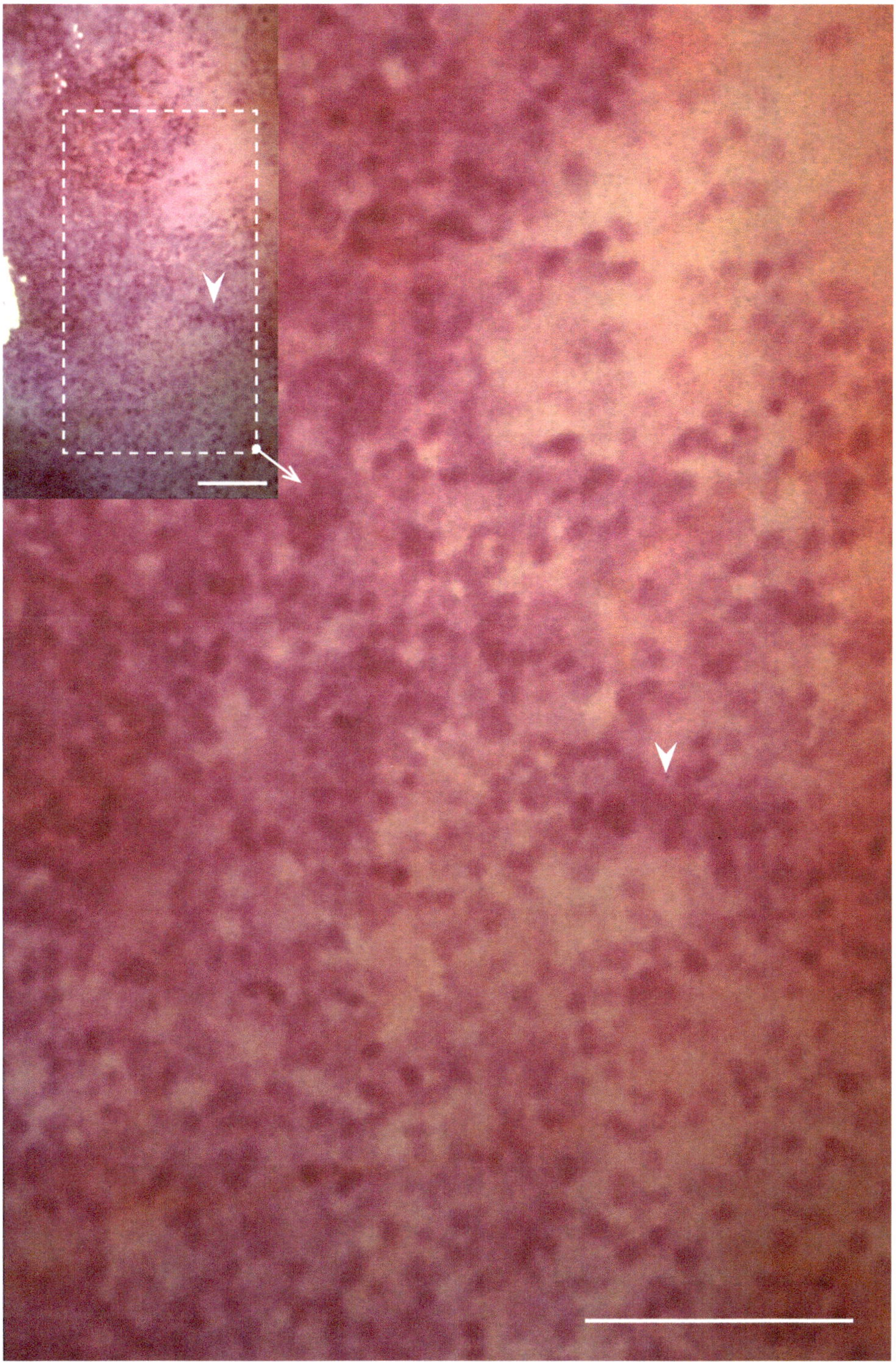

Fig. 3.17 *Inset*: Survey. The area in frame shows many variously shaped and more or less deeply stained surface cells (*arrowheads*) in apposition; the pattern is partly confluent. Whether or not some deeply stained dots might represent cell nuclei is uncertain. (A different area of the same conjunctiva as in Fig. 3.16; the arrowheads are placed in corresponding locations)

4 Case Reports

The cases presented in this chapter reflect some of the various combinations of symptoms and findings encountered in clinical practice.

Acute onset of KCS or a bout of disease activity, both simulating infections, may be more common than realized because what is attributed to a beneficial effect of antibiotics may be a spontaneous regression of symptoms occurring within a short period of time. In combination with general symptoms, an ophthalmologist recognizing KCS ocular surface changes plays an important role by pointing out the possibility of autoimmune disease as a common denominator (Case 1). A KCS diagnosis and a referral for investigation of a possible autoimmune disease may save many a patient antibiotic treatments, both topical and p.o. (Case 6).

Fluctuations in KCS severity are known, but in some patients the improvements appeared almost spectacular (Cases 4 and 5); still, there was no other explanation. Case 4 additionally demonstrates a situation in which a strict application of (the used) KCS criteria was difficult; it is also notable that while the surface showed a dramatic improvement, the test values remained more or less unchanged.

In some patients, mucus sheets may be a prominent feature (Case 2), in others corneal flecks coming and going for many years without leaving any trace (Cases 3 and 6); in the latter two patients, no progression of the disease was observed during the observation period of 11 respectively 8 years.

Stromal infiltrates associated with KCS are not very common; the patient (Case 7) had no known KCS, and the resolution of the infiltrate within a week with a topical antibiotic was satisfactory. The finding of KCS after healing, however, was suggestive of a sterile infiltrate.

Case 8 diverged from the others in that the patient had atopic eczema. The KCS diagnosis was in agreement with the used criteria but the appearance of the surface was partly different. Mainly, diseased surface cells were more strongly light-reflecting, showed no nuclei, and fluorescein diffusion into the tissues was absent. Whether these differences might have reflected a different disease cause remains open.

The last patient (Case 9) had a combination of KCS, corneal hyp- or anaesthesia after stroke, and recurrent erosions in the involved cornea. Unusual was a bout of epitheliopathy occurring several years after the stroke (see also 'Final Remark').

Patients with KCS and filaments are presented in Part II.

H.M. Tabery, *Keratoconjunctivitis Sicca and Filamentary Keratopathy*,
DOI 10.1007/978-3-642-31028-7_4, © Springer-Verlag Berlin Heidelberg 2012

Case 1: Acute Onset of KCS and General Symptoms

Case Report

A 70-year-old woman with a sudden onset of severe bilateral conjunctivitis, and cystitis, was treated by a general practitioner with antibiotics, both topical and p.o. About 2 weeks after symptom onset, she was admitted in the Department of Infectious Diseases because of new symptoms such as fever and joint pain and swelling. Investigation revealed no infectious causes, and she was transferred to the Rheumatology Department. During the investigation, her general symptoms gradually subsided without treatment. At presentation (about 3 weeks after onset of ocular symptoms), both conjunctivae were injected and oedematous, and the corneae showed many small filaments. BUT was unmeasurable, Schirmer 1 test 0/0 and RBS 9/9. She was treated with lubricating eye drops.

Six weeks later, both eyes were white and the symptoms less severe. The lower part of the left cornea showed a few fine filaments. The test values were unchanged.

The photographs of the left eye were taken at presentation and 6 weeks later; at that stage, the diagnosis was of a so far unspecified connective tissue disease.

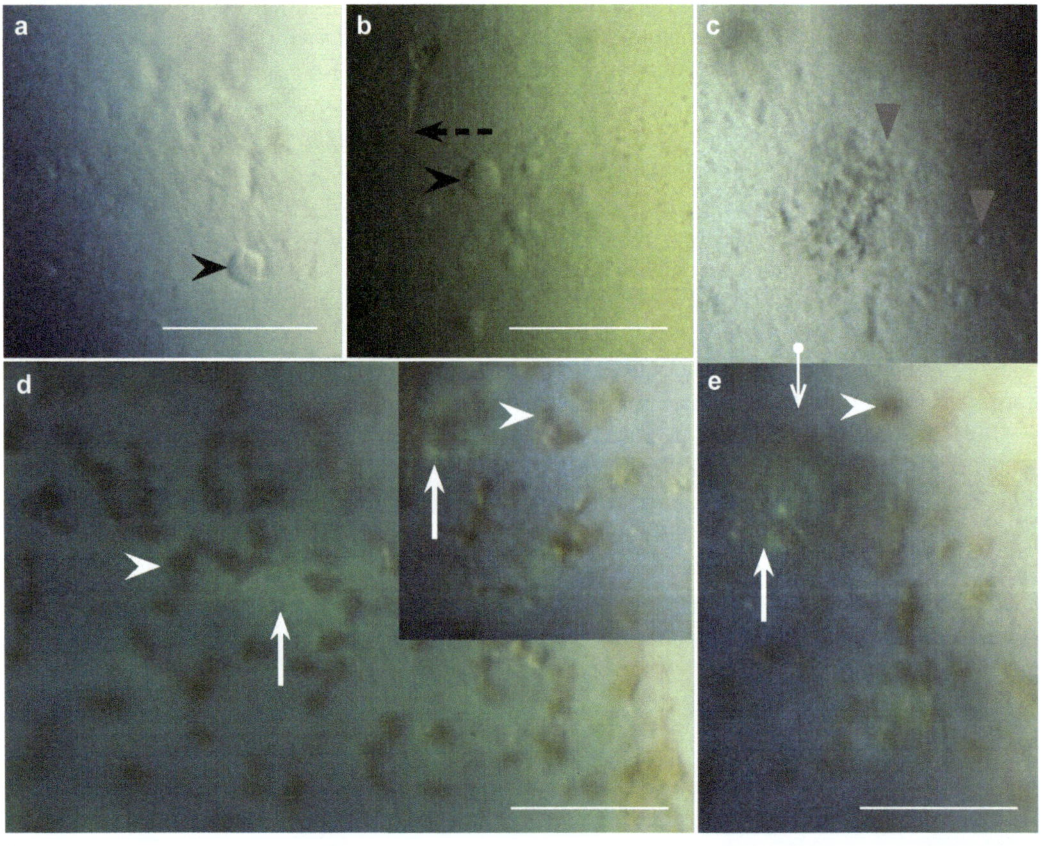

Fig. 4.1 Before staining were captured cystic spaces (**a**, **b**, *arrowheads*), a small filament (**b**, *arrow*), and an area showing rounded bodies (**c**, *arrowheads*; cf. Fig. 2.36). After the application of fluorescein are visible (**d**, inset in **d**, and **e**) non-fluorescent (yellow-brown) stained surface cells (*arrowheads*) and incipient fluorescein diffusion into the tissues (green, *arrows*). (**c**, **e**) show the same area

Case 1: Acute Onset of KCS and General Symptoms (cont.)

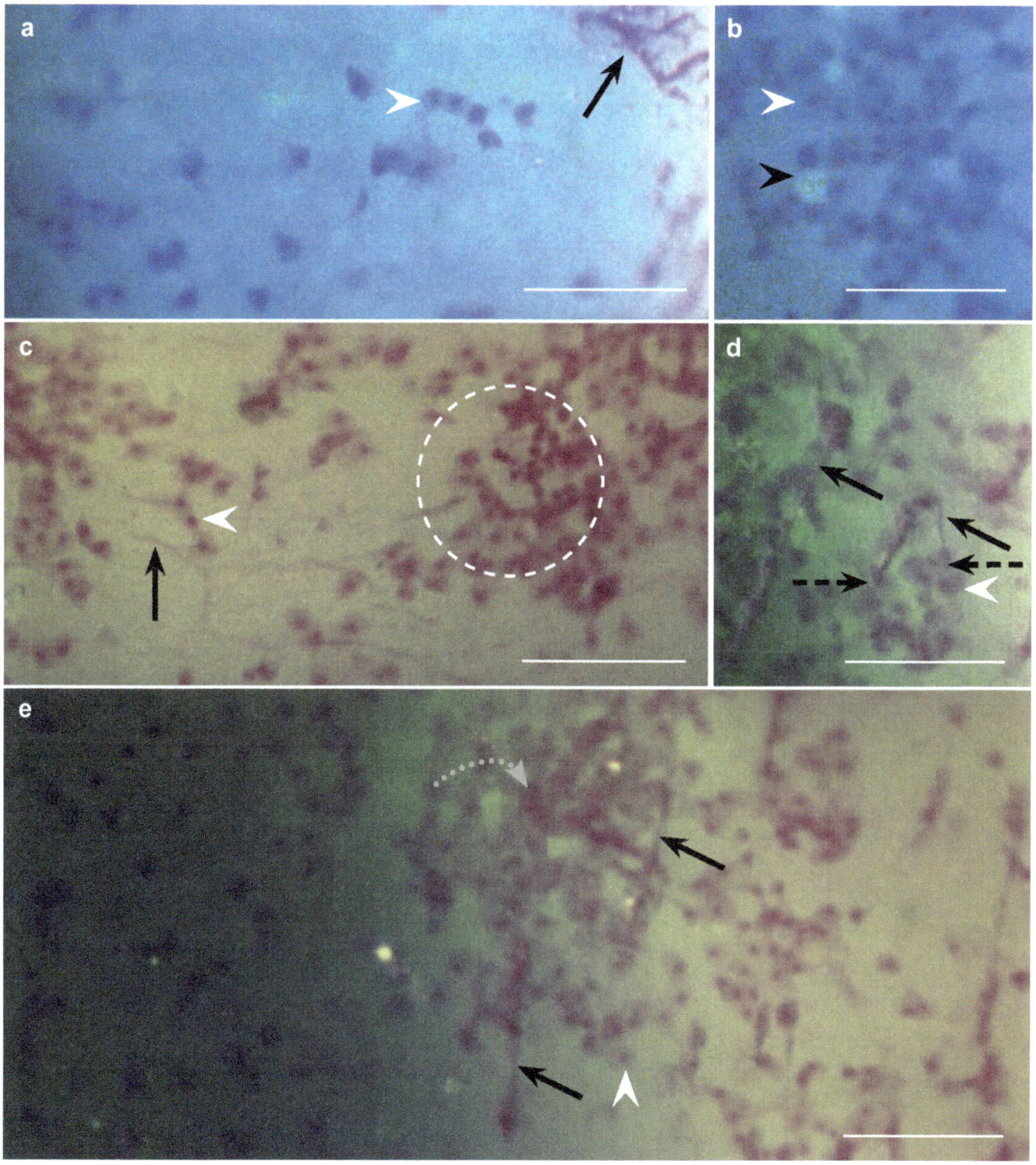

Fig. 4.2 (a–e) Many of the rose bengal stained surface cells (*white arrowheads*) show a distinct dark dot (nucleus). More or less deeply stained cells, larger and smaller, individual or grouped, are in places close to each other (c, in *frame*). In (c) are visible fine mucus threads (*arrow*) and in (a, d and e) thicker mucus threads with attached debris (*plain arrows*); one of these is attached at each end to a red stained cell (d, *dashed arrows*). The *bowed arrow* in (e) indicates an area showing mucus adhering to stained cells. The green background visible in (d, e) is caused by fluorescein diffusion into the tissues; the *black arrowhead* in (b) indicates a green stained cystic space

Case 1: Acute Onset of KCS and General Symptoms (cont.)

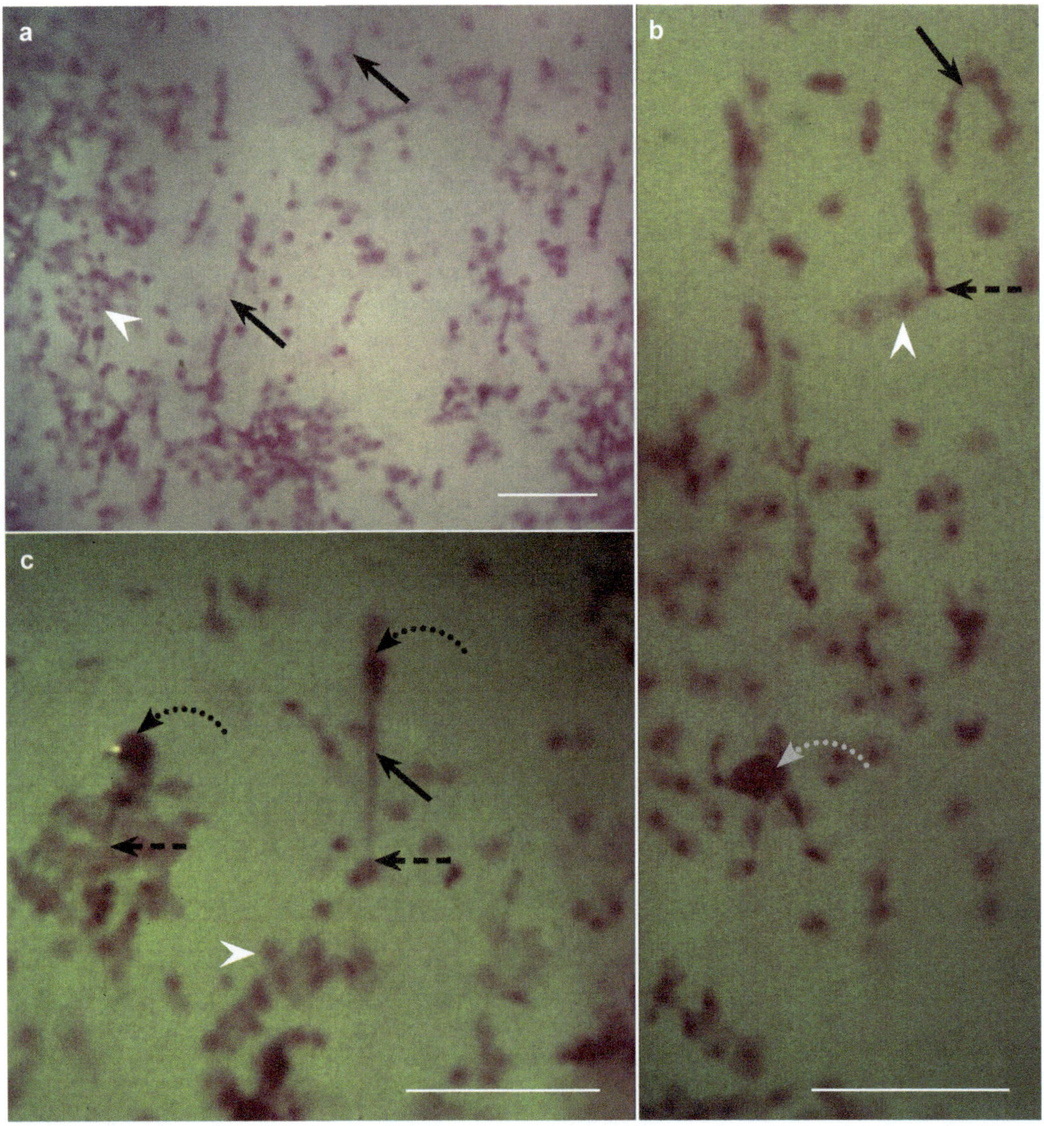

Fig. 4.3 (a) Survey of an area showing many rose bengal stained surface cells (*arrowhead*), individual or grouped, and several mucus threads apparently attached at their lower ends to red stained cells and stretching upwards after a blink (*arrows*). (b, c) Rose bengal stained cells (*arrowheads*) of which many show deeply stained dots (nuclei), and minifilaments, i.e. mucus threads (*plain arrows*) attached to the surface (*dashed arrows*) and carrying various amounts of material (*bowed arrows*); the thread in the right upper corner in (b, *plain arrow*), stretching upward like a bow, seems attached at both ends, and the lump of mucus (*bowed arrow*) seems attached to surface cells stretched upwards (cf. Part II)

Case 1: Acute Onset of KCS and General Symptoms (cont.)

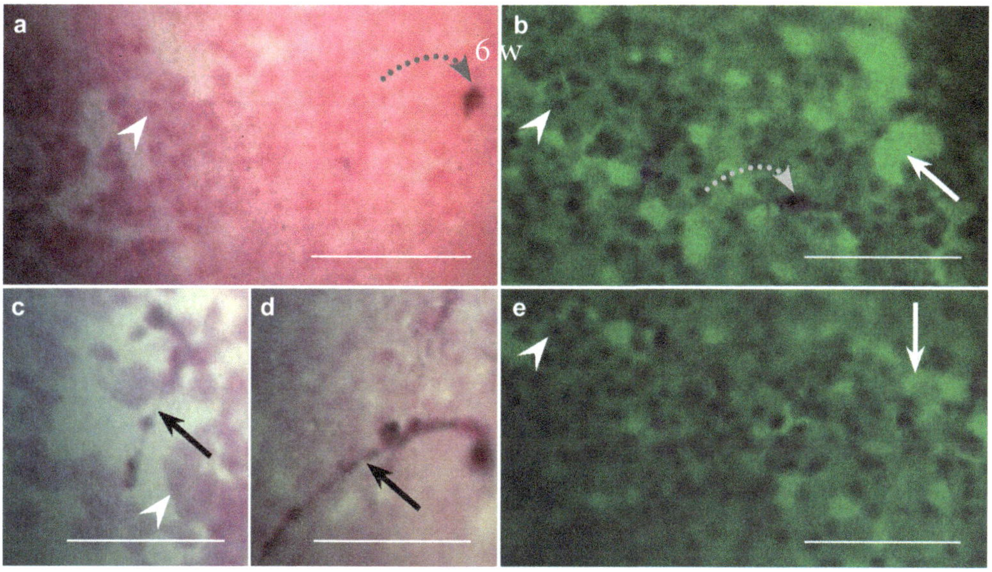

Fig. 4.4 (a–e) In this area are visible many rose bengal stained cells (*arrowheads*) in apposition, lumps of mucus (*bowed arrows*), and mucus threads and strands (*black arrows*). The brightly green staining (b and e, *white arrows*) reveals fluorescein diffusion into the tissues

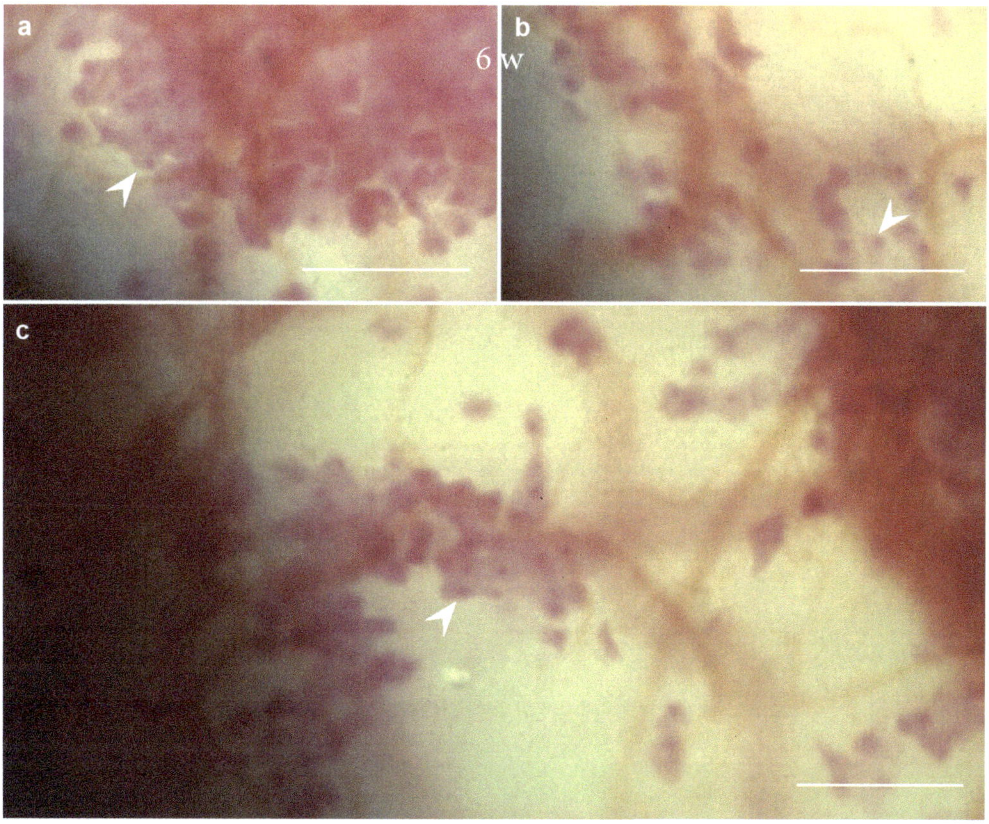

Fig. 4.5 (a–c) The conjunctival surface shows many rose bengal stained cells (*arrowheads*) some of which contain deeply stained dots (nuclei)

Case 2: Mucus Sheets

Case Report

A 68-year-old woman repeatedly presented with foreign body sensation in the right eye. No foreign body was found. The KCS diagnosis was made in connection with investigation for Sjögren's syndrome, later verified. At presentation, both eyes were slightly injected. Test values: BUT 0/0, Schirmer 1 test 0/2 and RBS 9/9.

The photographs of the right cornea were taken at presentation.

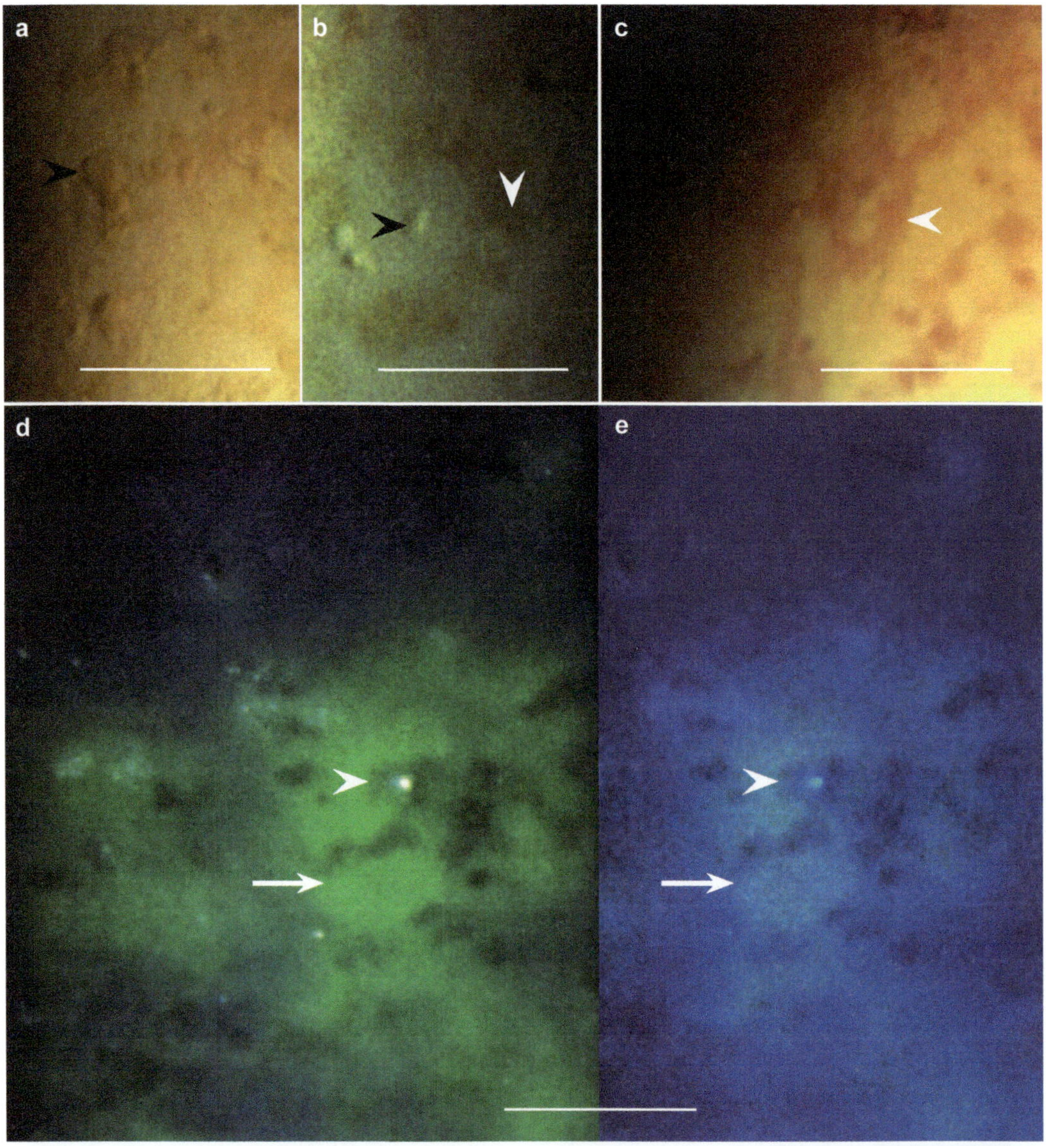

Fig. 4.6 The surface shows (**a**, **b**) cystic spaces (*black arrowheads*), (**b**) surface cells stained with non-fluorescent fluorescein (*white arrowhead*) and (**c**) with rose bengal (*arrowhead*). (**d**, **e**) Surface cells stained with non-fluorescent fluorescein (*arrowheads*) and confluence of fluorescent flecks caused by fluorescein diffusion into the tissues (green/bright, *arrows*). (The markers in **d** and **e** are placed in corresponding locations; **d**: blue filter; **d** and **e** Adapted from [9])

Case 2: Mucus Sheets (cont.)

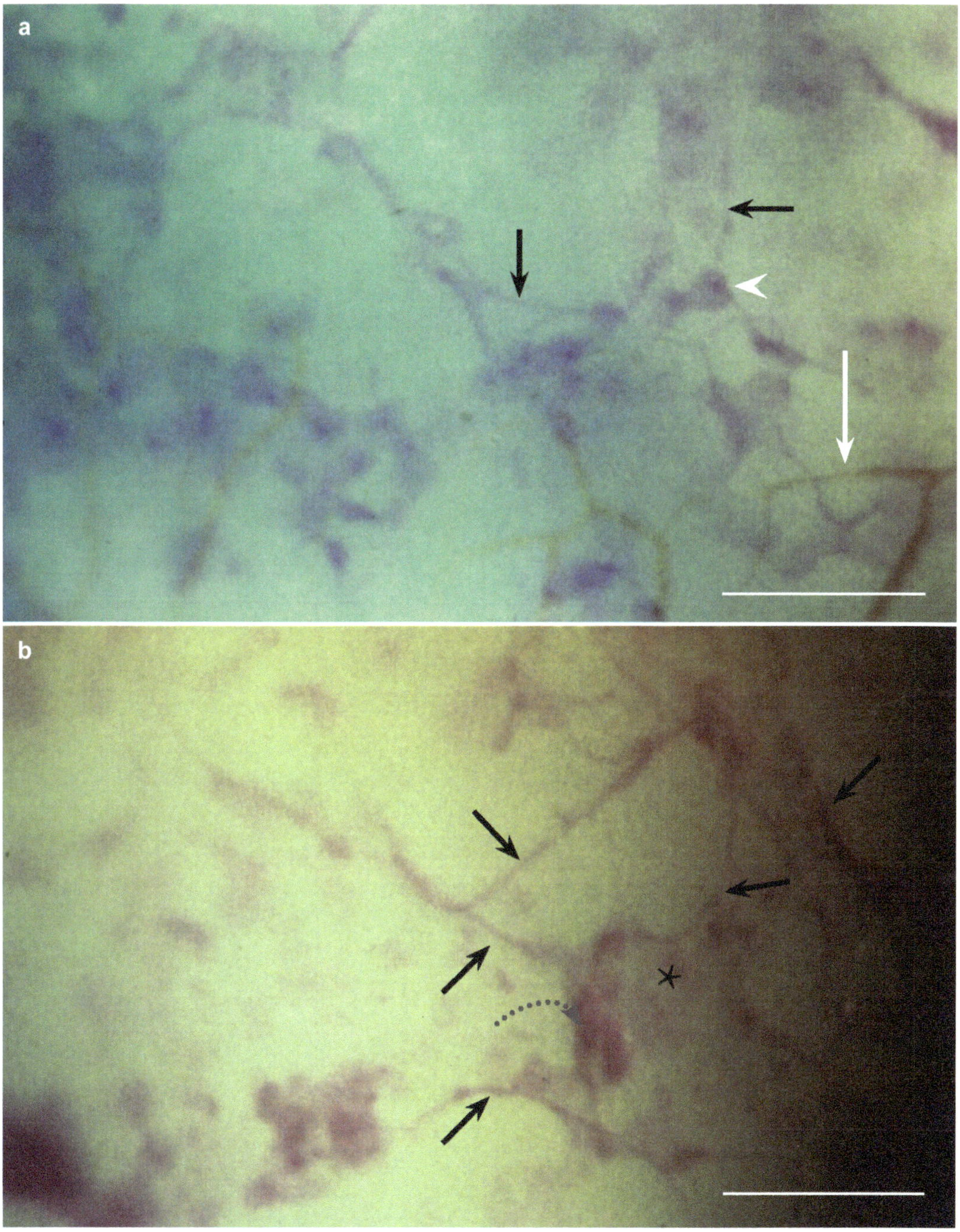

Fig. 4.7 In (a) are visible surface cells stained red with rose bengal (*arrowhead*), curved mucus strands (*black arrows*) and vessels (*white arrow*), here indicating proximity of the area to the corneal limbus. (b) shows mucus strands (*straight arrows*) and probably entrapped mucus/cell debris (*bowed arrow*). Rose bengal haze between some bowed strands (*asterisk*) implies that these strands represent rolled-up edges of torn mucus sheets (cf. Fig. 4.8, overleaf)

Case 2: Mucus Sheets (cont.)

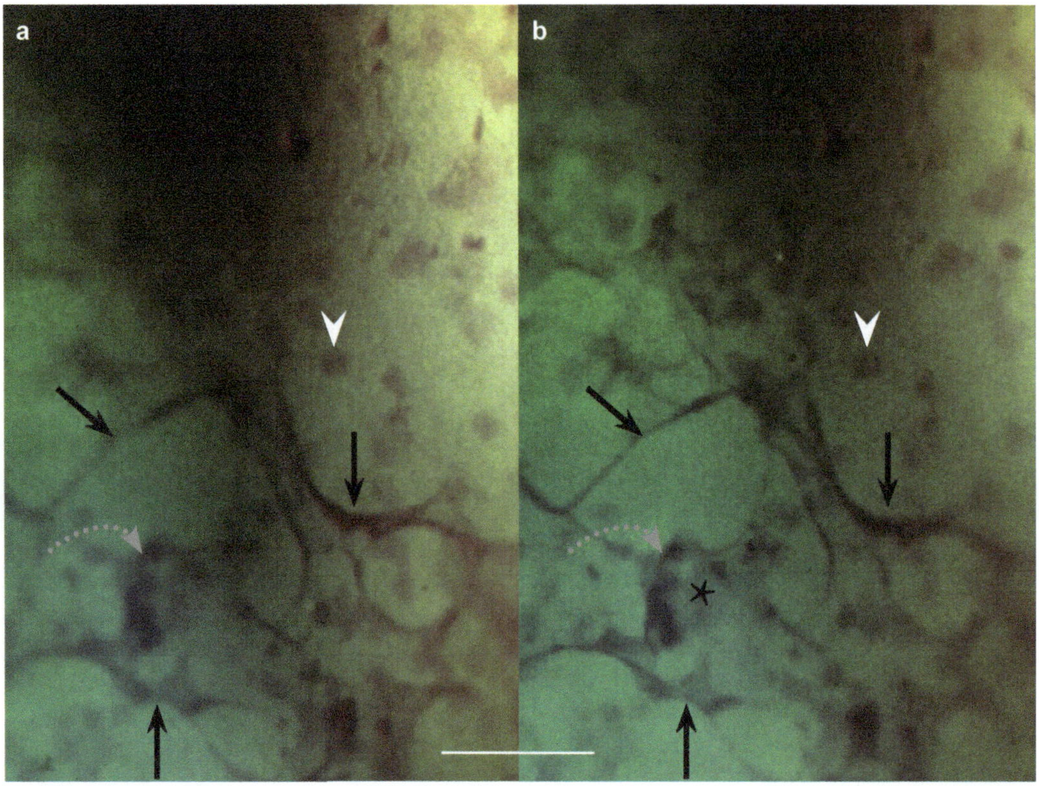

Fig. 4.8 Two consecutive photographs. Variously thick mucus strands (*straight arrows*), in places thicker as if folded (*arrows to the right*) and in places apparently interconnected by a thin sheet (*asterisk*) capturing cell debris (*bowed arrows*). The *arrowheads* indicate rose bengal stained surface cells. (The markers are placed in corresponding locations. (**a**) Adapted from [3])

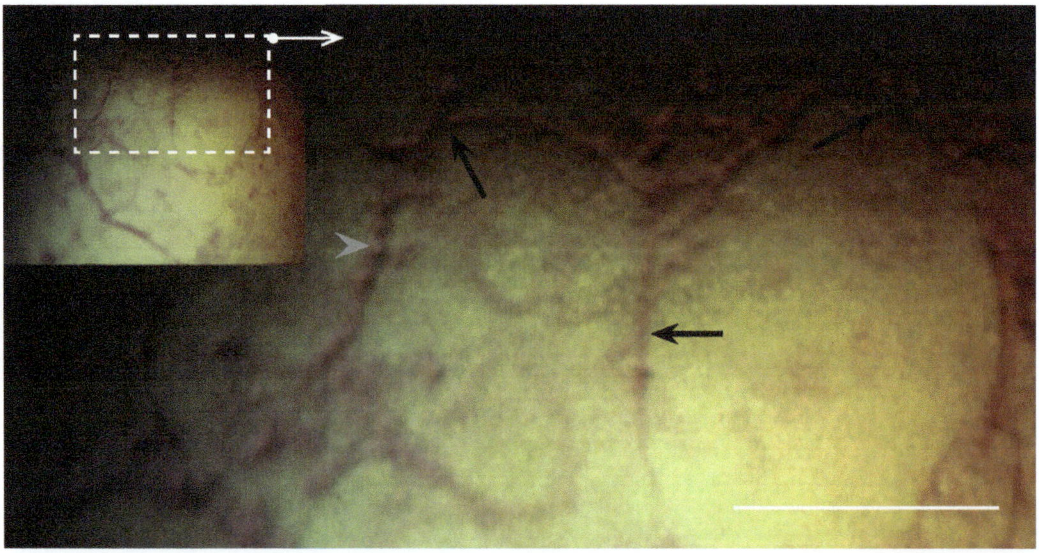

Fig. 4.9 The area indicated by *frame* in the inset shows thick mucus strands (*arrows*) with partly granular appearance (*arrowhead*)

Case 2: Mucus Sheets (cont.)

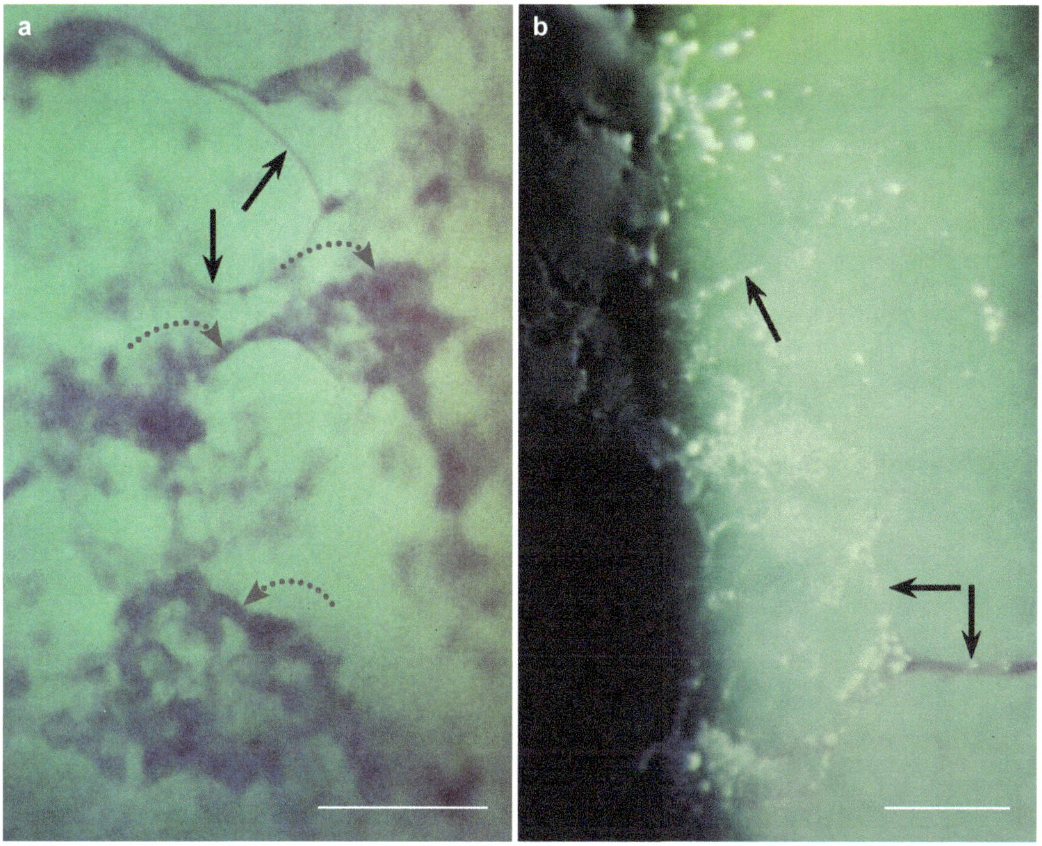

Fig. 4.10 (a) Mucus strands (*straight arrows*) and conglomerates of material, presumably mucus and cell debris (*bowed arrows*). (b) shows the light-reflecting property of mucus strands (*arrows*)

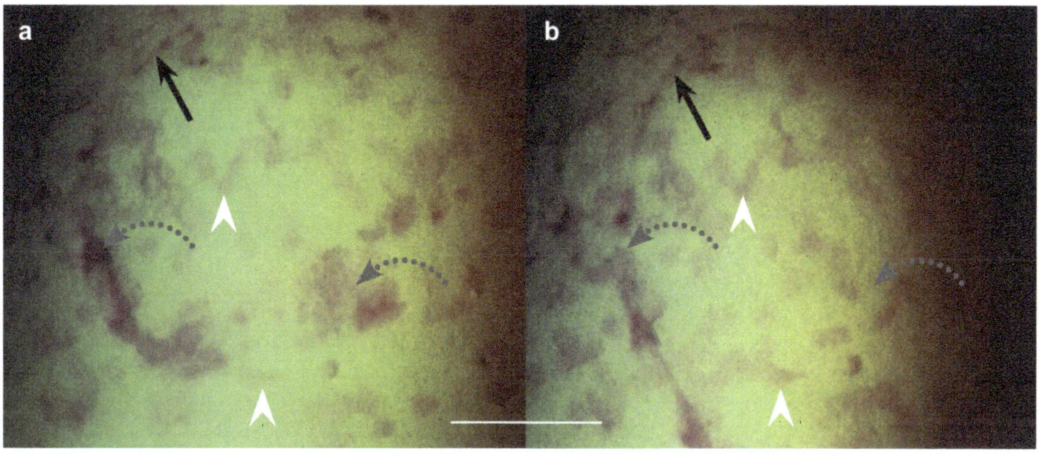

Fig. 4.11 Two consecutive photographs, cf. (a) and (b). (a) Mucus strands (*straight arrows*), mucus/cell debris (*bowed arrows*) and rose bengal stained surface cells (*arrowheads*). (b) Some of the mucus has disappeared or was displaced between the photographs. (The markers are placed in corresponding locations)

Case 3: Recurrent Corneal Flecks

Case Report

A 53-year-old woman with xerostomia was referred for KCS tests. She had no eye symptoms except for an occasional slight grittiness which she did not experience as a problem. Both eyes were white, the tear film showed a moderate amount of debris and the corneae a few flecks. Her test values were BUT 3/4, Schirmer 1 test 0/1, and RBS 8/6. Because symptom-free, she declined treatment.

The photographs of the right cornea were taken at presentation, and 9 months and 11 years later.

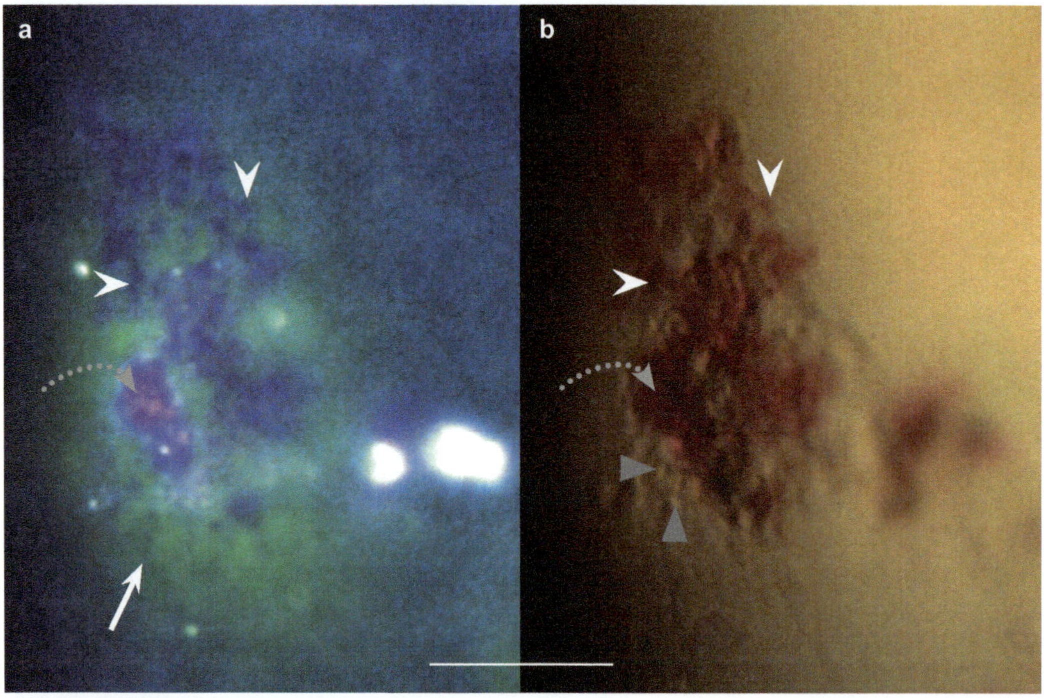

Fig. 4.12 (**a**) In the green fleck (*straight arrow*) caused by fluorescein diffusion into the tissues are visible rose bengal stained surface cells (*white arrowheads*) and an adherent lump of mucus (*bowed arrow*). In (**b**) showing the same fleck are additionally visible many rounded bodies (*grey arrowheads*). (The white arrowheads and the bowed arrows are placed in corresponding locations)

Case 3: Recurrent Corneal Flecks (cont.)

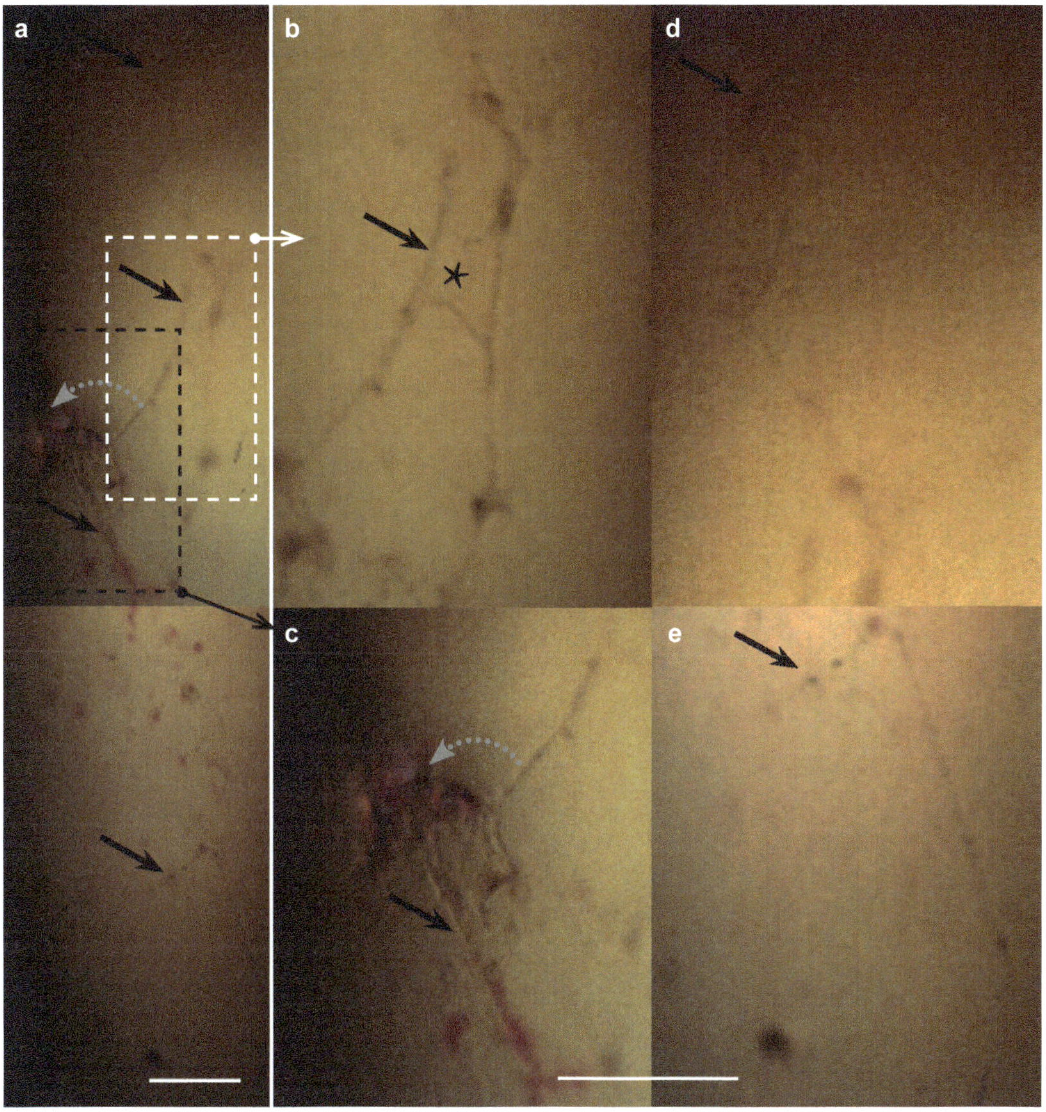

Fig. 4.13 (a) Survey photograph of mucus strands (*straight arrows*) and a lump (*bowed arrow*) adhering to the surface (composed photograph). The area in *white frame* is shown in (b) and that in *black frame* in (c). (b) The mucus strand (*arrow*) seems to be an edge of a sheet (*asterisk*) located between strands, cf. Figs. 4.7 and 4.8. (c) A rose bengal stained lump of mucus (*bowed arrow*) adhering to the surface and mucus strands (*straight arrow*). (d, e) In the upper (d) and the lower (e) part of the figure shown in (a) are visible fine mucus strands (*arrows*). (The markers in b and e are placed in locations corresponding to (a); (b) Adapted from [3])

Case 3: Recurrent Corneal Flecks (cont.)

The patient was diagnosed with primary Sjögren's syndrome. *Nine months after presentation*, she had minimal symptoms but had chosen to use lubricating eye drops. The eyes were white; the tear film showed debris and the cornea a few flecks. BUT was 1/1, Schirmer 1 test 0/0 and RBS 8/8.

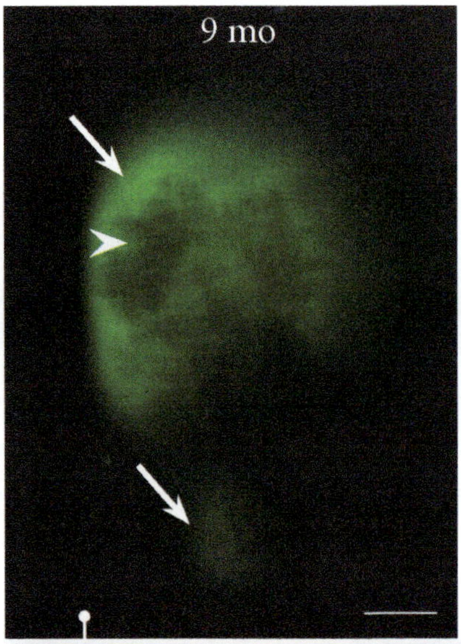

Fig. 4.14 Partially confluent green flecks (*arrows*) caused by fluorescein diffusion into the tissues; the dark areas within them (*arrowhead*) visualise non-fluorescent fluorescein staining of surface cells

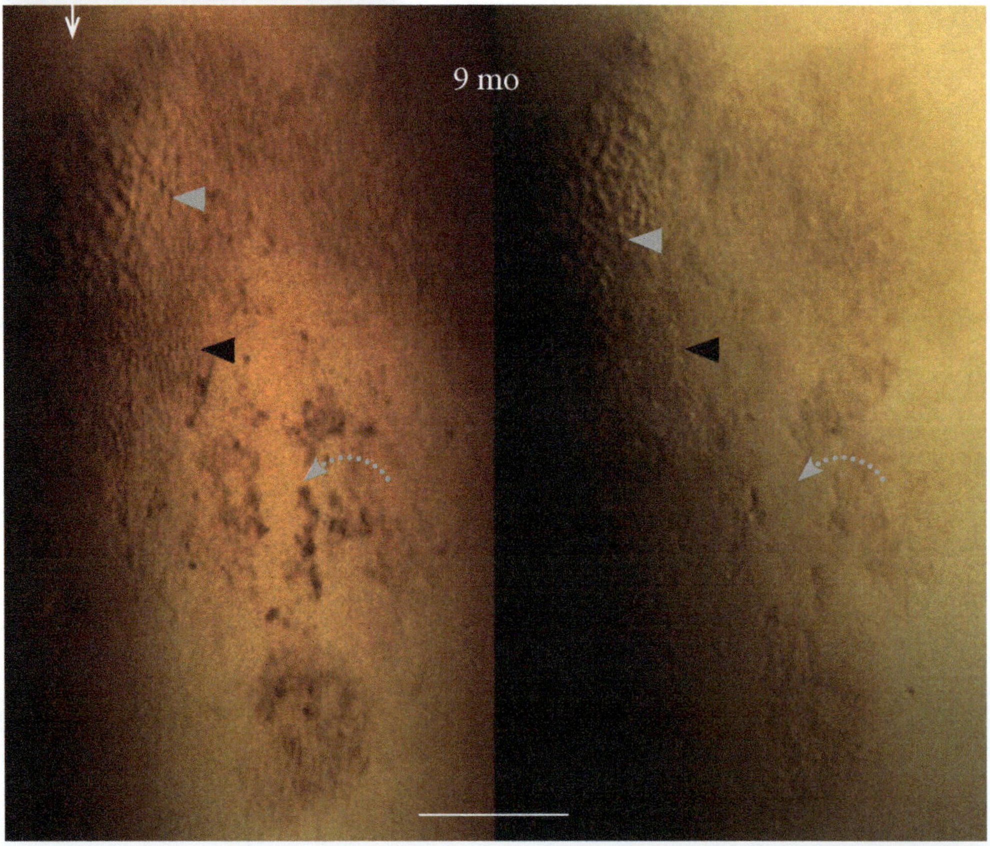

Fig. 4.15 The same flecks as in Fig. 4.14. Two consecutive photographs showing a fine granularity in the area of the flecks. In places are visible rounded bodies (*grey arrowheads*); the *black arrowheads* indicate areas suggestive of epithelial basal cell oedema. A structure implying mucus (**a**, *arrow*) has disappeared between the photographs. (The black arrowheads and the arrows are placed in corresponding locations)

Case 3: Recurrent Corneal Flecks (cont.)

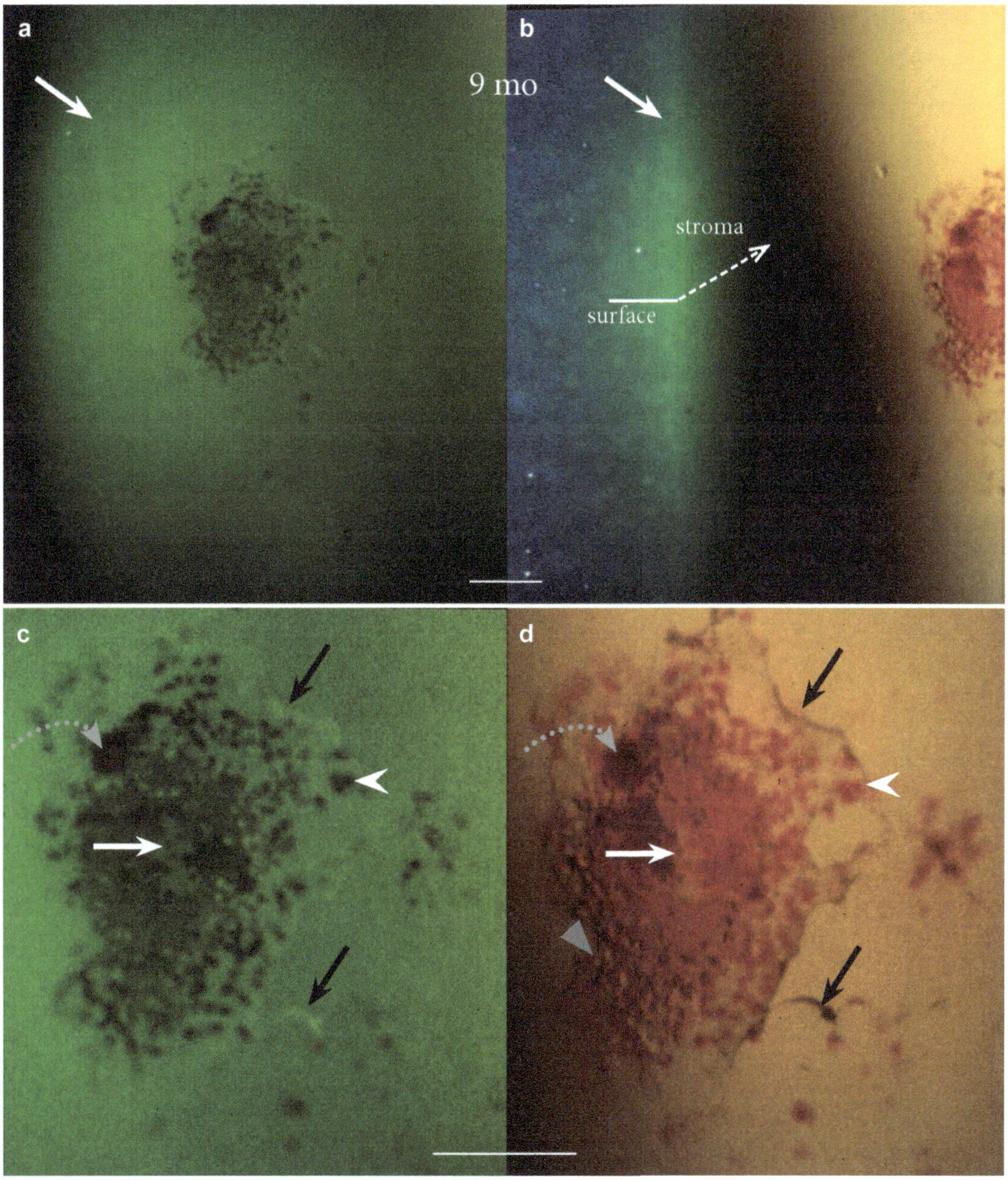

Fig. 4.16 Another green fleck. In (a, b) is visible extensive fluorescein diffusion into the tissues (*arrows*). (c, d) The fleck shows many small rose bengal stained cells (*white arrowheads*), adherent mucus lumps (*bowed arrows*) and mucus strands (*black arrows*), at the edges of the fleck implying rolled-up edges of a sheet. The dirty green hue of fluorescein staining in the centre (c, *white arrow*) is caused by rose bengal haze (d, *white arrow*). The area adjacent to it shows confluent rose bengal staining. (The markers are placed in corresponding locations.) In (d) are additionally visible rounded bodies (*grey arrowhead*)

Case 3: Recurrent Corneal Flecks (cont.)

Eleven years after the first visit, the patient was referred for examination because of fluctuating vision. Her optician had noted changing astigmatism in the right eye. At presentation, the patient's symptoms had already disappeared and her vision returned to normal. She had no problems whatsoever but she was using lubricating eye drops. The right cornea showed several flecks but none was located centrally. The left cornea was clear. KCS tests were not performed.

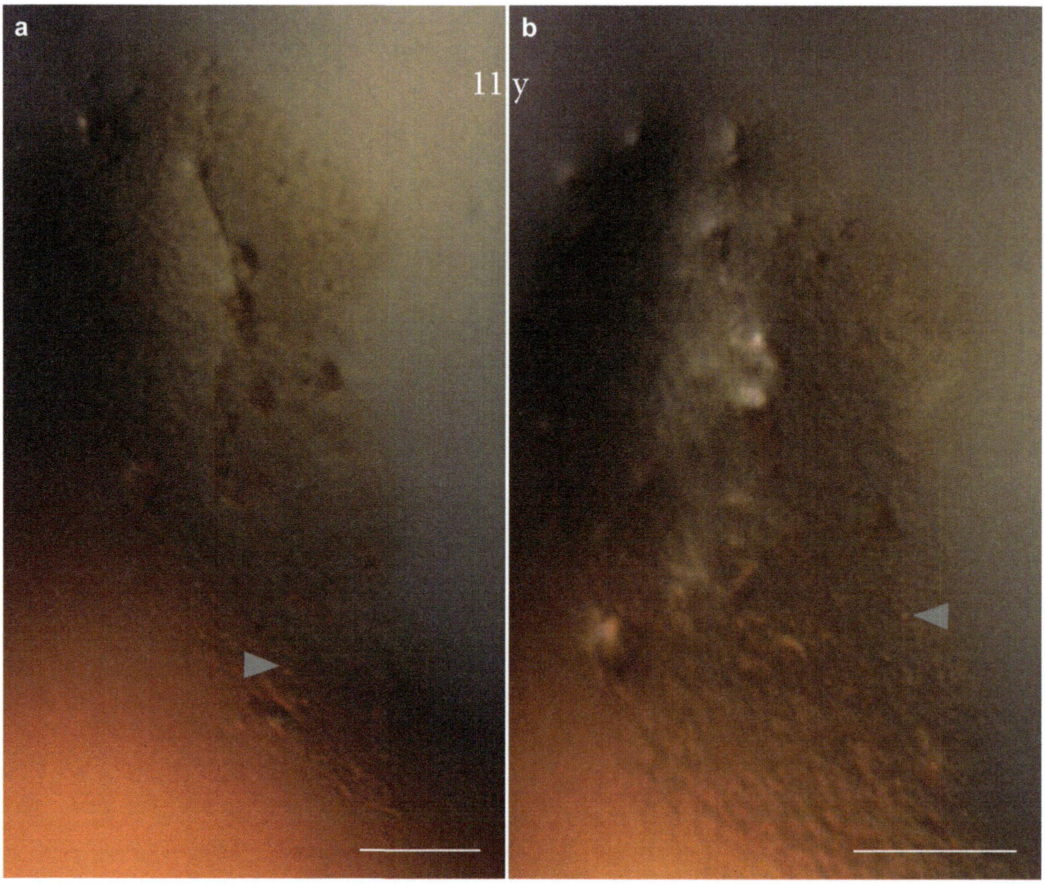

Fig. 4.17 A fleck located in the paracentral temporal lower cornea; it shows many rounded bodies (*arrowheads*)

Fig. 4.18 Nasal cornea close to the limbus shows (a) green stained flecks (*arrow*) caused by fluorescein diffusion into the tissues which in (b), by confluence, form a green background (*arrow*) against which are visible rose bengal stained surface cells (*arrowhead*). (The arrows are placed in corresponding locations.) (c, d) A different area showing small rose bengal stained surface cells (*arrowheads*) and mucus adhering to the surface (*bowed arrows*). (The markers are placed in corresponding locations.) (e) Additional green flecks (*arrows*) showing rose bengal stained cells. (f) Rose bengal stained conjunctival surface cells (*arrowhead*). (g) Punctate fluorescent conjunctival staining (*arrowheads*) (g: blue filter)

Case 4: When Findings and Tests Do Not Match

Case Report

A 38-year-old healthy woman with irritation in both eyes for several weeks had noted a greyish fleck on her right cornea. At presentation, the right eye was slightly injected, the cornea showed several greyish flecks and the conjunctiva patches of fluorescein and rose bengal staining. The left eye was white, the cornea clear and the conjunctiva showed a few patches similar to those present in the right eye. BUT was >15 in both eyes and Schirmer 1 test 7/6. RBS was difficult to estimate because the staining pattern diverged from the usual one.

The patient was treated with lubricating eye drops. Three weeks later, she had less symptoms but the findings were unchanged. Test values: BUT >15 in both eyes, Schirmer 1 test 4/7.

During the next 6 months, she was using the drops only sporadically because her symptoms had almost disappeared. Both corneae showed only a few areas of punctate fluorescein staining, and a few were present also on the conjunctivae. Test values: BUT >15 in both eyes, Schirmer 1 test 6/5.

She presented again after a further year and a half. During that time, her symptoms had entirely disappeared without treatment, and the only finding was a discrete punctate fluorescein staining of the nasal conjunctivae. Test values: BUT >15 in both eyes, Schirmer 1 test 7/6.

The photographs of the right cornea were taken at presentation.

Comment

In this patient, the ocular surface findings were well in agreement with KCS but she had not really fulfilled the used criteria. She recovered spontaneously, had no other symptoms and thus no investigation was performed.

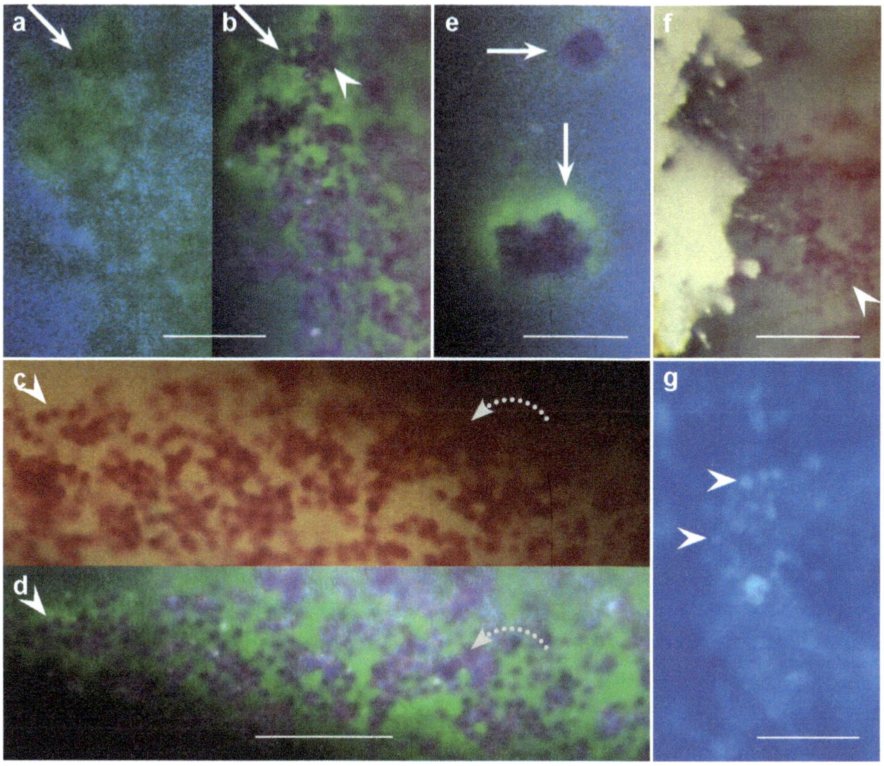

Case 5: A Case of Spontaneous Regression

Case Report

A 53-year-old woman with irritation in both eyes for about six years was diagnosed elsewhere with KCS (BUT 2/3, Schirmer 1 test 6/10 and RBS 7/4). Two years later, already diagnosed with primary Sjögren's syndrome, she was referred for a new evaluation. She had minimal symptoms but was using lubricating eye drops once a day; both eyes were white, the BUT 3/4, Schirmer 1 test 4/5 and RBS 0/0. Three years later, her symptoms were still minimal and her use of eye drops sporadic. Both eyes were white but both corneae showed large numbers of greyish surface cells. Test values: BUT 1/2, Schirmer 1 test 1/1 and RBS 4/3. The photographs of the right cornea were taken at that occasion.

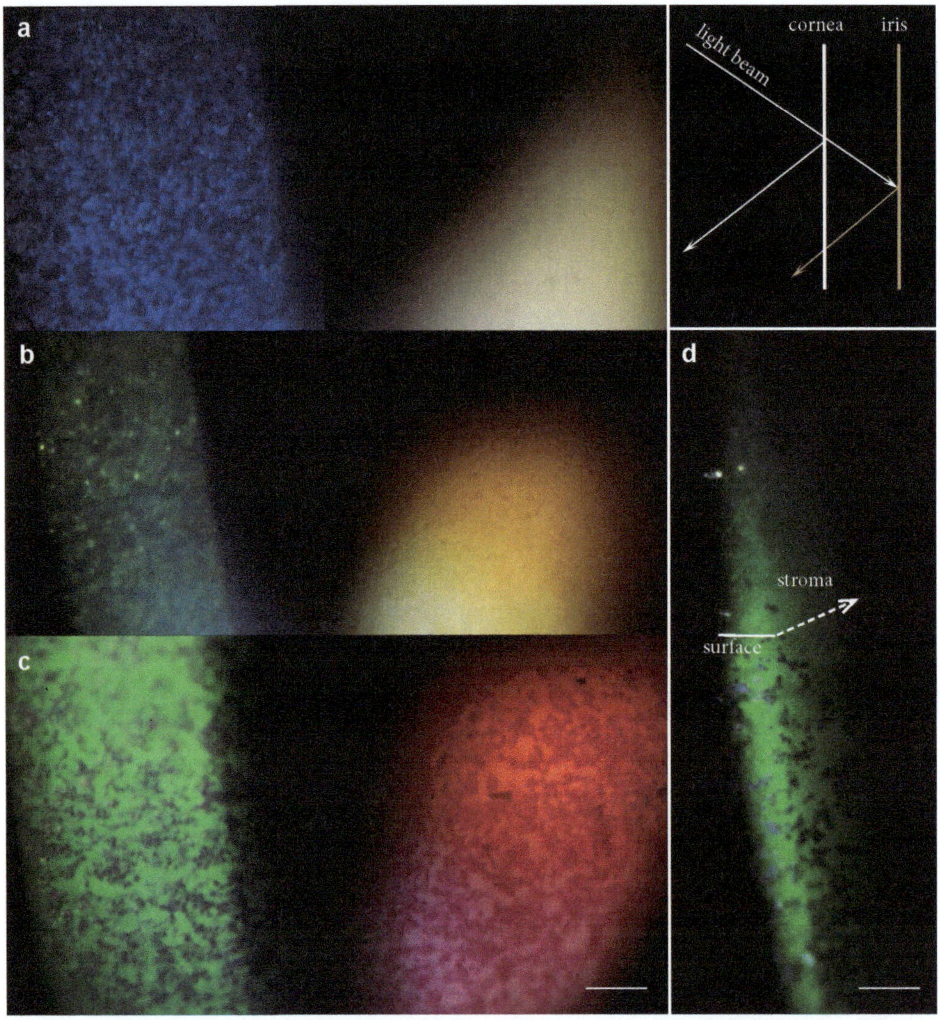

Fig. 4.19 (a–c) The left part of the photographs is visualised by light reflected from the cornea and the right one by light reflected from the iris (cf. *inset*). The photographs show (a) many greyish cells; (b) early punctate fluorescein staining; (c) heavy rose bengal staining the hue of which varies with illumination, and green fluorescein staining caused by diffusion of the dye into the tissues; the latter is shown in (d) in a narrower light beam

Case 5: A Case of Spontaneous Regression (cont.)

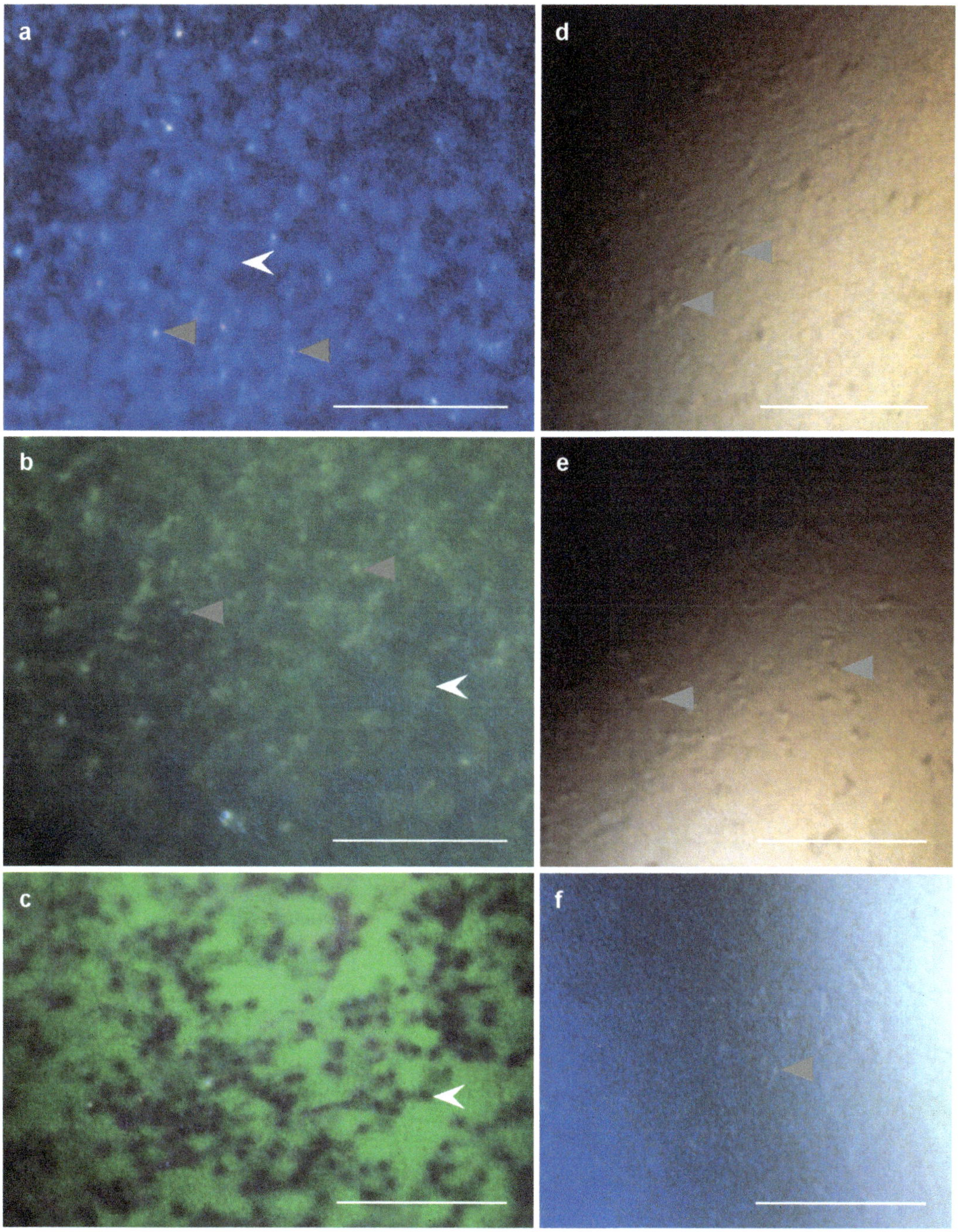

Fig. 4.20 (a–c) A partly confluent pattern of surface cells (*white arrowheads*), in (a) greyish and light-reflecting, in (b) staining faintly green with fluorescein and in (c) staining with rose bengal; this area shows small cells with prominent dark dots (nuclei) here visualised against green background caused by fluorescein diffusion into the tissues. Additionally are visible many small bright dots (a and b, *grey arrowheads*). (d, e) Many rounded bodies (*arrowheads*) captured before staining in different areas of the same cornea

Case 5: A Case of Spontaneous Regression (cont.)

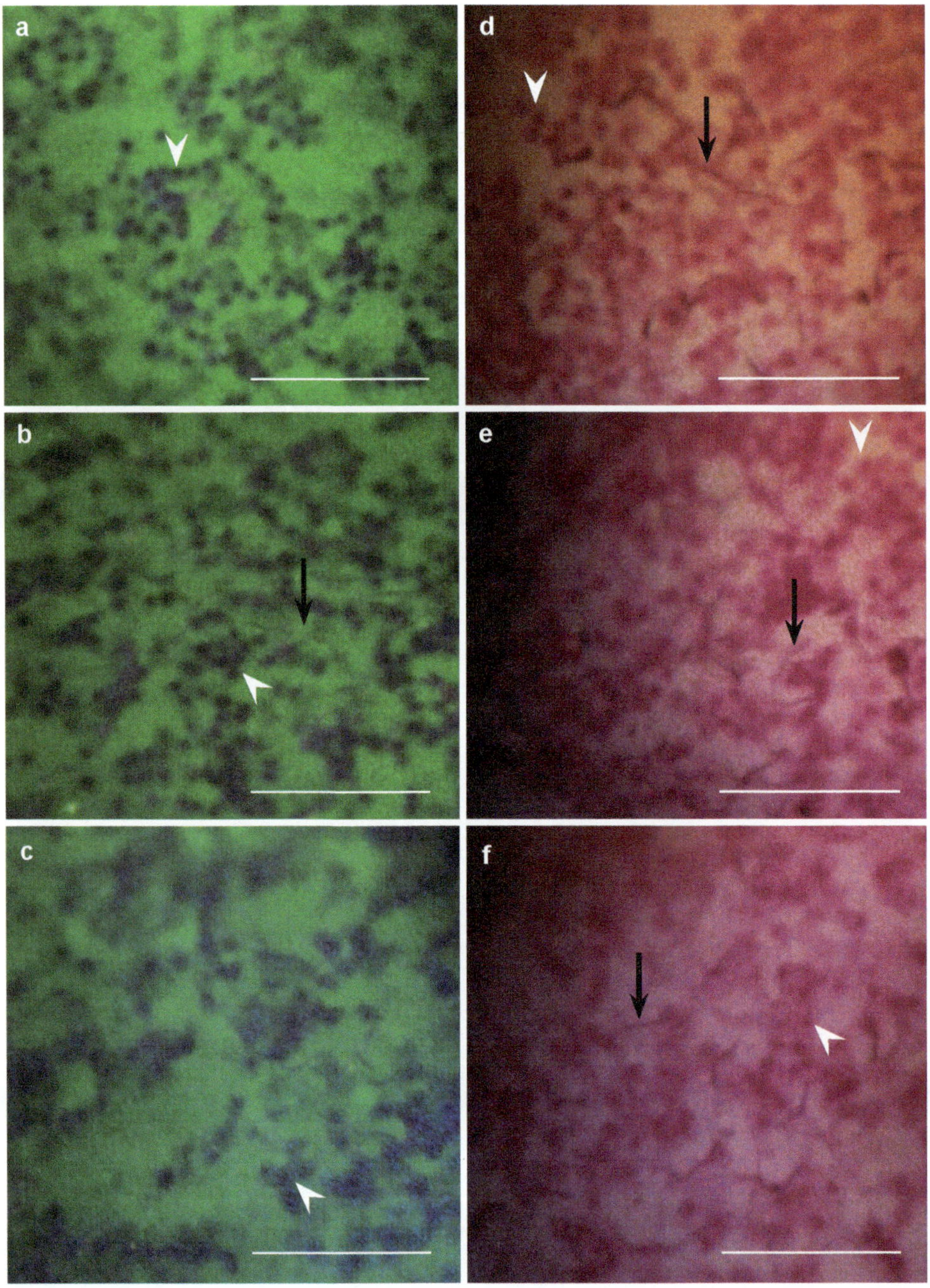

Fig. 4.21 (**a–c**) Rose bengal stained surface cells (*arrowheads*), individual, in groups or rows, with or without a dark dot (nucleus); in (**b**) are visible fine threads (*arrow*) in the in-between areas. (**d–f**) The same phenomena captured in retroillumination. The nuclei are better discernible against the green background, the threads in retroillumination. (The nature of the threads is uncertain; some might be the result of cell exfoliation.) Cf. Fig. 4.22

Case 5: A Case of Spontaneous Regression (cont.)

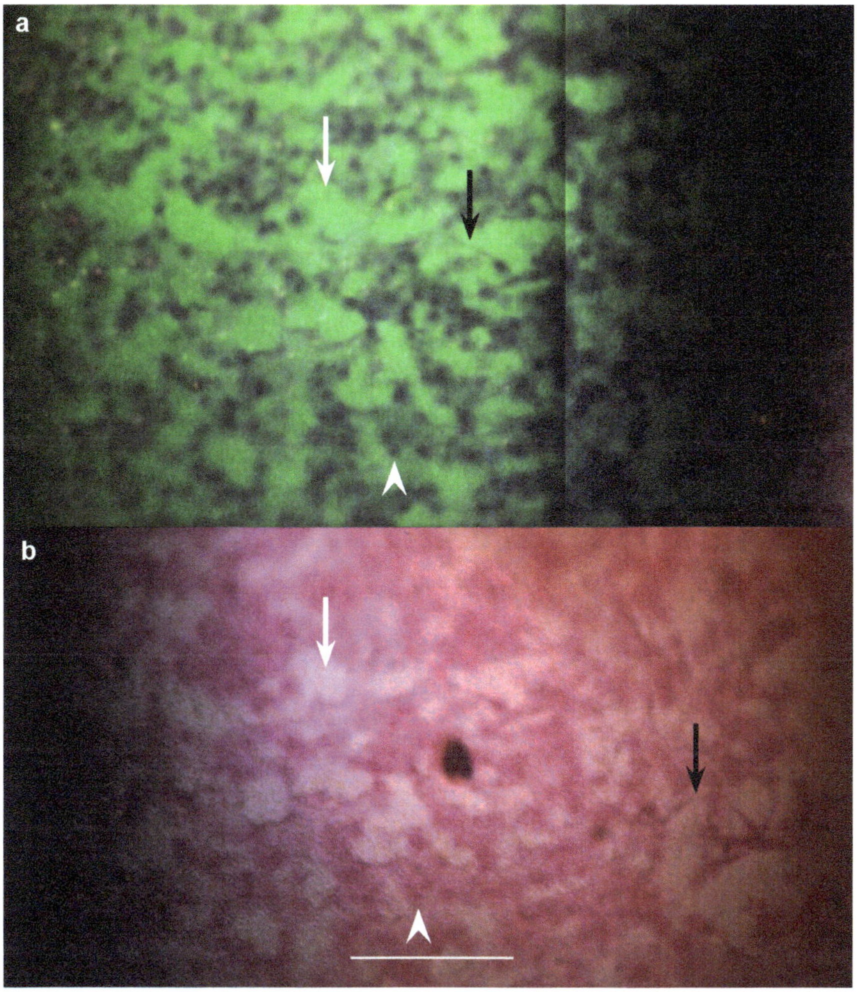

Fig. 4.22 Another area, captured after staining with fluorescein and rose bengal in different illumination modes. Similarly to Fig. 4.21, it shows small rose bengal stained surface cells (*arrowheads*) with or without dark dots (nuclei), threads (*black arrowhead*) and (a) green background (*white arrow*) caused by fluorescein diffusion into the tissues. (The white arrows and the arrowheads are placed in corresponding locations; (a) is a composed photograph)

Addendum

The patient was treated with lubricating eye drops. Seven weeks later, when next seen, both corneae were clear, and the only finding was a discrete punctate fluorescein staining in the lower part of the right cornea. (BUT 1/2, Schirmer 1 test 5/5). The condition was unchanged after a further 5 months when last seen (BUT 3/3, Schirmer 1 test 1/3).

Comment

The patient had KCS in agreement with the used criteria, and the findings were in agreement with the diagnosis. Fluctuations of symptoms are known but a bout of such a severe epithelial disturbance seems rare. Yet, there were neither signs nor history suggestive of other causes.

Case 6: A Peculiar Keratitis

Case Report

A 34-year-old woman with (presumed) recurrent eye infections treated with topical antibiotics, all for about 1,5 years, was referred to the Eye Clinic because of peculiar corneal flecks. The eyes were white; the right cornea showed 1 and the left one 3 greyish flecks. BUT was 0/0, Schirmer 1 test 5/4 and RBS 9/8. The findings in combination with a history of recurrent throat infections (?), repeatedly treated with antibiotics p.o., were suggestive of Sjögren's syndrome.

The photographs of the left cornea were taken at presentation and 8 years later.

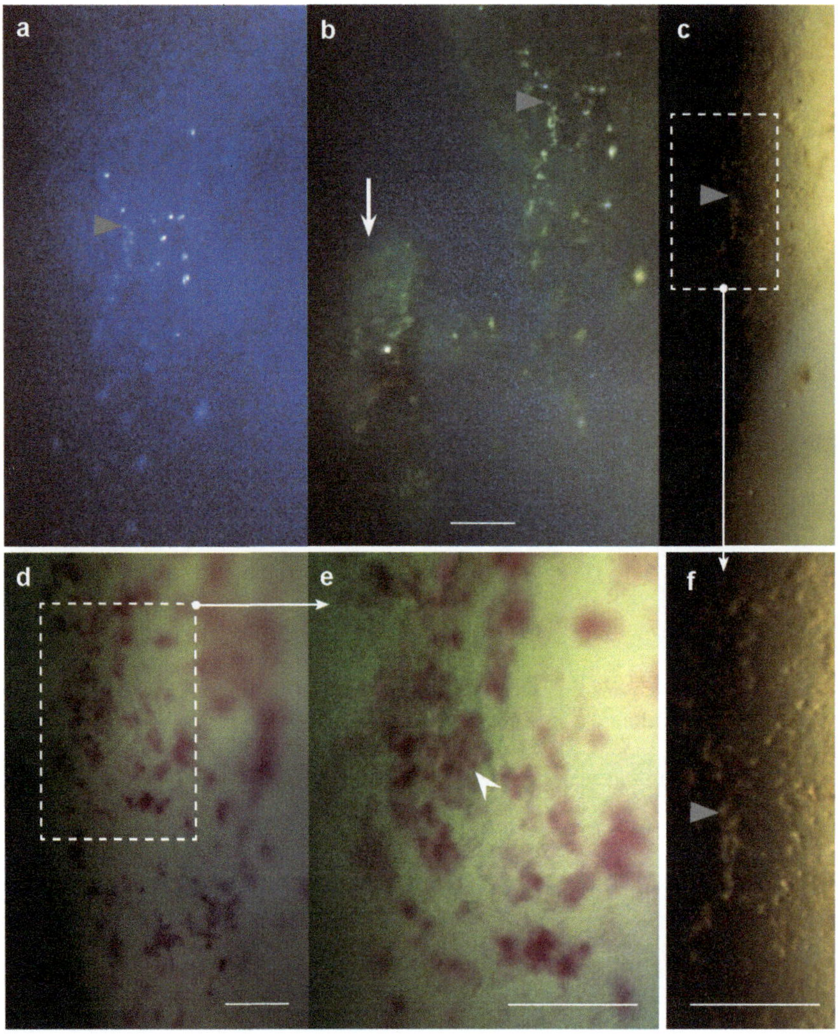

Fig. 4.23 (a–c) Survey of a fleck showing many light-reflecting dots (*arrowheads*) visible against (a) grey background, (b) incipient fluorescein diffusion into the tissues (green, *straight arrow*) and (c) in retroillumination. (f) The area in *frame* in (c) at higher magnification; some of the light reflections in (a and b) are caused by rounded bodies (*arrowhead*). (The arrowheads are placed in corresponding locations.) (d) Survey of rose bengal staining captured approximately in the same location. (e) The area in *frame* at higher magnification. In the red stained areas, individual cells are difficult to discern; the more deeply red dots (*arrowhead*) probably represent cell nuclei

Case 6: A Peculiar Keratitis (cont.)

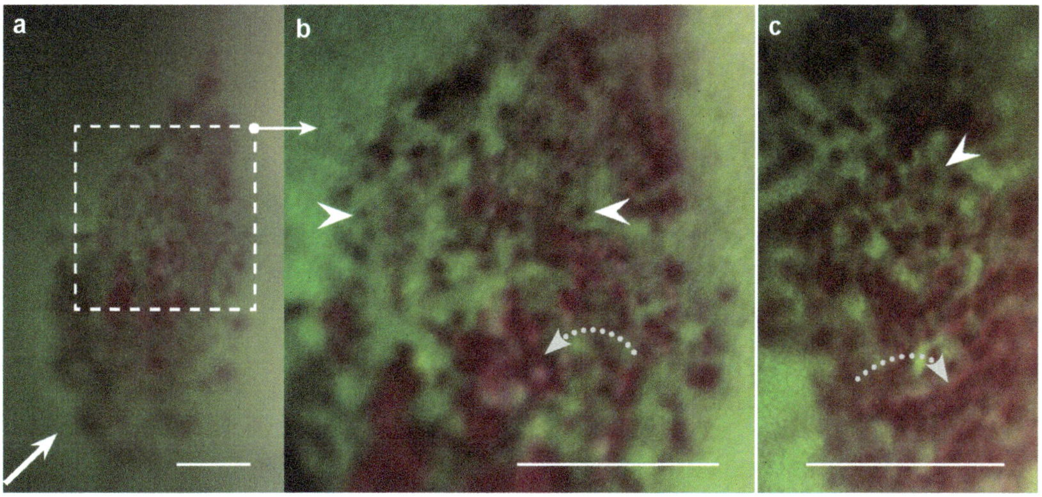

Fig. 4.24 (a) Survey of another fleck showing rose bengal staining and fluorescein diffusion into the tissues (green, *arrow*). (b) In the area in *frame* in (a) are visible many small rose bengal stained surface cells (*arrowheads*) with deeply stained dots (nuclei) and brighter red stained areas (*arrow*) implying mucus adherence. (c) A different area of the same fleck with the same features as in (b)

Investigation revealed primary Sjögren's syndrome. The patient was helped by lubricating eye drops. At her yearly visits, the flecks were sometimes present and other times absent. *Eight years* after the first visit, when last seen, the right cornea showed 3 and the left one 1 fleck.

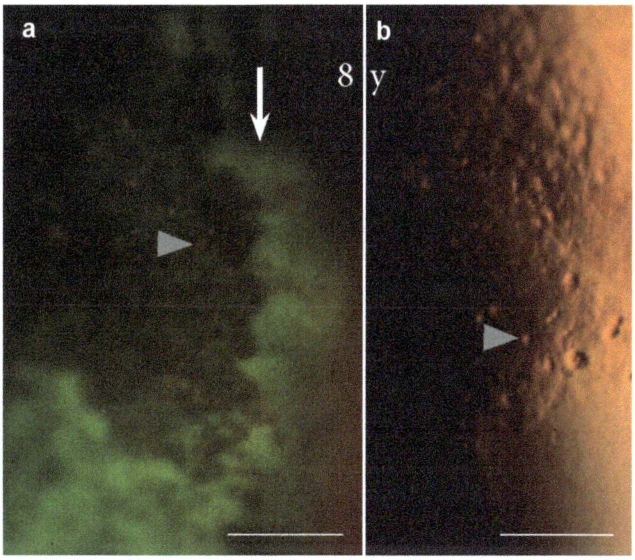

Fig. 4.25 (a) A corneal fleck captured 8 years after the first visit. In the central area stained dark with non-fluorescent fluorescein are visible brighter dots (*arrowhead*); the surroundings show fluorescein diffusion into the tissues (green, *arrow*). In (b) are visible many rounded bodies (*arrowhead*), cf. Fig. 4.23

Case 7: KCS and Stromal Infiltrate

Case Report

A 54-year-old woman presented with pain and redness in the left eye for about 10 days. The right eye was white. The left eye was injected and the temporal upper part of the cornea showed a whitish subepithelial infiltrate with disrupted surface. She was treated with a topical antibiotic; 3 days later, the infiltrate was much smaller and after further week it was healed leaving a small scar. At that occasion, the patient mentioned irritation in both eyes. KCS tests showed BUT 3/5, Schirmer 1 test 0/0 and RBS 7/5. She was treated with lubricating eye drops; investigation revealed primary Sjögren's syndrome. During the 4 years of follow-up, she had episodes of irritation in both eyes but no new infiltrates or corneal scars were observed.

The photographs of the left cornea were taken at presentation and 3 days later and of the conjunctiva in conjunction with KCS tests.

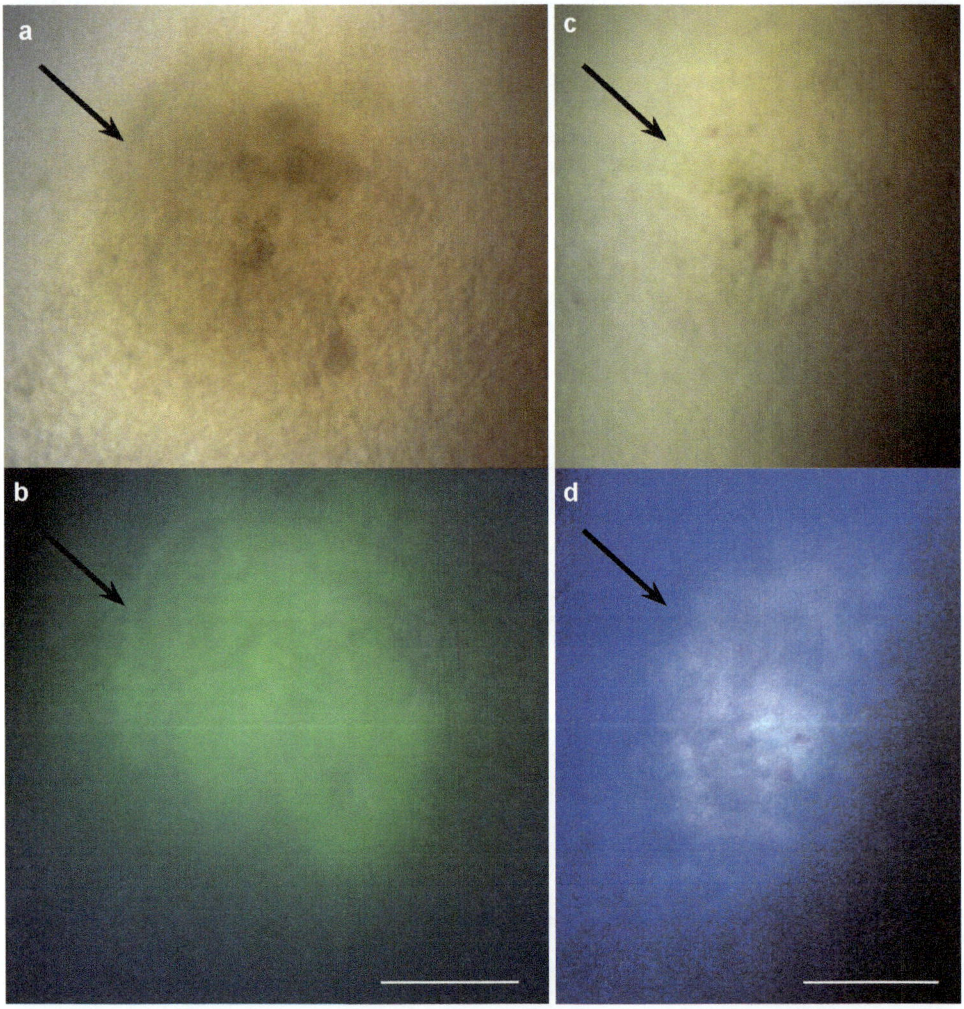

Fig. 4.26 (**a, b**) Corneal subepithelial infiltrate (*arrows*) in (**b**) staining green with fluorescein. (**c, d**) The same infiltrate 3 days later. (**d**) The area of the infiltrate is light-reflecting

Case 7: KCS and Stromal Infiltrate (cont.)

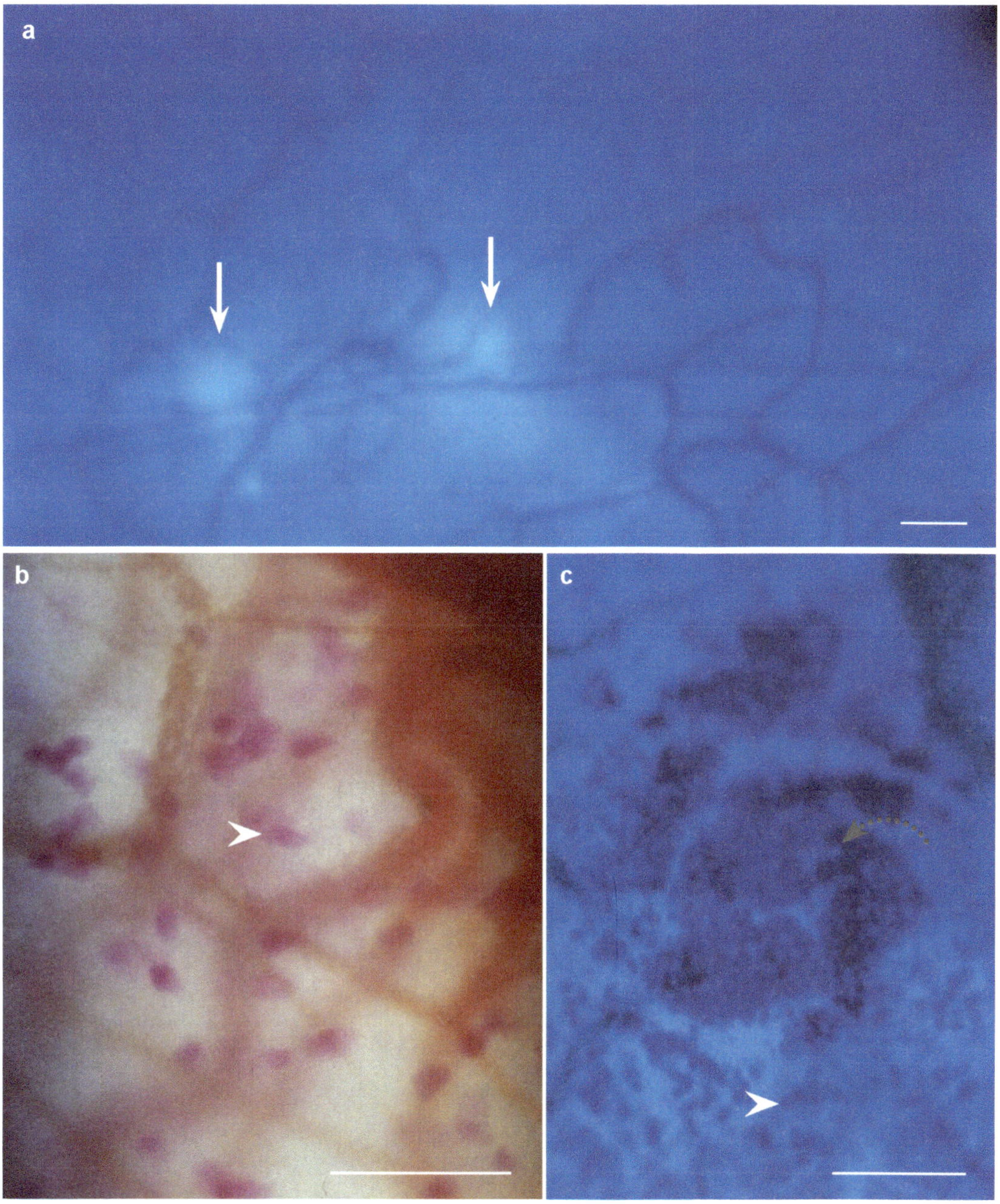

Fig. 4.27 The conjunctiva shows (a) fluorescent flecks (*arrows*) caused by fluorescein diffusion into the tissues and (b, c) rose bengal stained surface cells (*arrowheads*); in (c) is additionally visible a lump of cell debris (*arrow*) ((a) blue filter, (c) green filter)

Case 8: KCS and Atopic Eczema

Case Report

A 23-year-old woman with atopic eczema since childhood and dry eye symptoms for 3 years. At presentation, the lid skin was dry and she had difficulties to close her eyes. The eyes were white; both corneae showed many greyish-whitish dots. BUT was not measured; Schirmer 1 test 1/0 and RBS 4/4. She was treated with an emollient and lubricating eye drops.

The photographs of the right cornea were taken at presentation and 6 weeks later.

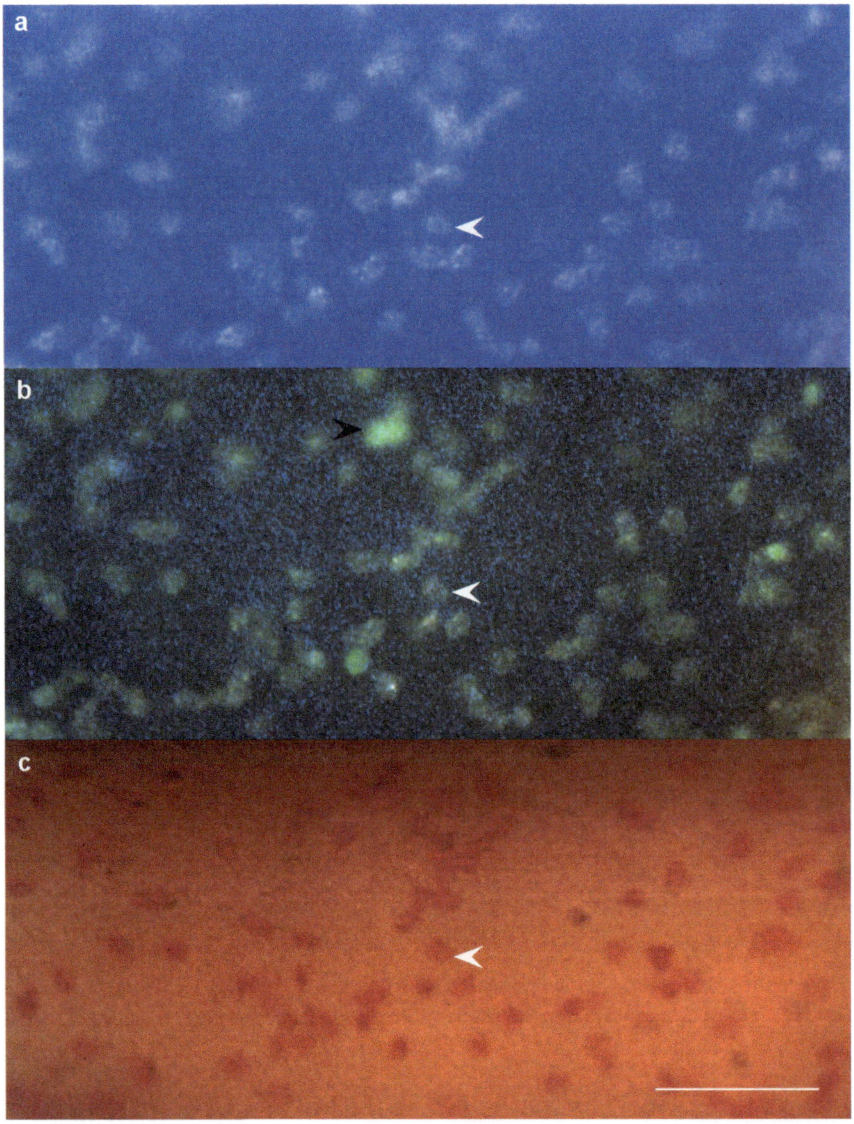

Fig. 4.28 (a–c) The cornea shows (a) many greyish surface cells (*white arrowhead*) stained (b) weakly green with fluorescein and (c) red with rose bengal. The *black arrowhead* in (b) indicates a more brilliantly green stained cystic space. There is no fluorescein diffusion into the tissues. (The white arrowheads are placed in corresponding locations)

Case 8: KCS and Atopic Eczema (cont.)

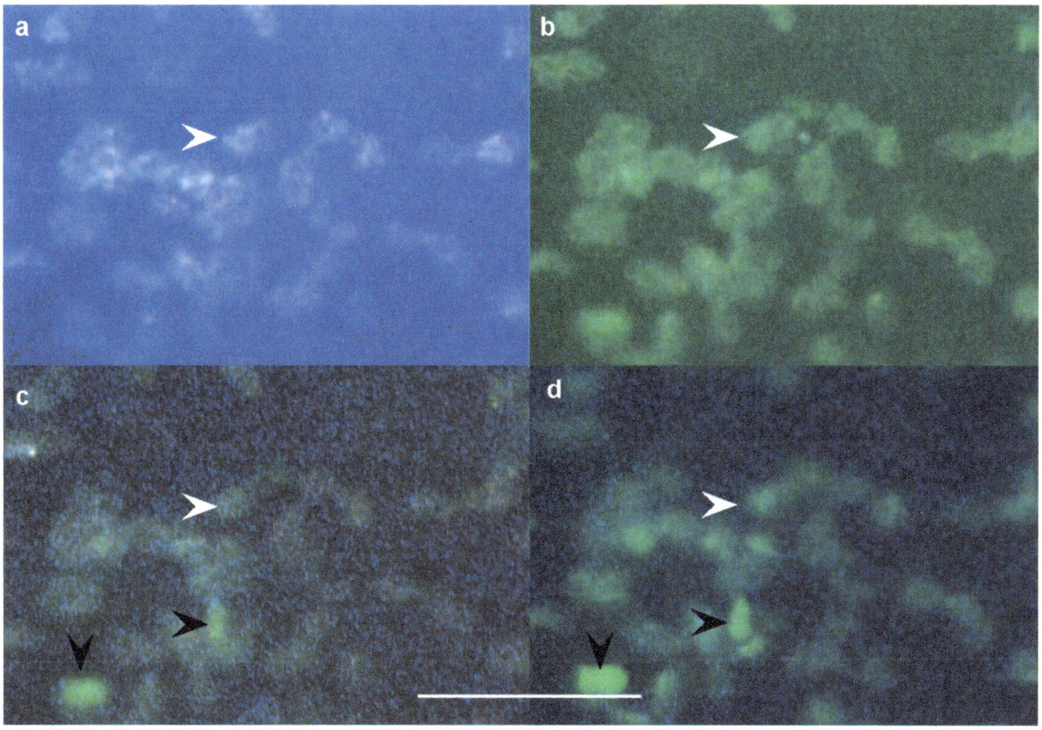

Fig. 4.29 This area shows (a) greyish surface cells (*arrowhead*) which (b) are visible (*arrowhead*) through the tear film stained green with fluorescein. Only slowly (c and d), the cells (*white arrowheads*) start to stain green. The *black arrowheads* in (c) and (d) indicate brilliantly green stained cystic spaces. Cf. Fig. 2.5. (The markers are placed in corresponding locations)

Six weeks later, the symptoms were less pronounced, the lid skin softer and she had no problems with lid closure. The corneal findings were more or less the same; test values: BUT >15 o.a., Schirmer 1 test 2/1 and RBS 5/4.

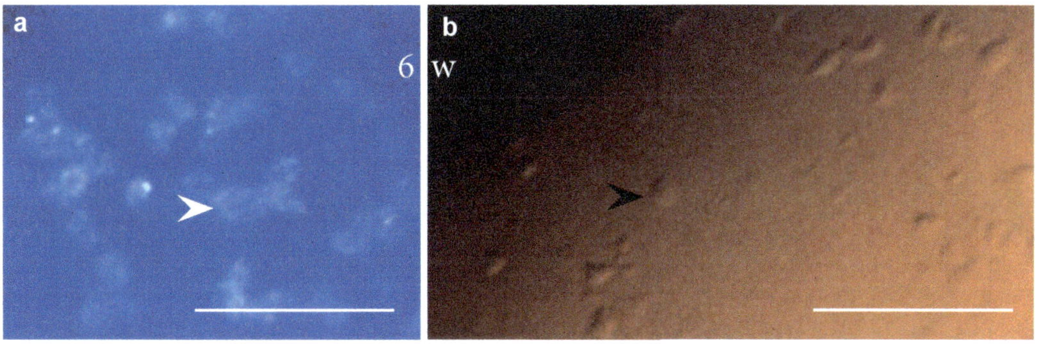

Fig. 4.30 (a) Greyish surface cells (*arrowhead*) and (b) cystic spaces (*arrowhead*)

Case 9: KCS and Corneal Anaesthesia

Case Report

A 64-year-old man presented with a red left eye; he had no history of trauma. About 2 years previously, while abroad, he had had a stroke, attributed to arterial hypertension, with transient right-sided motoric symptoms and persisting left-sided facial pain. The left eye was injected and the central cornea showed a clean erosion. The healing was very slow. Almost 3 weeks after presentation, the central epithelium was still defect but it healed within a further week; the corneal sensitivity was impaired. Three months later, the corneal sensitivity seemed absent; KCS tests showed BUT 0/0, Schirmer 1 test 2/1 and RBS 2/3. He was treated with lubricating eye drops. During the following 7 years, the left cornea suffered several spontaneous erosions.

About 8 years after onset the patient presented again, this time because of hazy vision in the left eye for a couple of weeks. The right eye was white and the cornea clear. In the left eye, the central cornea showed large numbers of greyish cells. One month later, greyish cells were spread over the upper and central cornea but the lower part was clear. Within a further month, the number of the greyish cells had diminished and the visual acuity substantially increased. He was not seen thereafter.

The photographs of the left cornea were taken after testing the corneal sensitivity, and at two occasions during the period of hazy vision, at presentation and 1 month later (at the two latter occasions without the aid of rose bengal).

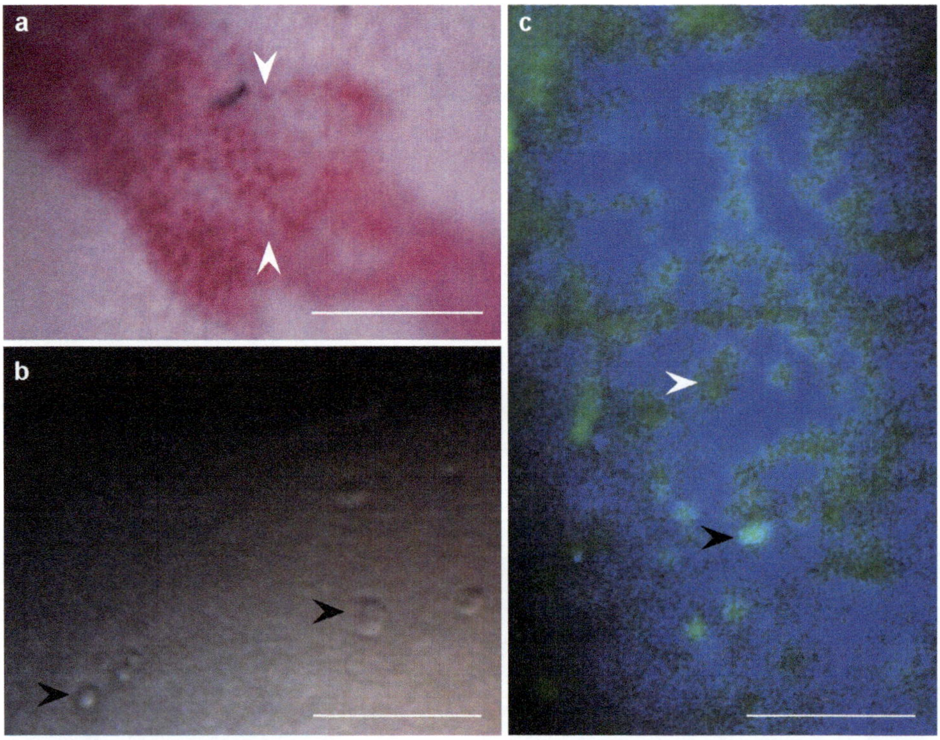

Fig. 4.31 (a) Rose bengal staining after touch of a cotton thread; the red stained dots (*arrowheads*) seem to represent nuclei of small surface cells (this photograph was taken when corneal sensitivity was tested 4 months after the first erosion). (b) shows cystic spaces (*arrowheads*) and (c) fluorescein staining of surface cells (*white arrowhead*) and cystic spaces (*black arrowhead*), captured early after the application of the dye (cf. Fig. 2.5)

Case 9: KCS and Corneal Anaesthesia (cont.)

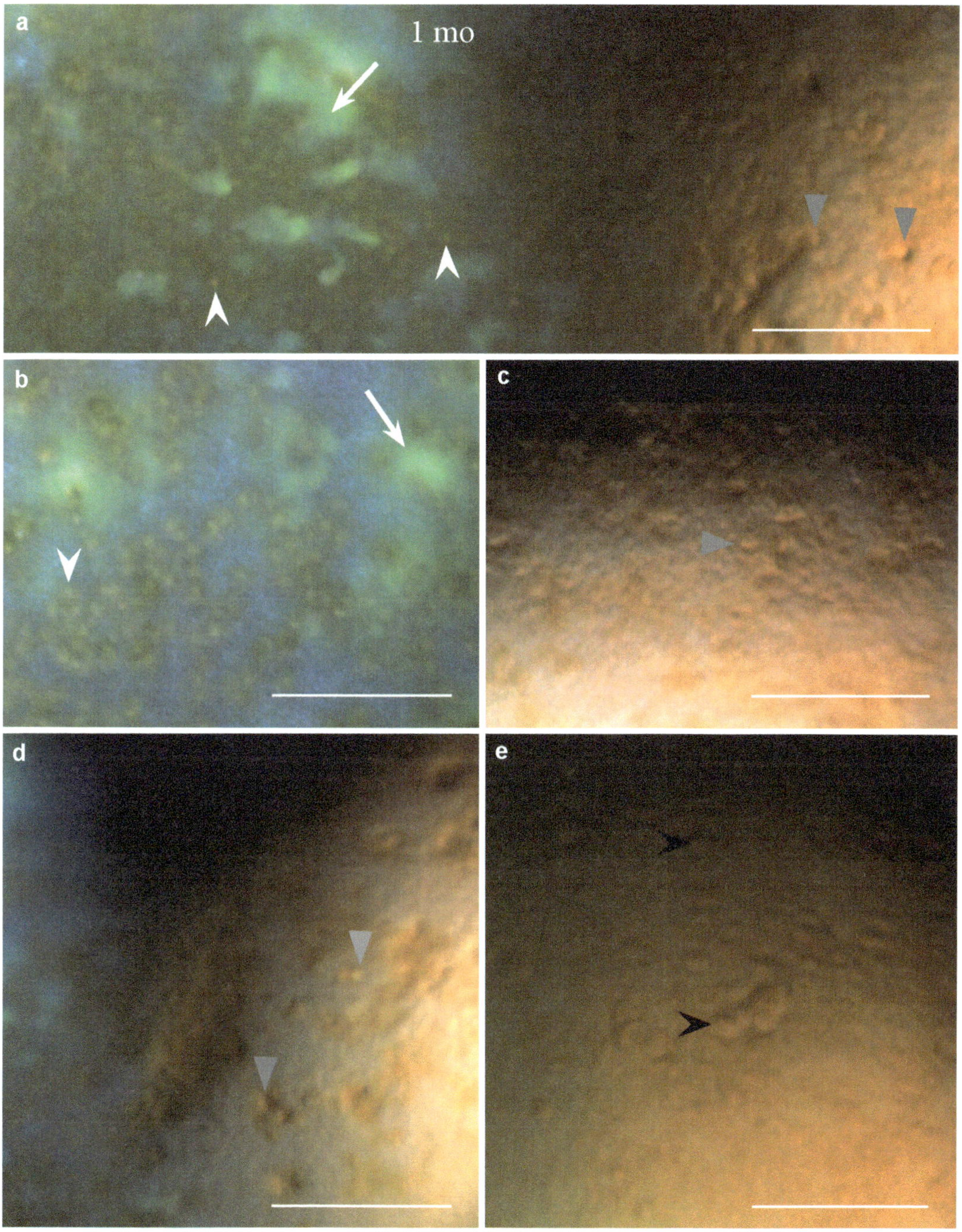

Fig. 4.32 (a) Heavy, confluent staining of surface cells with non-fluorescent fluorescein; in the left part of the picture are visible many brighter dots (*white arrowheads*) and in the right part many rounded bodies (*grey arrowheads*). The *arrows* indicate incipient fluorescein diffusion. (b–d) Different areas showing the same phenomena as in (a) (cf. Figs. 4.33 and 5.2, and 5.4). (e) shows cystic spaces (*arrowheads*)

Case 9: KCS and Corneal Anaesthesia (cont.)

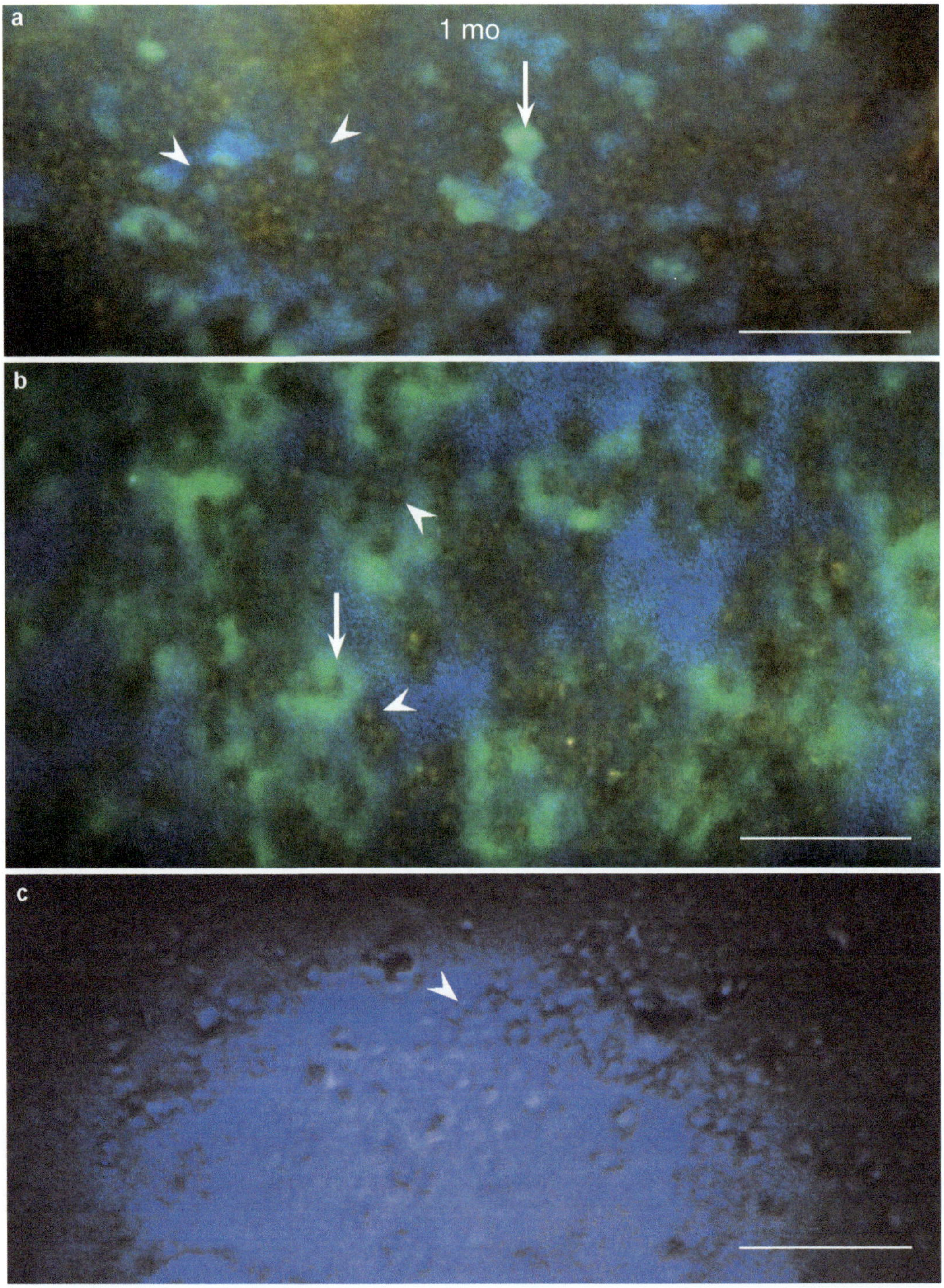

Fig. 4.33 (a–b) The brighter brown/yellowish dots (*arrowheads*) are surrounded by a thin, darker rim (cf. also Fig. 4.34b). The *arrows* indicate incipient fluorescein diffusion into the tissues (green). (c) The rounded bodies (*arrowhead*) visible in light reflected from the lens might represent the same phenomenon as the dots in (a) and (b)

Case 9: KCS and Corneal Anaesthesia (cont.)

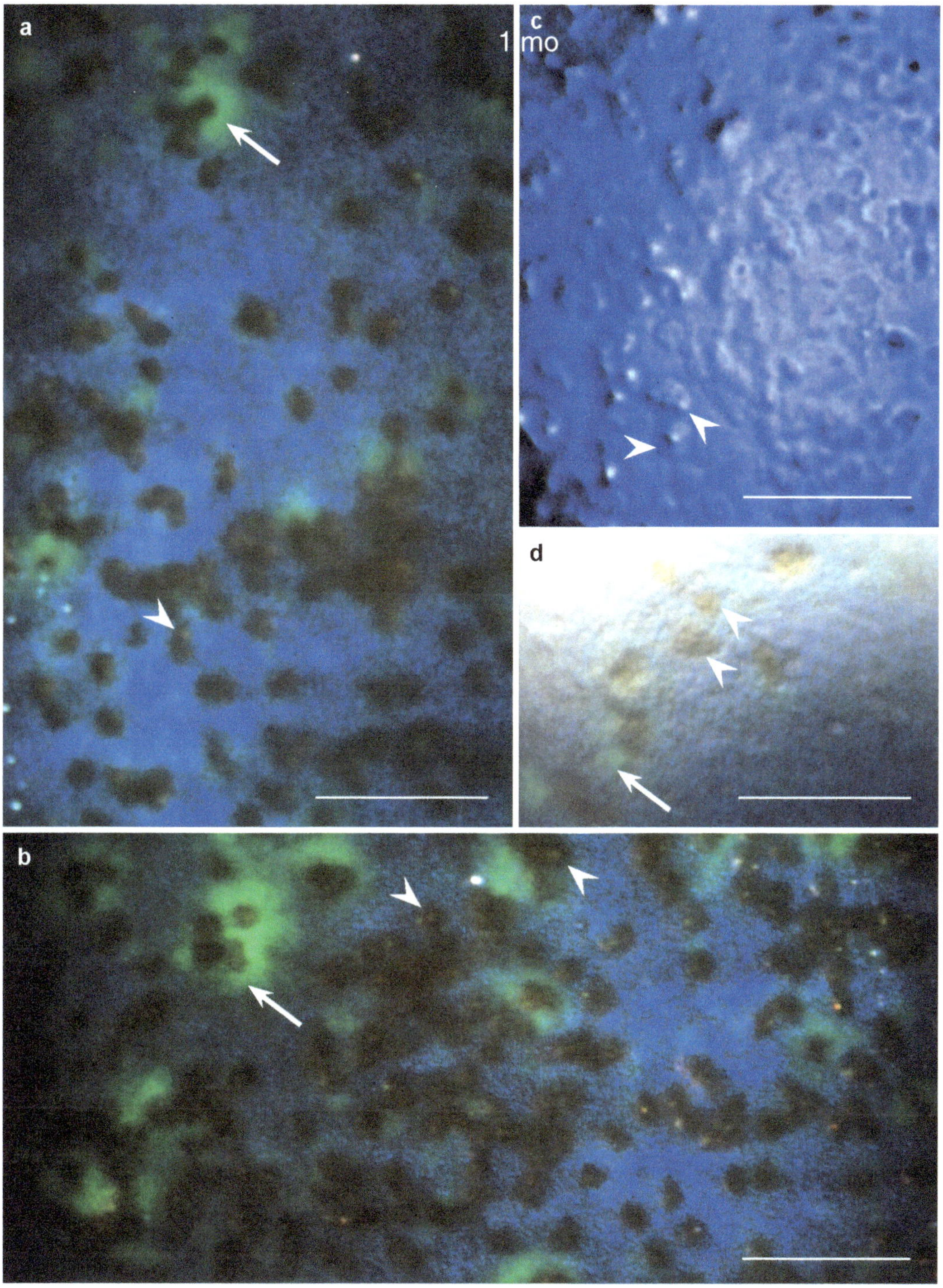

Fig. 4.34 (a, b) Some of the surface cells stained with non-fluorescent fluorescein (*arrowheads*) show a brighter dot; the *arrows* indicate incipient fluorescein diffusion into the tissues (green). (c) In light reflected from the lens, the surface appears rough; the structures indicated by *arrowheads* imply distorted and slightly protruding surface cells (cf. Fig. 5.18). (d) Another area showing surface cells visualised with non-fluorescent fluorescein (*arrowheads*) and incipient fluorescein diffusion into the tissues (green, *arrow*)

5 Corneal Epitheliopathy After Herpes Zoster Ophthalmicus

The four patients presented in this chapter had in common a severe herpes zoster ophthalmicus (HZO) with corneal epitheliopathy as one of sequels. Three of them had *bilateral KCS* (Case 2 not tested) and three *corneal hyp- or anaesthesia* (Case 3 not tested), both conditions diagnosed some time after the infection had subsided. One more patient with impaired corneal sensitivity after HZO and, additionally, filamentary keratopathy is presented in Part II (Chap. 7, Case 5).

The epitheliopathy showed partly basic KCS features (such as greyish surface cells, cystic spaces, fluorescein diffusion indicating surface disruptions, non-fluorescent fluorescein and rose bengal staining of diseased surface cells, surface-adherent mucus, and occasional minifilaments) and partly features strikingly diverging from it.

In comparison with KCS, the epithelial derangement was more pronounced. Staining with *non-fluorescent fluorescein* was in places very heavy, in some areas confluent with no discernible details; in others it revealed surface cells but often in groups or aggregates in which individual cells were difficult or impossible to discern. A peculiar phenomenon were areas showing brighter dots surrounded by thin, darker rim (Case 1; cf. also Chap. 4, Case 9).

Also *rose bengal* staining was very heavy, in places reminding of thick paint applied to the surface with a brush. Similarly to non-fluorescent fluorescein, it revealed areas with no discernible details, and groups or aggregates in which individual cells were difficult or impossible to discern; structures possibly representing individual cells measured about 25–30 μm in diameter. Rose bengal stained the same cells as non-fluorescent fluorescein; in places, some cells seemed to stain only with non-fluorescent fluorescein or showed a hue compatible with a mixture of dyes. Rose bengal, showing a better contrast than non-fluorescent fluorescein, visualised *additional phenomena*, such as *cell distortions*; many larger or smaller *fragments*, presumably cell fragments attached to the surface; and peculiar *lines* surrounding small spaces of about 25–40 μm in diameter, i.e. with dimensions perhaps compatible with cells sizes. Striking was a general absence in the captured areas of cells showing deeply stained central dots (nuclei) similar to those so amply represented in KCS, with only few exceptions (Case 1, Figs. 5.15 and 5.16, and Case 3, Fig. 5.26).

H.M. Tabery, *Keratoconjunctivitis Sicca and Filamentary Keratopathy*,
DOI 10.1007/978-3-642-31028-7_5, © Springer-Verlag Berlin Heidelberg 2012

Case 1: 2, 5–22 Months After Onset

Case Report

An 82-year-old woman presented a week after onset of left-sided HZO. Because of severe symptoms, she was admitted in the Department of Infectious Diseases and treated with acyclovir, both p.o. and topically. The left eye suffered epithelial keratitis, anterior uveitis and a dilated pupil. During the observation period of almost 2,5 years was diagnosed impaired corneal sensitivity in the left eye and KCS in both eyes (test values: BUT 3/4, Schirmer 1 test 3/2, RBS 1/4). She was treated with lubricating eye drops.

The photographs of the left cornea were taken at several occasions (2,5; 4,5; 6,5; 9,5; 12,5; 16,5; and 22 months after onset).

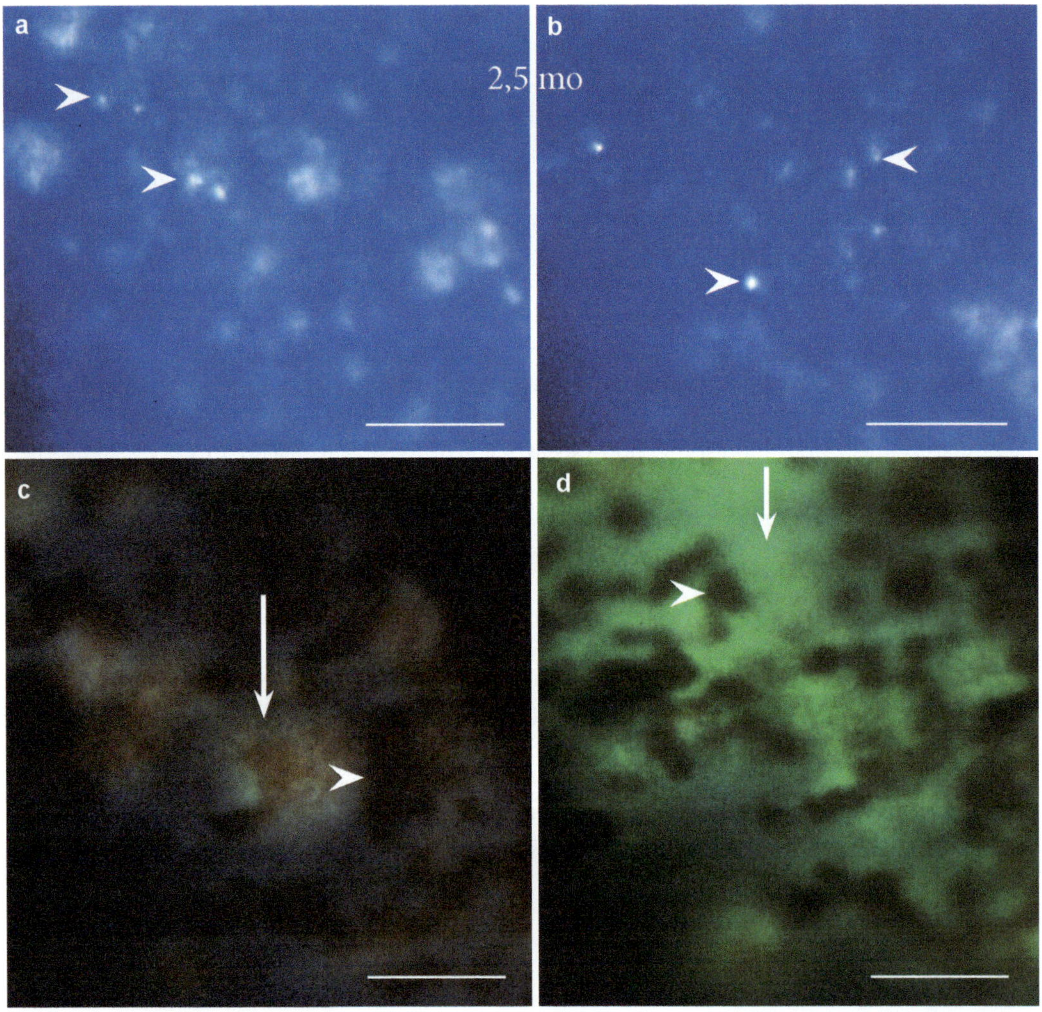

Fig. 5.1 (**a**, **b**) Before staining are visible greyish surface cells or cell aggregates many of which show strongly light-reflecting dots (*arrowheads*). (**c**) shows non-fluorescent fluorescein staining of surface cells (*arrowhead*); its brownish hue is better discernible against a bright background, here due to light reflected from endothelial precipitates (*arrow*). (**d**) Non-fluorescent staining of surface cells (*arrowhead*) is well visible against the green background caused by fluorescein diffusion into the tissues (*arrow*)

Case 1: 2, 5–22 Months After Onset (cont.)

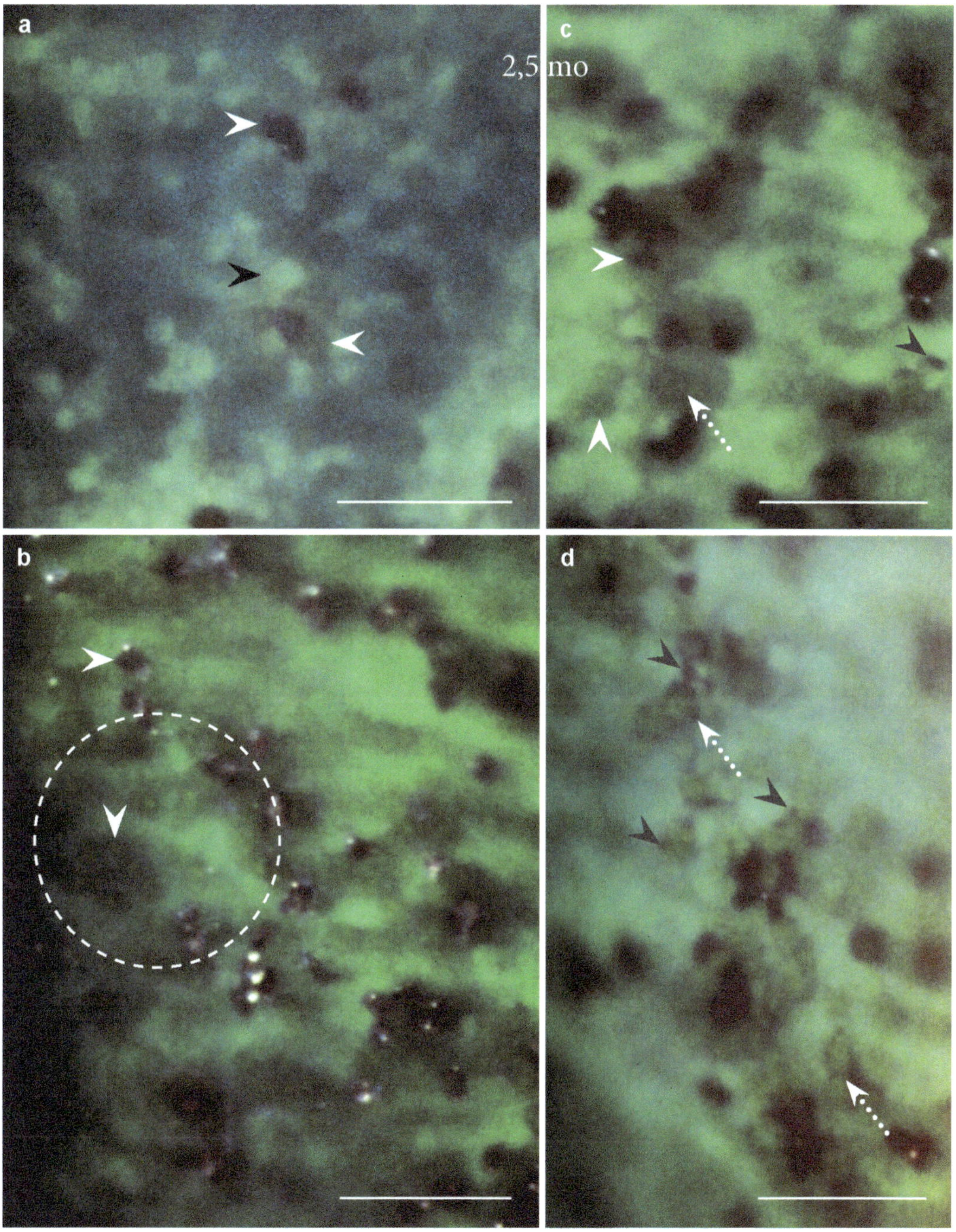

Fig. 5.2 (a) Surface cells stained with non-fluorescent fluorescein and rose bengal (*white arrowheads*) and green stained cystic spaces (*black arrowhead*) in apposition. (b–d) Against the green background caused by fluorescein diffusion into the tissues are visible non-fluorescent fluorescein and rose bengal stained distorted surface cells, individual (*white arrowheads*) or in groups and rows, and cell fragments (*grey arrowheads*). In (b), in the area in *frame*, are additionally visible bright spots (*arrowhead*) surrounded by a darker rim, and in (c, d) dark lines surrounding small spaces (*arrows*)

Case 1: 2, 5–22 Months After Onset (cont.)

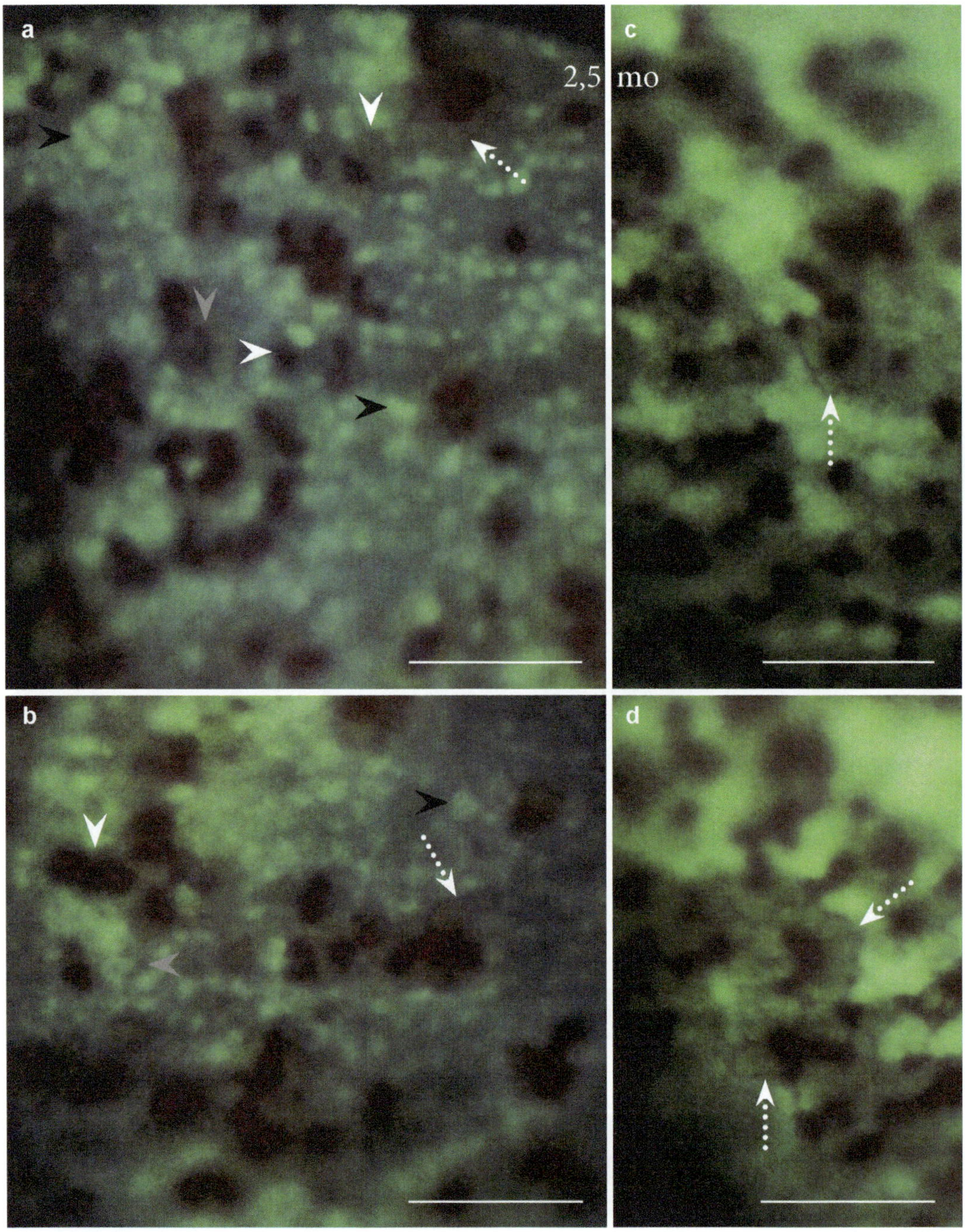

Fig. 5.3 (a, b) Variously large cystic spaces (green, *black arrowheads*); non-fluorescent fluorescein and rose bengal stained distorted surface cells (*white arrowheads*), individual or in groups and rows, and cell fragments (*grey arrowheads*). The *arrows* indicate dark lines surrounding small spaces; this phenomenon is particularly well visible in (c, d) against the green background caused by fluorescein diffusion into the tissues

Case 1: 2, 5–22 Months After Onset (cont.)

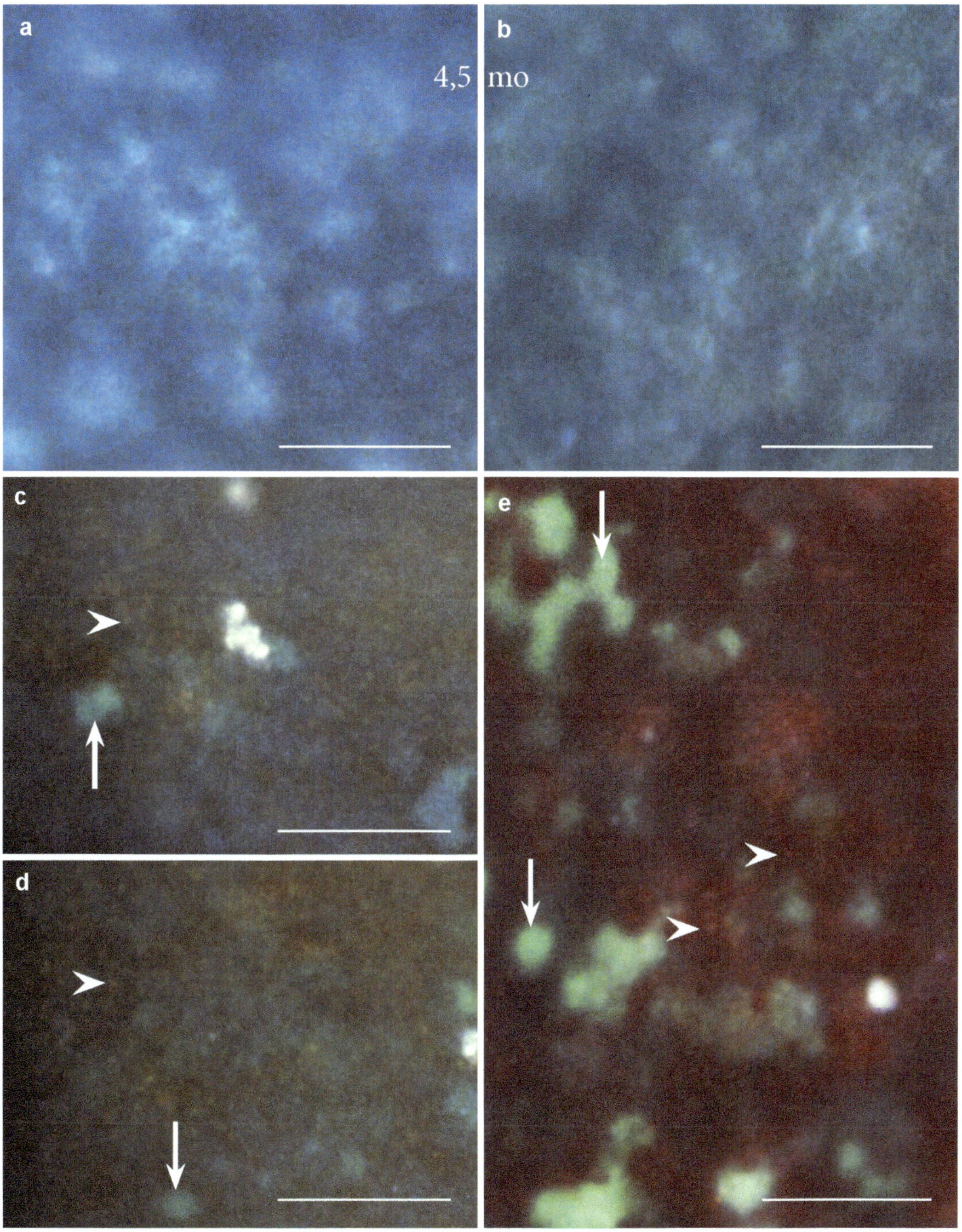

Fig. 5.4 (a, b) Net-like surface reflections in which individual cells are difficult to distinguish; (c, d) heavy non-fluorescent fluorescein staining showing many brighter dots (*arrowheads*) and clear in-between spaces starting to stain green with fluorescein (*arrows*) (cf. Figs. 4.32 and 4.33); (e) heavy rose bengal staining showing brighter dots (*arrowheads*), and green staining of in-between areas (*arrows*) caused by fluorescein diffusion into the tissues (not the same areas)

Case 1: 2, 5–22 Months After Onset (cont.)

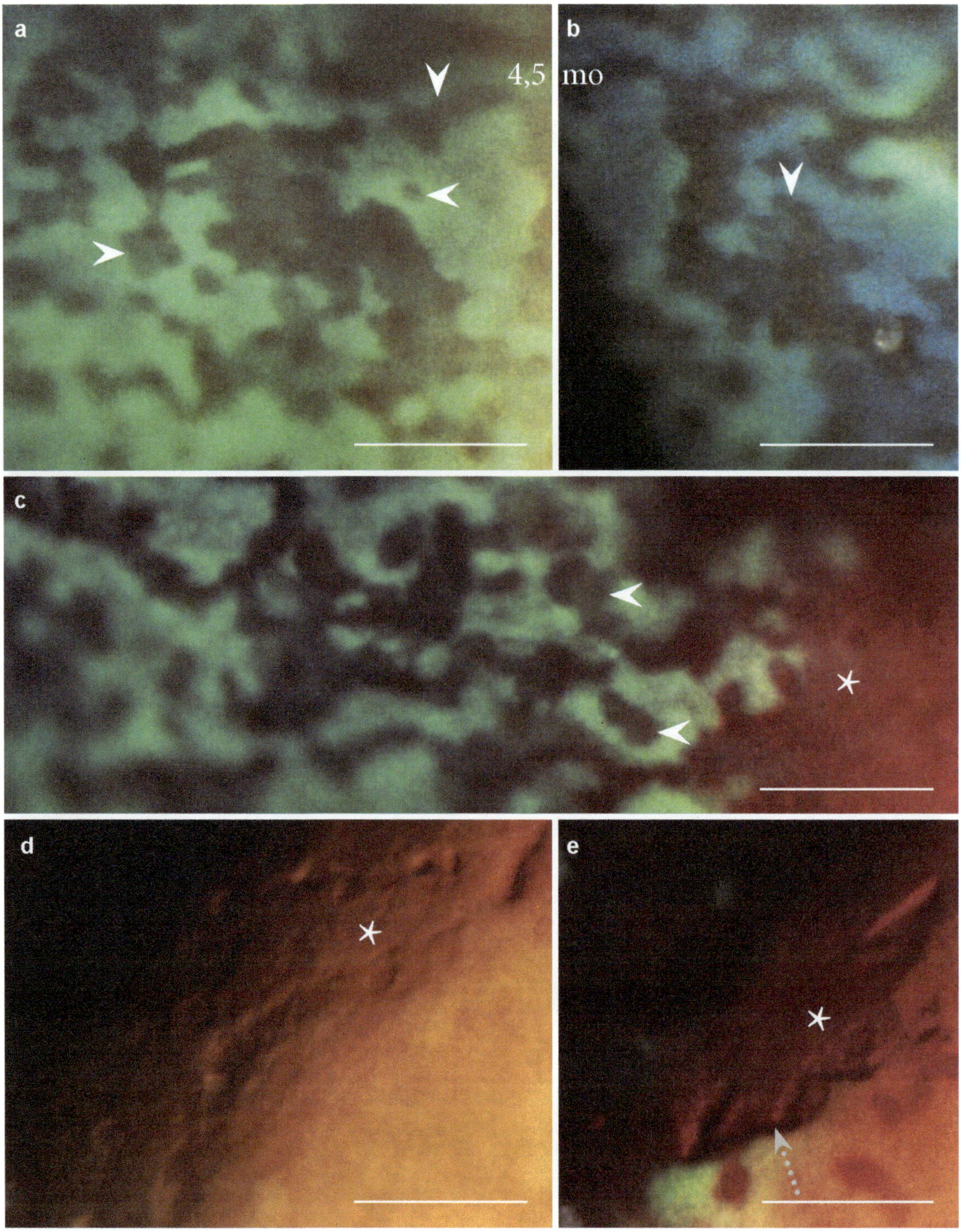

Fig. 5.5 (**a**) Surface cells stained yellow-brown with non-fluorescent fluorescein (*arrowheads*), individual, in groups and rows; the staining density varies. In (**b**) are additionally visible brighter dots within the brown staining. (**c**) Stained surface cells (*arrowheads*) in rows and groups adjacent to an area of confluent rose bengal staining (*asterisk*). (**d**) An area showing heavy staining with non-fluorescent fluorescein (*asterisk*) and (**e**) a different one showing heavy staining with rose bengal (*asterisk*); in (**d**), the surface appears rough and in (**e**) the red stained area seems to represent an elevated plaque casting a shadow (*arrow*)

Case 1: 2, 5–22 Months After Onset (cont.)

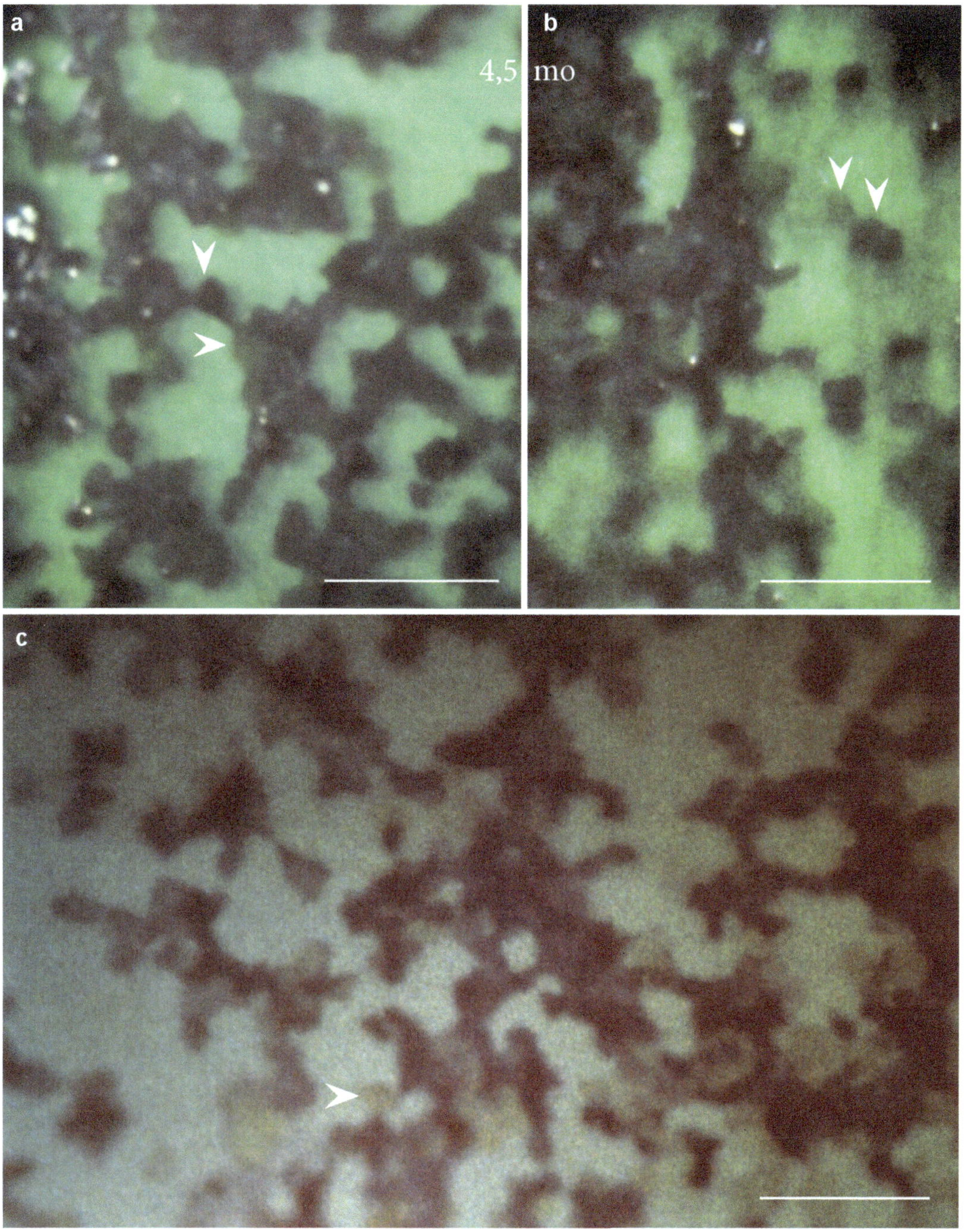

Fig. 5.6 (a, b) Deeply stained distorted surface cells (*arrowheads*), in groups, rows and individual ones seen against a brightly green background caused by fluorescein diffusion into the tissues; the hues of non-fluorescent fluorescein and rose bengal are difficult to distinguish from each other. (c) In this illumination is visible the varying staining intensity of rose bengal and the yellow hue of fluorescein (*arrowhead*) (cf. Fig. 5.7, overleaf)

Case 1: 2, 5–22 Months After Onset (cont.)

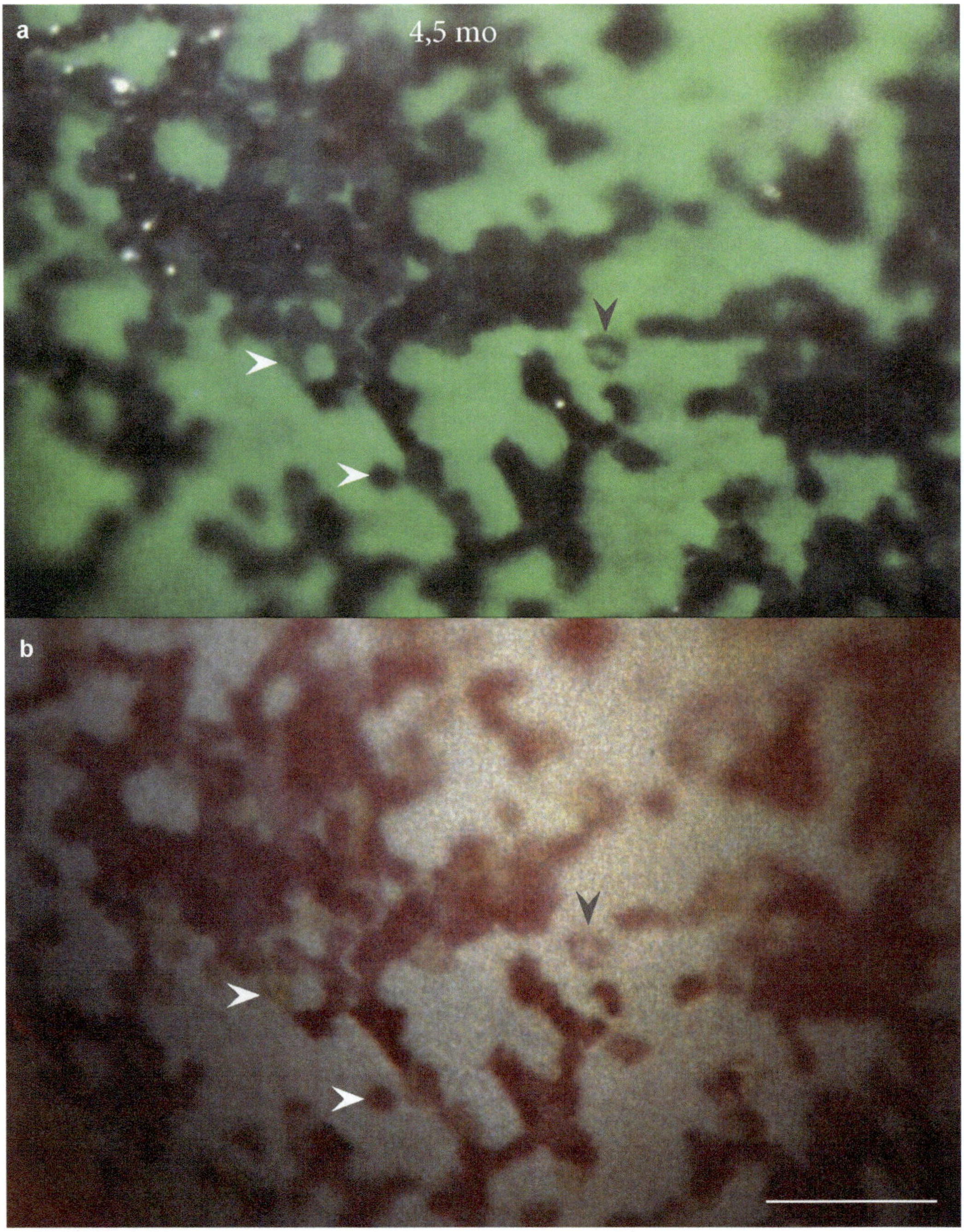

Fig. 5.7 (a, b) The same area. (a) More or less deeply stained distorted surface cells, individual or grouped (*white arrowheads*) and cell fragments (*grey arrowheads*) seen against green background caused by fluorescein diffusion into the tissues. The varying staining density is visible but the yellowish hue of non-fluorescent fluorescein and the red one of rose bengal are better discernible in (b). (The arrowheads are placed in corresponding locations)

Case 1: 2, 5–22 Months After Onset (cont.)

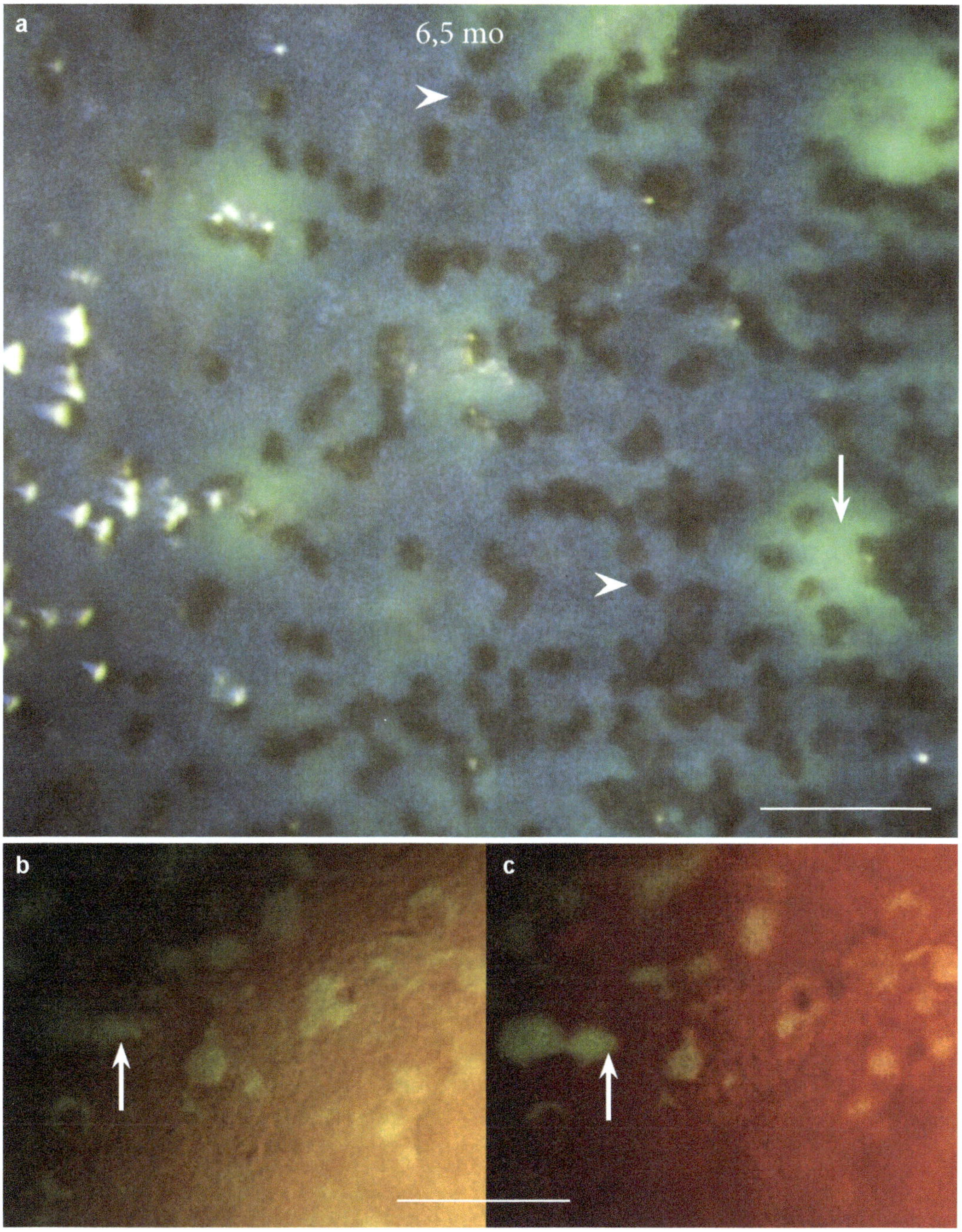

Fig. 5.8 (a) Many surface cells staining yellow-brown with non-fluorescent fluorescein (*arrowheads*) and incipient fluorescein diffusion into the tissues (*arrow*). (Cf. Fig. 4.34.) (b, c) show an area staining heavily with (a) non-fluorescent fluorescein and (b) with rose bengal. The *arrows* indicating areas of green staining caused by fluorescein diffusion into the tissues are placed in corresponding locations

Case 1: 2, 5–22 Months After Onset (cont.)

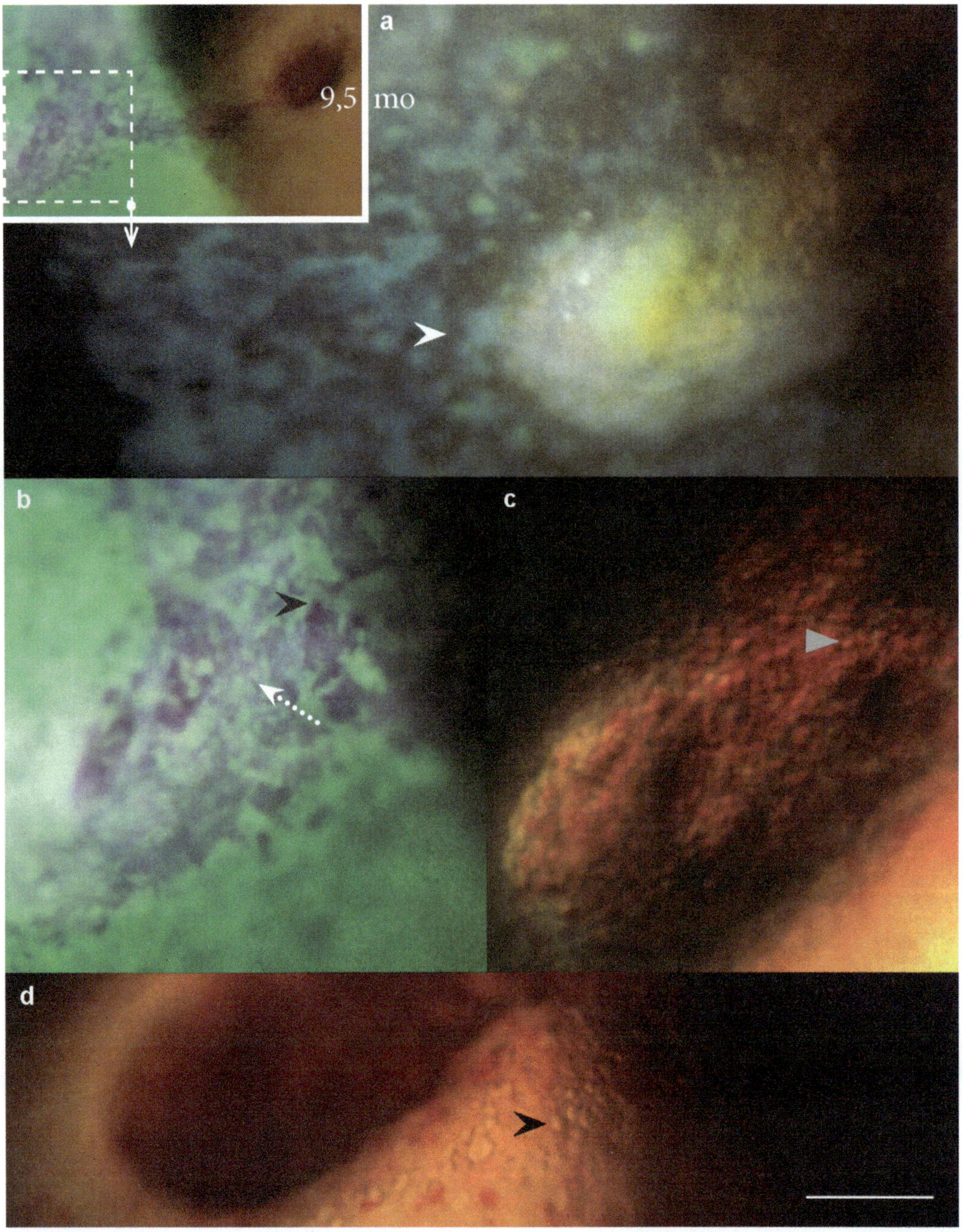

Fig. 5.9 At this occasion was captured a figure shown in the *inset*. (**a**–**d**) The area in *frame* is (**a**) strongly light reflecting; it shows (**b**) cell fragments staining with rose bengal (*arrowhead*) and lines surrounding small spaces (*arrow*; cf. Figs. 5.2 and 5.3); (**c**) a granular component (*arrowhead*); and (**d**) adjoining cystic spaces (*arrowhead*). (**a**) additionally shows non-fluorescent fluorescein staining of surface cells (*arrowhead*) in the surroundings

Comment

The figure was not an expression of HZO recurrence, such figures sometimes form in a deranged epithelium; it disappeared spontaneously with no consequence.

Case 1: 2, 5–22 Months After Onset (cont.)

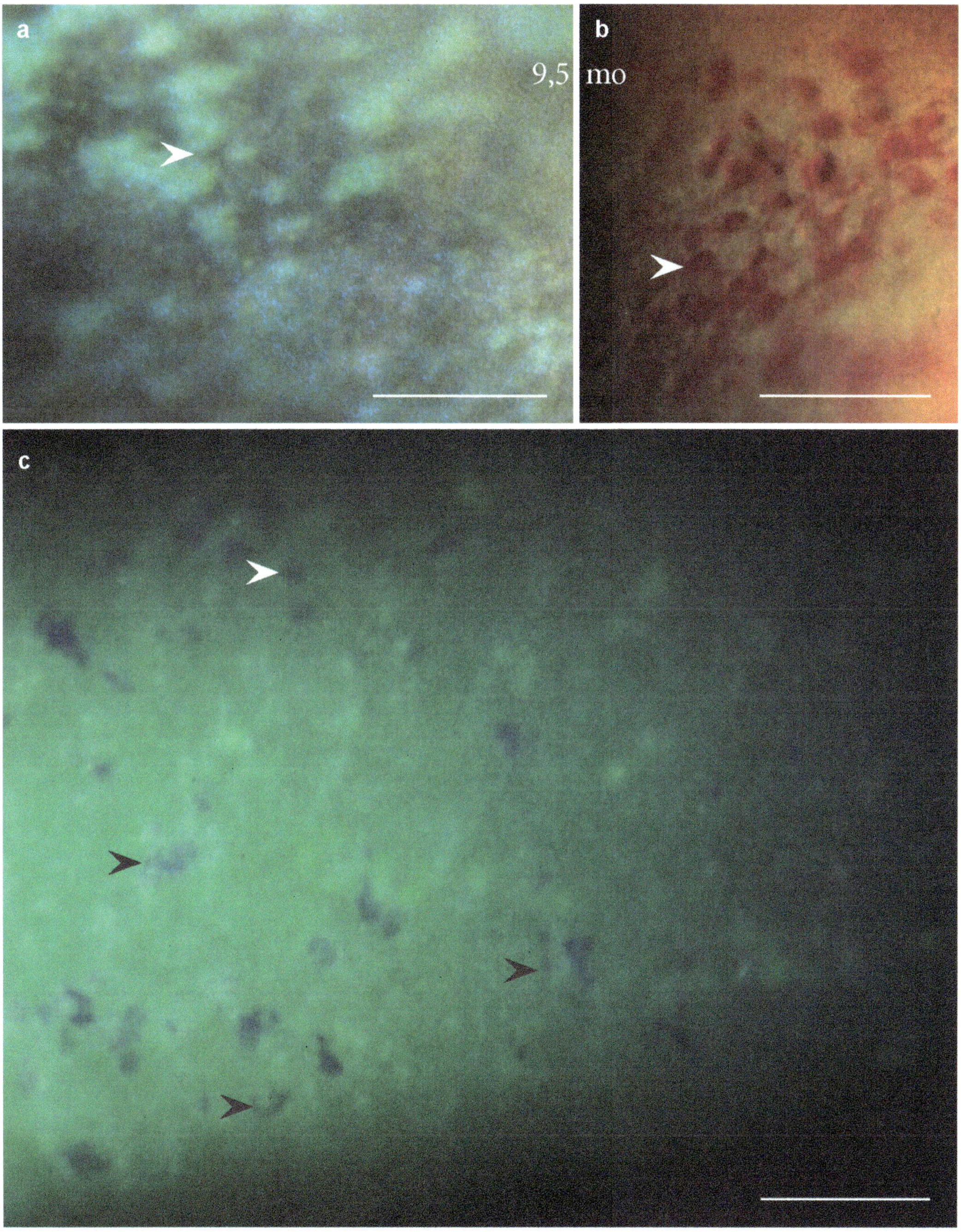

Fig. 5.10 Three different areas showing (a) a partly confluent non-fluorescent staining of surface cells (*arrowhead*); (b, c) rose bengal staining of surface cells (*white arrowheads*); and (c) cell fragments (*grey arrowheads*) seen against green background caused by fluorescein diffusion into the tissues

Case 1: 2, 5–22 Months After Onset (cont.)

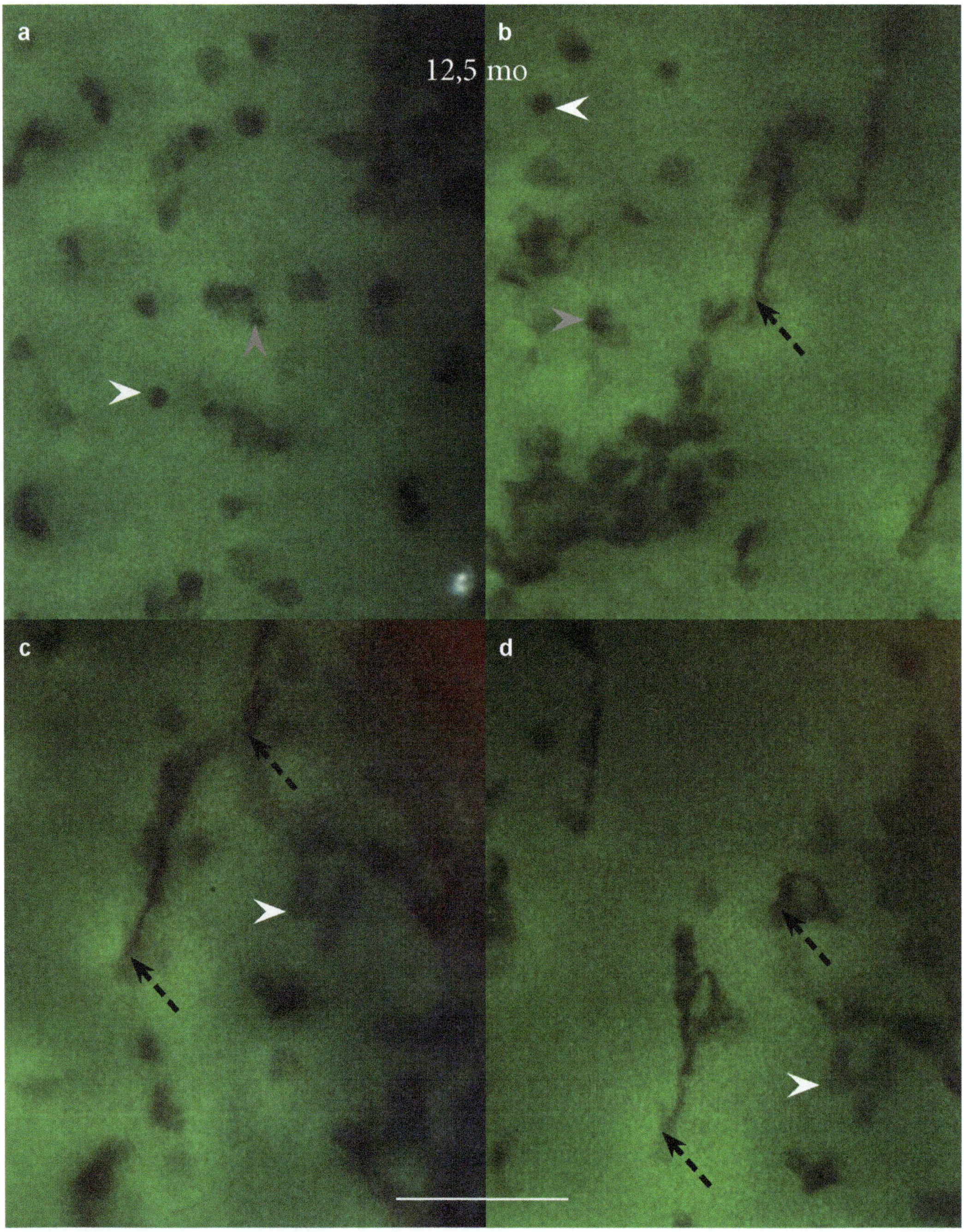

Fig. 5.11 More or less densely rose bengal stained surface cells (*white arrowheads*) and cell fragments (*grey arrowheads*) seen against green background caused by fluorescein diffusion into the tissues. In (**b**–**d**) are additionally visible small filaments with attachment points indicated by *arrows*. The upper one in (**c**) is coiled in (**d**). (The markers in **c** and **d** are placed in corresponding locations)

Case 1: 2, 5–22 Months After Onset (cont.)

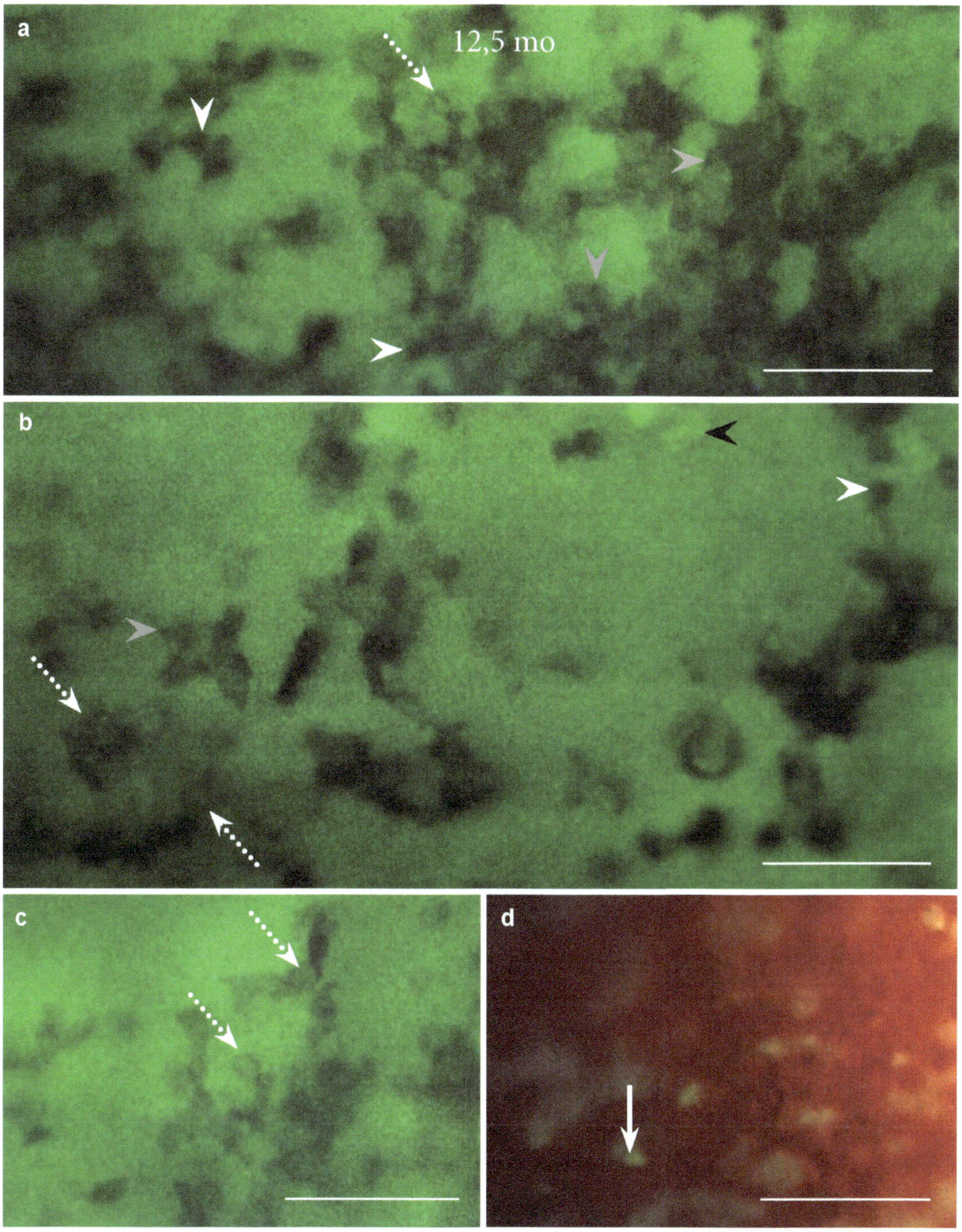

Fig. 5.12 (a–c) Rose bengal stained surface cells (*white arrowheads*), cell fragments (*grey arrowheads*), brilliantly green cystic spaces (*black arrowhead*) and lines surrounding small spaces (*arrows*), all seen against green background caused by fluorescein diffusion into the tissues. (d) shows an area of heavy rose bengal staining with incipient fluorescein diffusion (*arrow*) visible in the in-between areas

Case 1: 2, 5–22 Months After Onset (cont.)

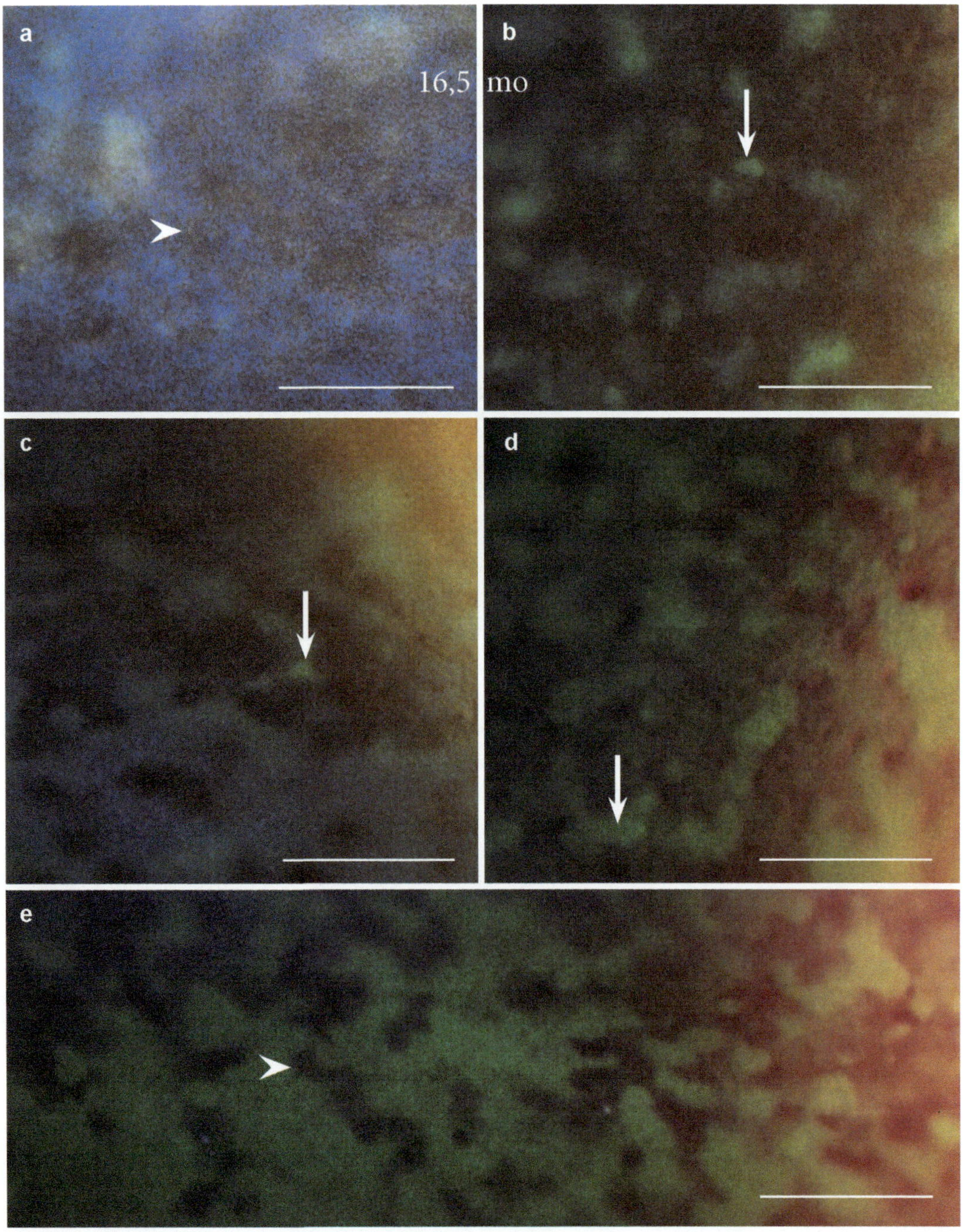

Fig. 5.13 (**a**) Patches of surface cells stained with non-fluorescent fluorescein (*arrowhead*); (**b, c**) heavy, partly confluent non-fluorescent fluorescein surface staining and green staining of in-between areas (*arrows*) visualising fluorescein diffusion into the tissues; (**d**) rose bengal staining with small green in-between areas (*arrow*); and (**e**) a different area showing rows of rose bengal stained surface cells (*arrowhead*) against a green background and, to the right, a more confluent red staining

Case 1: 2, 5–22 Months After Onset (cont.)

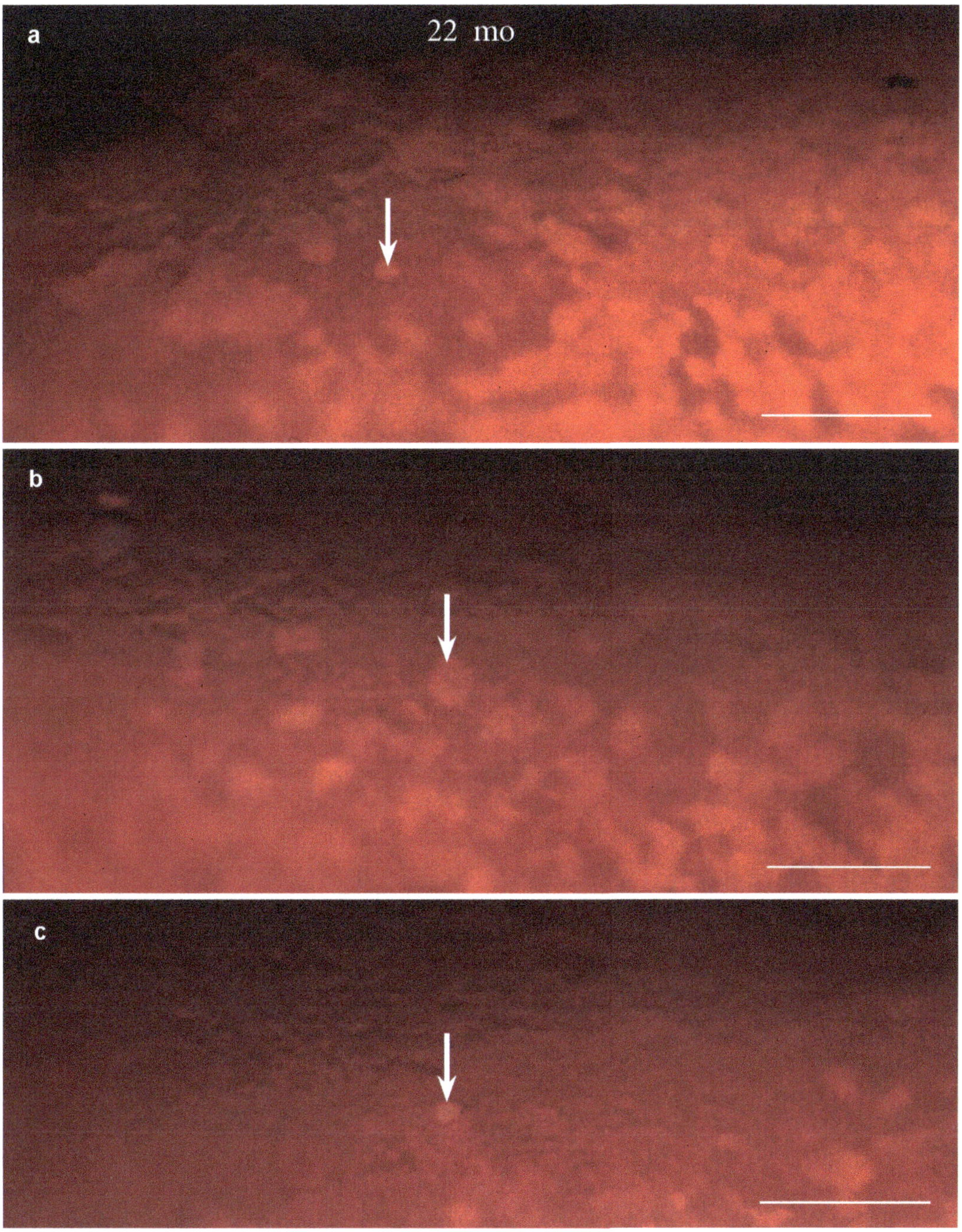

Fig. 5.14 (a–c) Three areas showing heavy rose bengal surface staining and brighter in-between areas (*arrows*; no fluorescein used)

Case 1: 2, 5–22 Months After Onset (cont.)

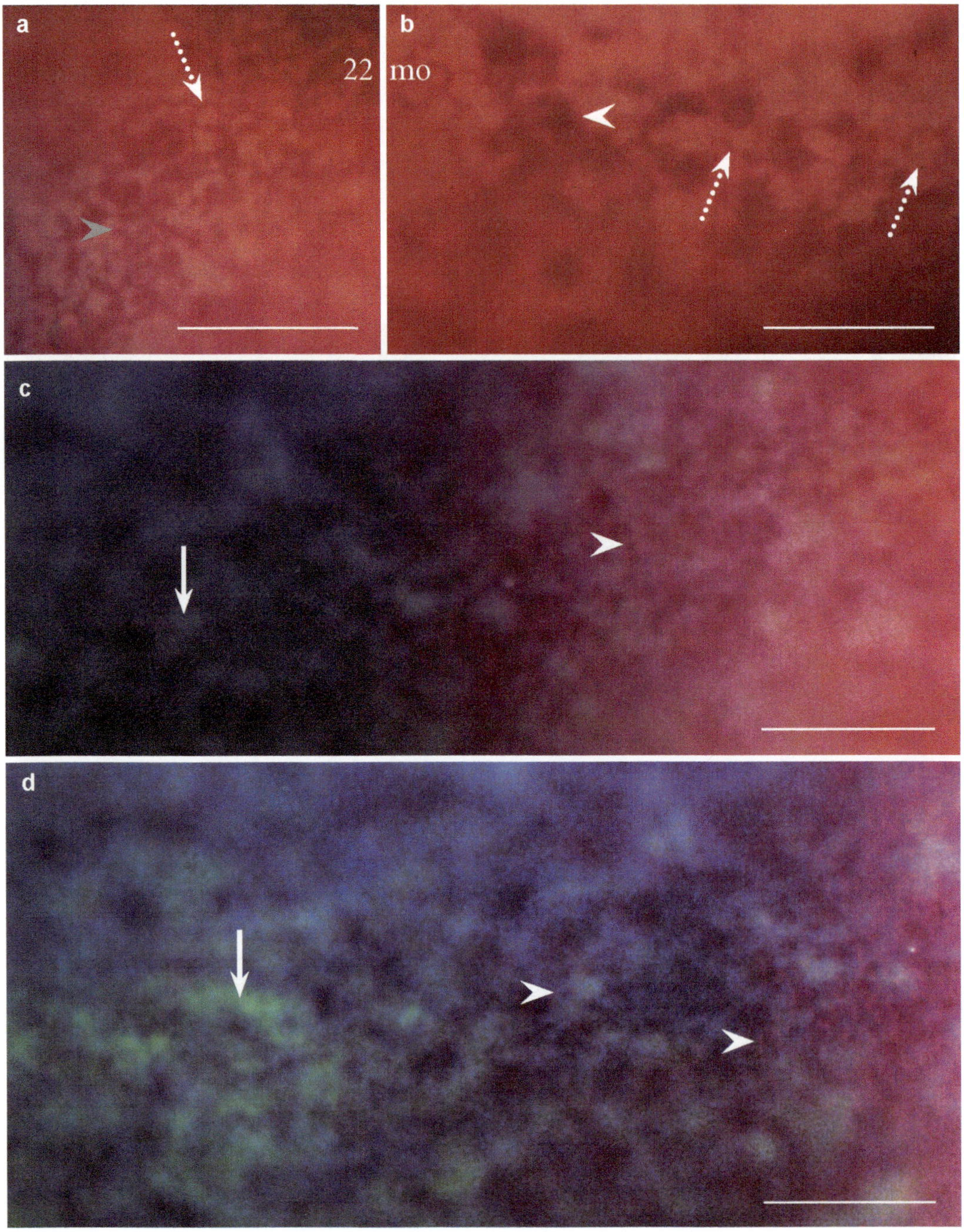

Fig. 5.15 (**a, b**) With rose bengal only are visible cell fragments (*grey arrowhead*), surface cells/cell aggregates (*white arrowhead*), and red stained lines (*arrows*) surrounding small spaces (cf. Fig. 5.27). (**c, d**) After the application of fluorescein, the in-between areas (*arrows*) start to stain green. The small more deeply stained dots (*arrowheads*) seem to represent cell nuclei

Case 1: 2, 5–22 Months After Onset (cont.)

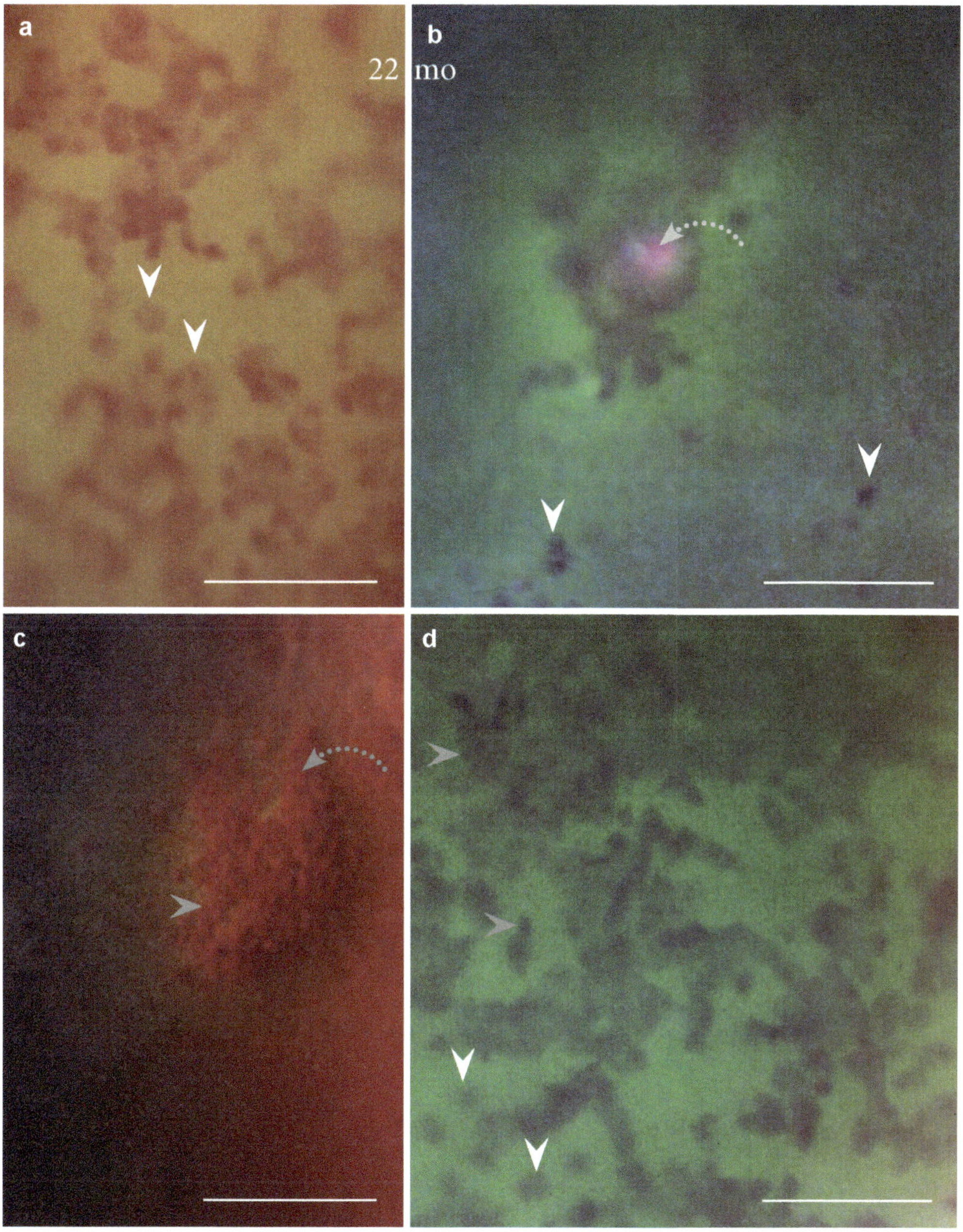

Fig. 5.16 (a, b) Rose bengal stained surface cells (*arrowheads*) with or without a deeply stained dot (nucleus) and (b) light-reflecting mucus (*arrow*). (c) A lump (*arrow*) of cell debris (*arrowhead*) lying on the surface. (d) Rose bengal stained surface cells (*white arrowheads*) in groups, rows or individual, and cell fragments (*grey arrowheads*) visualised against green background caused by fluorescein diffusion into the tissues; the staining density varies

Comment

Changes shown in Fig. 5.15 (c, d) and Fig. 5.16 (a–c) are common in KCS, cf. Chap. 2.

Case 2: 2–5 Years After Onset

Case Report

A 74-year-old woman had a severe right-sided HZO with keratitis and anterior uveitis and sequels such as corneal anaesthesia, epitheliopathy, recurrent erosions, subepithelial scarring and posterior synechiae. KCS was not tested.

The photographs of the right cornea were taken at various occasions between 2 and 5 years after the infection.

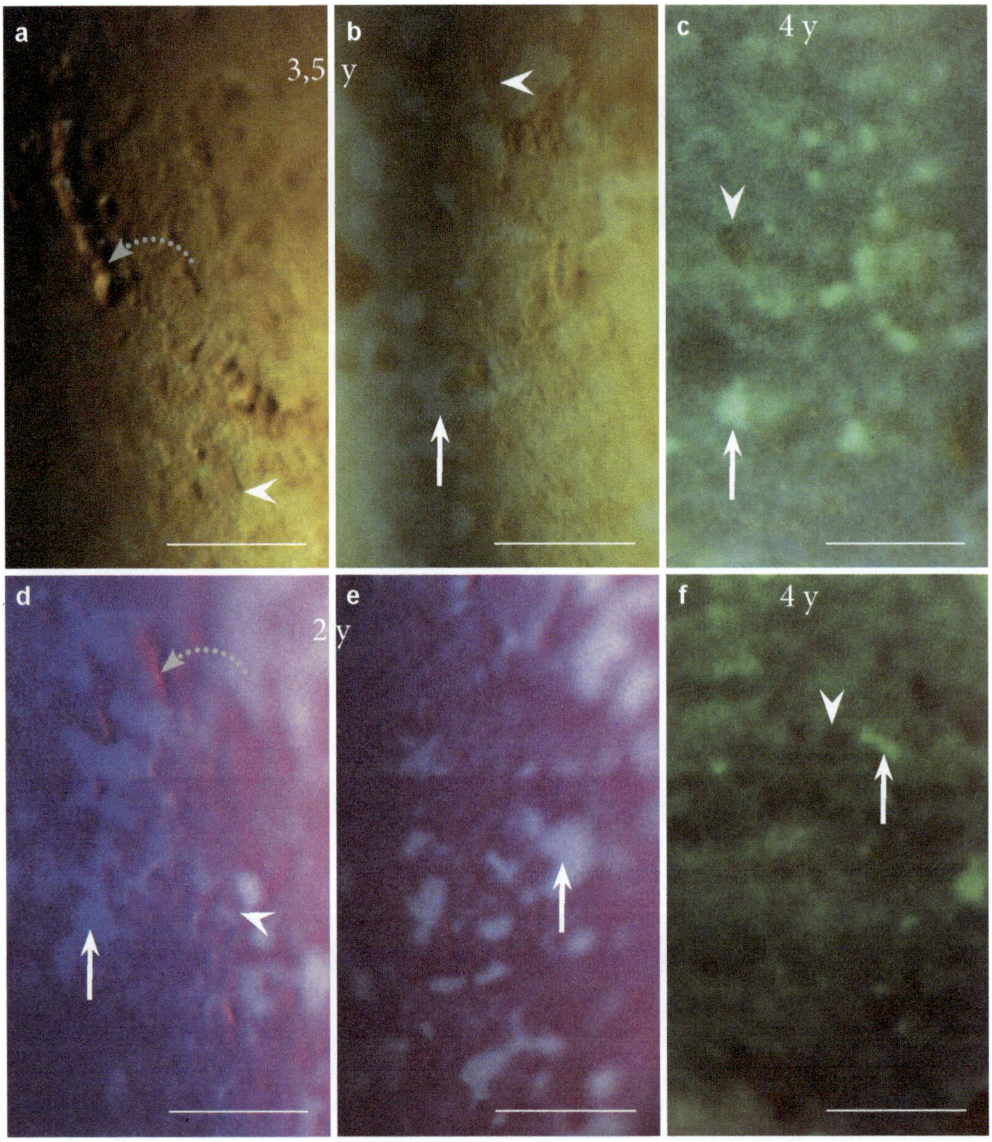

Fig. 5.17 Heavy surface staining with (**a, b, c** and **f**) non-fluorescent fluorescein and (**d, e**) rose bengal. The staining is largely confluent and individual cells (*arrowheads*) difficult to discern; the surface appears rough (cf. Fig. 5.18). In (**b, d** and **e**) are visible clear in-between spaces (*straight arrows*), and in (**c** and **f**) in-between spaces stained green with fluorescein (*arrows*). (Fluorescein was not used in (**d**) and (**e**).) The *bowed arrows* in (**a**) and (**d**) indicate structures probably representing mucus lying on the surface

Case 2: 2–5 Years After Onset (cont.)

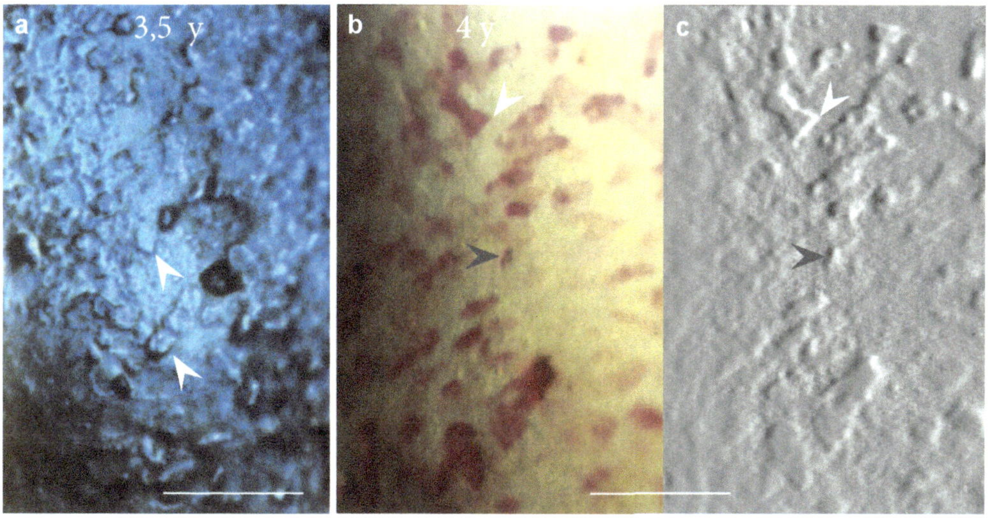

Fig. 5.18 The surface, captured in light reflected from the lens, appears rough; arrowheads indicate structures implying distorted surface cells (cf. Fig. 4.34). (**b**) An area showing distorted red stained surface cells (*white arrowhead*) and cell fragments (*grey arrowhead*). (**c**) The same area in computer-produced relief simulating a 3-D image. (The markers are placed in corresponding locations)

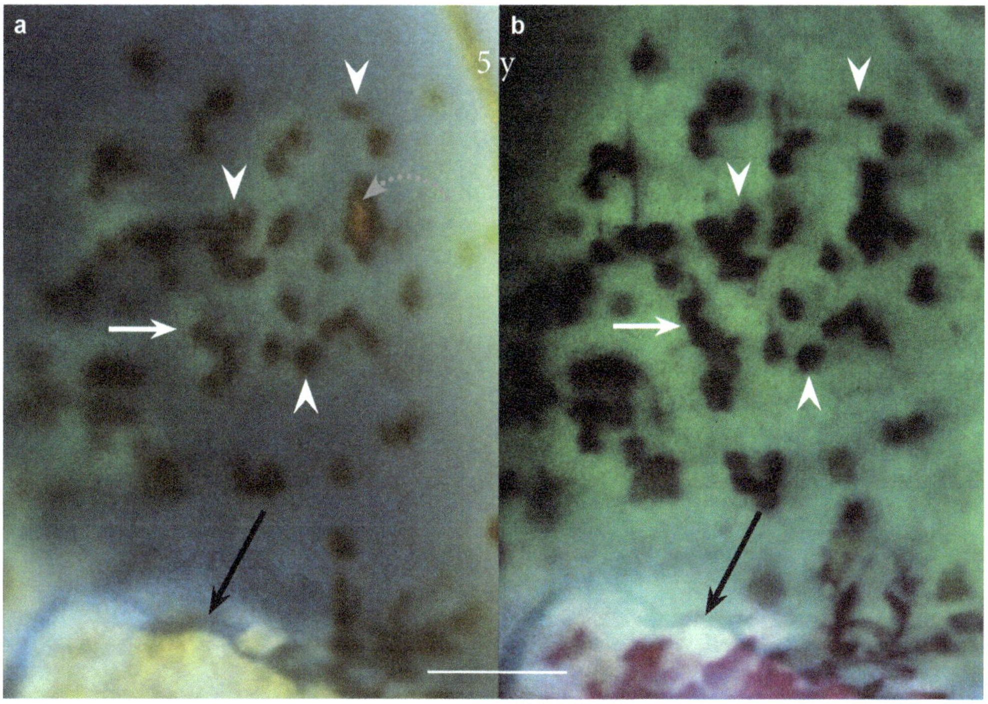

Fig. 5.19 (**a**, **b**) An area showing surface cells (*arrowheads*) staining (**a**) with non-fluorescent fluorescein and (**b**) with rose bengal; the patterns are not exactly the same because of cell displacements between the photographs. In (**a**) is visible incipient fluorescein diffusion into the tissues (green, *white arrow*); with time (**b**) the green staining becomes confluent. The brighter spot in (**a**, *bowed arrow*) implies adhering mucus. The *black arrows* indicate a subepithelial scar. (The markers are placed in corresponding locations)

Case 2: 2–5 Years After Onset (cont.)

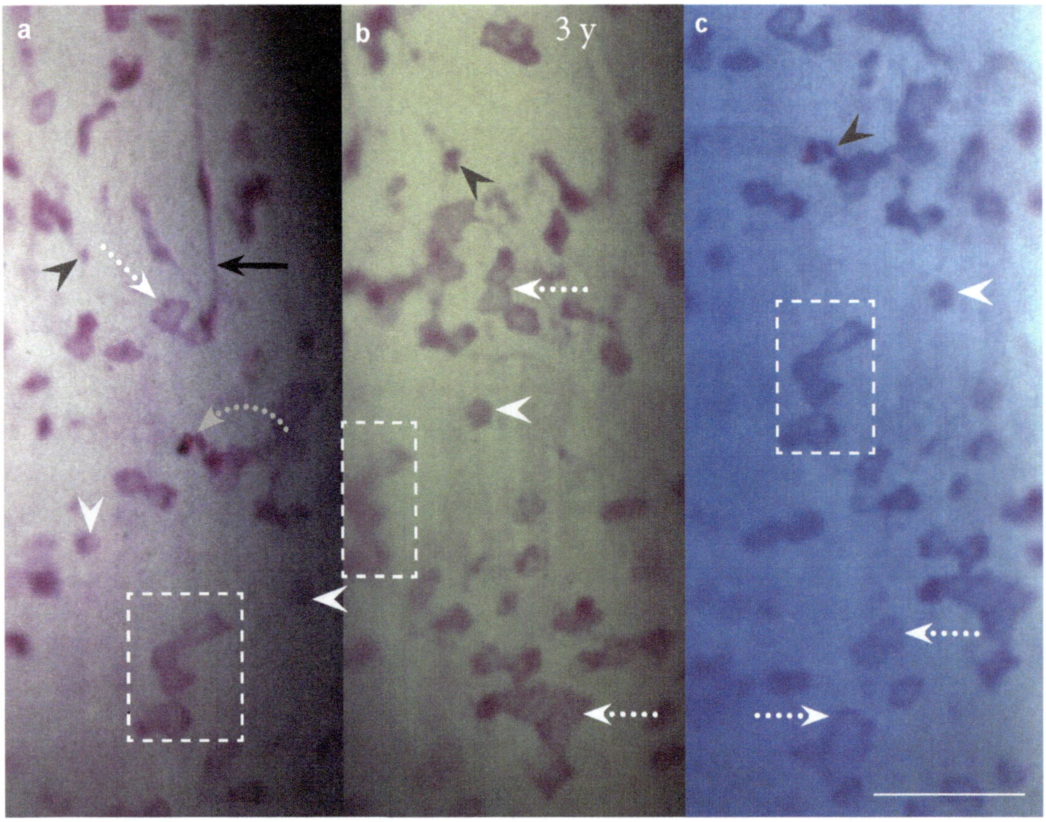

Fig. 5.20 (a–c) With rose bengal only are visible red stained cells (*white arrowheads*), cell fragments (*grey arrowheads*), lines (*dotted straight arrows*) surrounding small weakly red stained spaces, and in (a) a mucus thread (*black arrow*). In places is visible a more brightly red hue of rose bengal implying mucus adhering to the surface (a, *bowed arrow*). The *frames* indicate a configuration visible in all three photographs

Case 2: 2–5 Years After Onset (cont.)

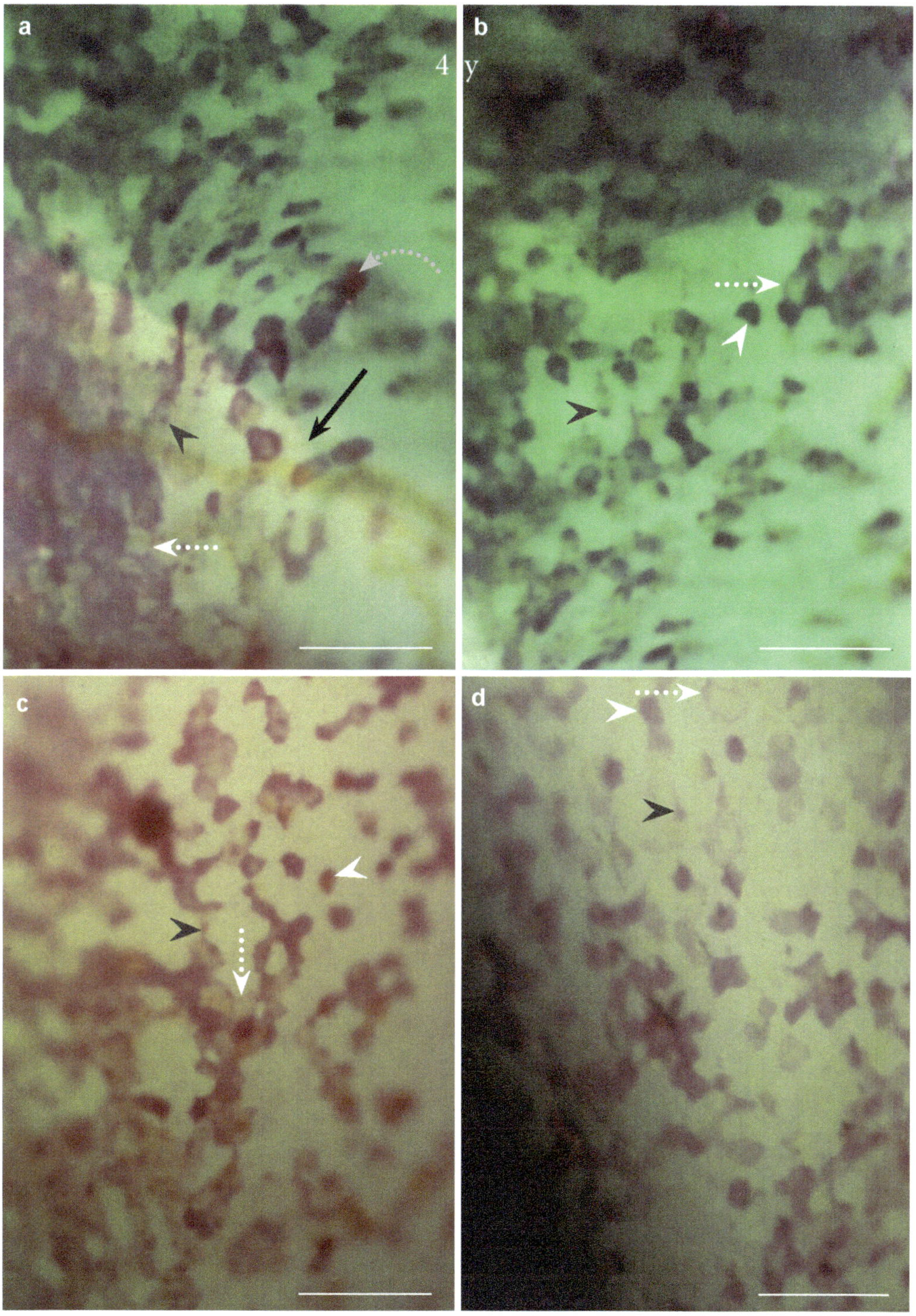

Fig. 5.21 (a–d) Rose bengal stained cells (*white arrowheads*), cell fragments (*grey arrowheads*) and lines (*dotted arrows*) surrounding small spaces, in (a, b) visualised against green background caused by fluorescein diffusion into the tissues. The staining density of rose bengal varies; the more brightly red hue of rose bengal (a, *bowed arrow*) implies mucus adhering to the surface. The *black arrow* in (a) indicates an edge of a subepithelial scar

Case 3: 2 Weeks–4 Months After Recurrence of HZO

Case Report

An 84-year-old diabetic woman with left-sided HZO complicated by relapsing anterior uveitis, epitheliopathy and a recurrence of an HZO pseudodendrite 6 months after the first episode. KCS tester were performed 6 months later: BUT 2/2, Schirmer 1 test 3/4 and RBS 4/7. Corneal sensitivity was not tested.

The photographs of the left cornea were taken 2 weeks, 3 months and 4 months after the recurrent pseudodendrite had healed.

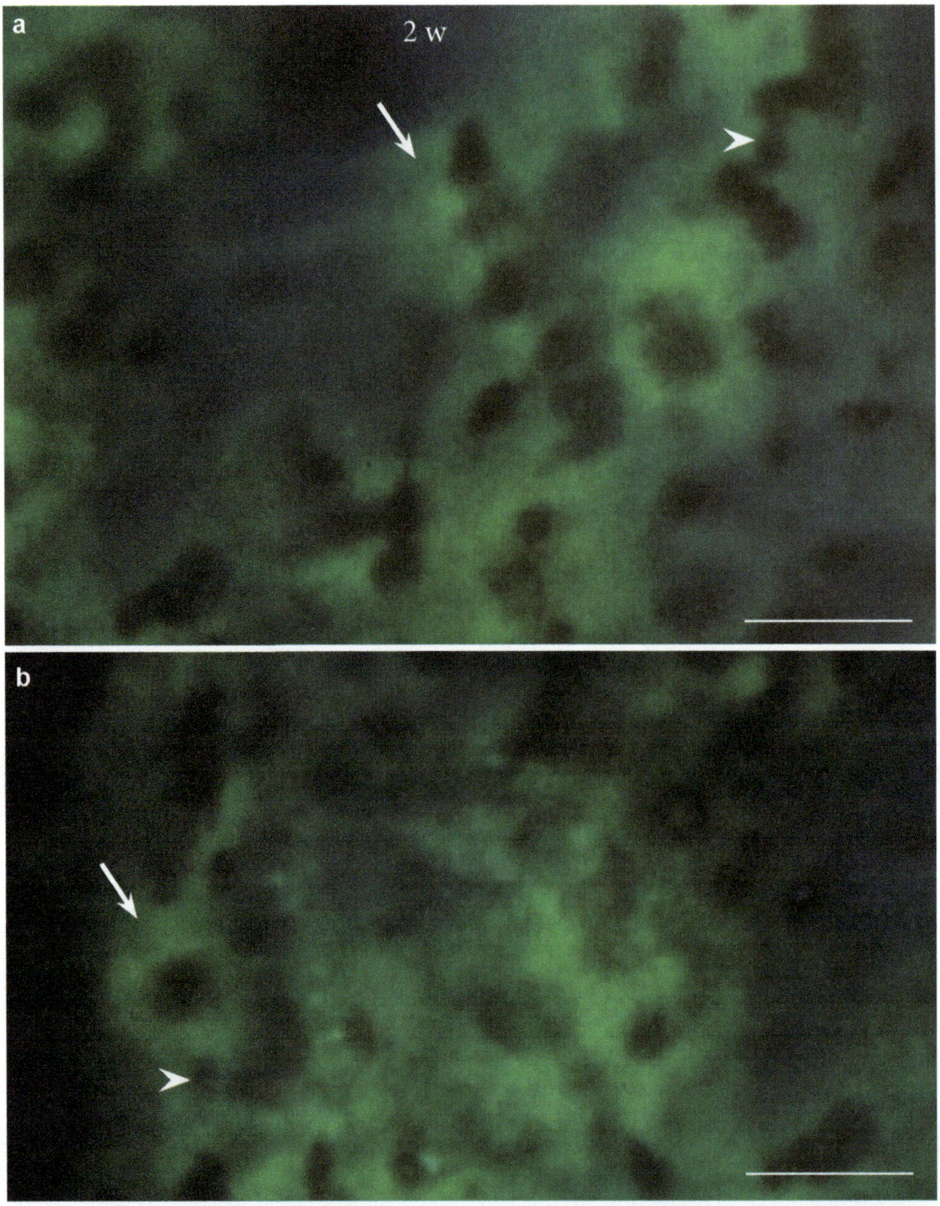

Fig. 5.22 (a, b) Individual or grouped surface cells (*arrowheads*) stained with non-fluorescent fluorescein and fluorescein diffusion into the tissues (green, *arrows*)

Case 3: 2 Weeks–4 Months After Recurrence of HZO (cont.)

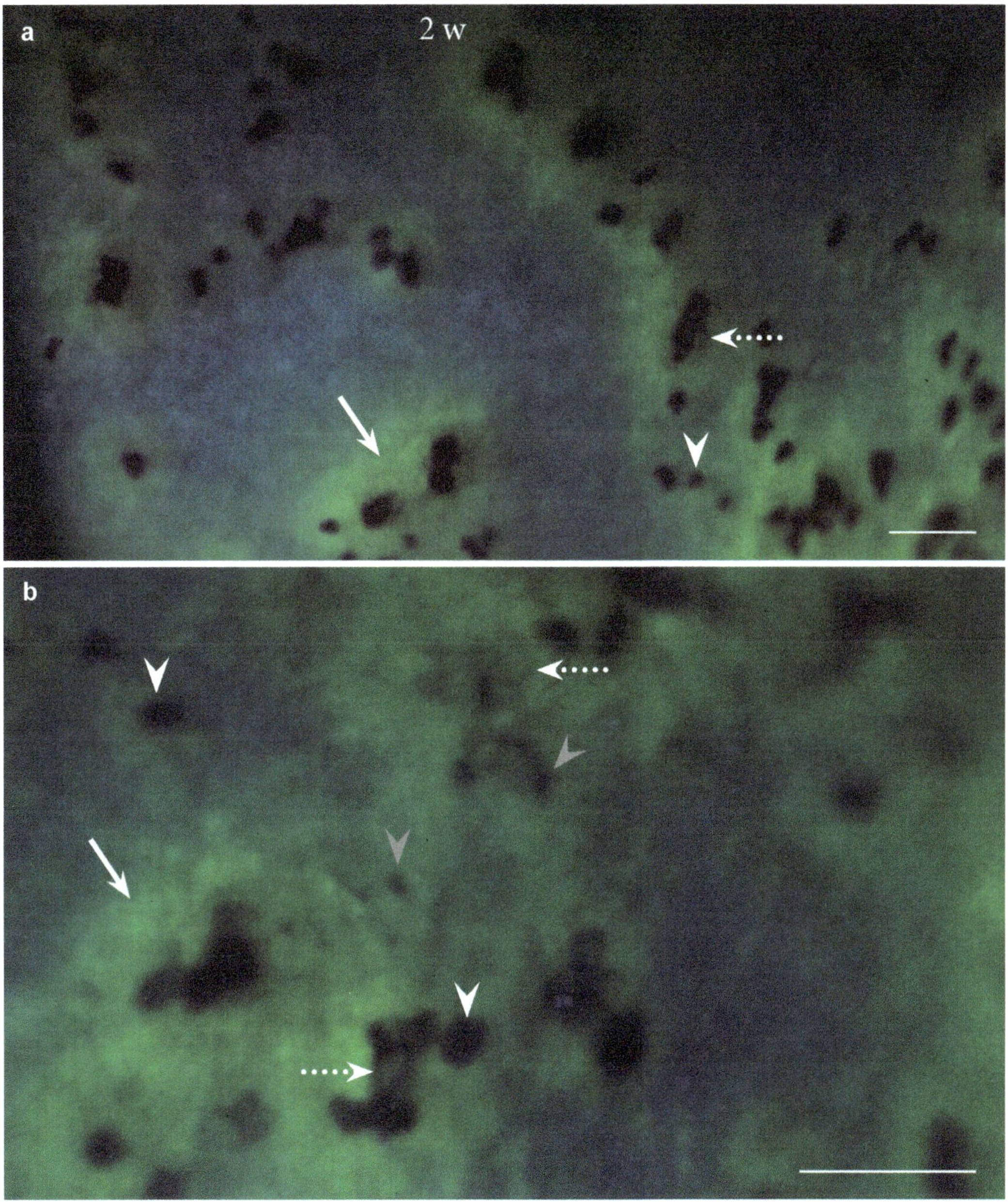

Fig. 5.23 (a, b) Two areas showing rose bengal stained surface cells (*white arrowheads*), individual or grouped, cell fragments (*grey arrowheads*), lines surrounding small spaces (*dotted arrows*), and fluorescein diffusion into the tissues (green, *plain arrows*) (cf. Fig. 5.3)

Case 3: 2 Weeks–4 Months After Recurrence of HZO (cont.)

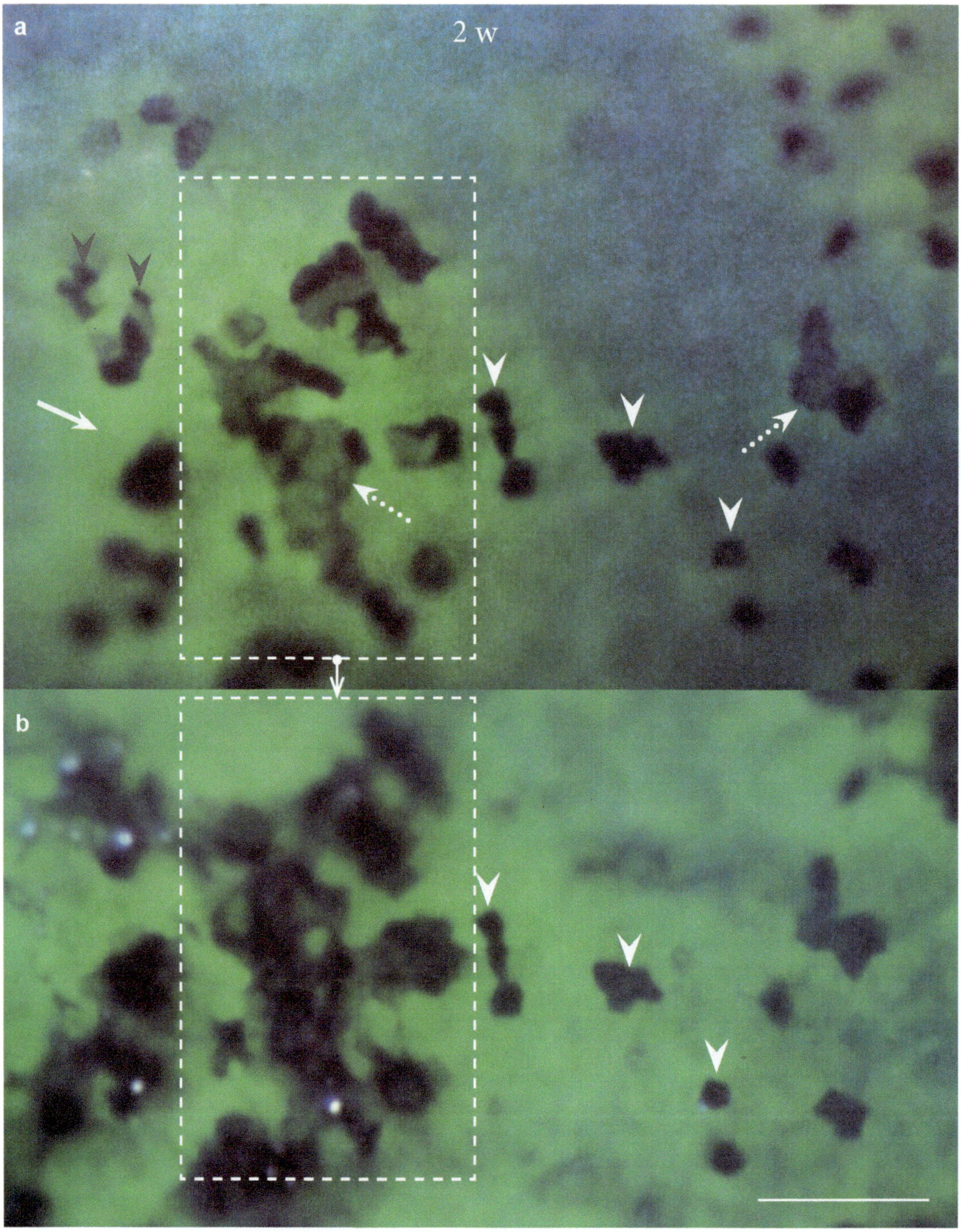

Fig. 5.24 (a) Rose bengal stained surface cells (*white arrowheads*), individual or grouped, cell fragments (*grey arrowheads*) and lines surrounding small spaces (*dotted arrows*); the *plain arrow* indicates incipient fluorescein diffusion into the tissues. (b) With time, the green staining has enlarged, and the area in frame in (a) has changed appearance; it is now largely covered by rose bengal stained material implying conglomerates of mucus and cell debris. Rose bengal stained cells in the right part of the picture have remained in place. (The white arrowheads in a and b are placed in corresponding locations)

Case 3: 2 Weeks–4 Months After Recurrence of HZO (cont.)

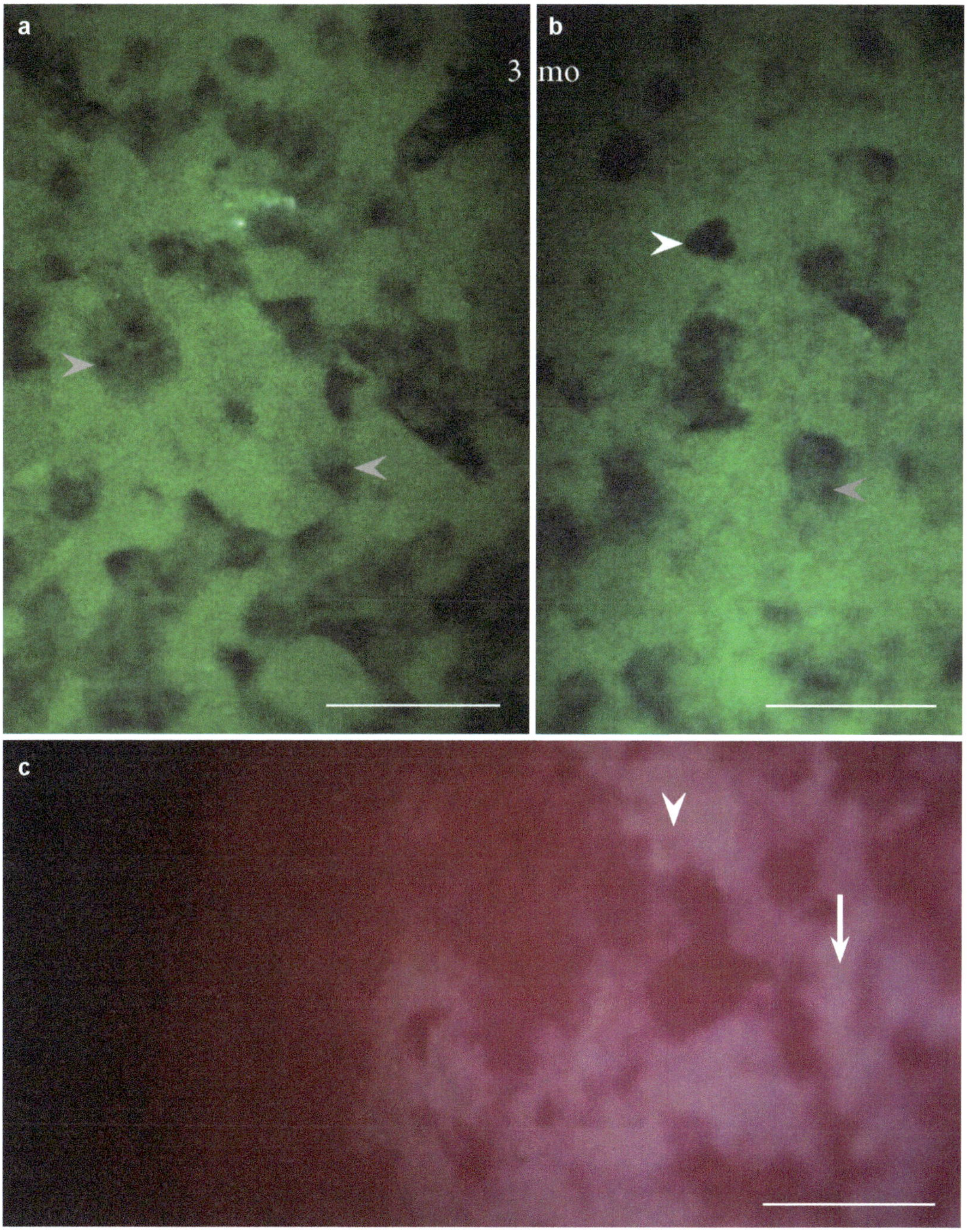

Fig. 5.25 (a, b) Rose bengal stained cells or groups of cells (b, *white arrowhead*) and cell fragments (*grey arrowheads*) seen against green background caused by fluorescein diffusion into the tissues. (c) An area showing heavy rose bengal staining; within the clearer spaces (*arrow*) in the right part of the picture are visible less densely stained structures (*arrowhead*) probably representing individual cells

Case 3: 2 Weeks–4 Months After Recurrence of HZO (cont.)

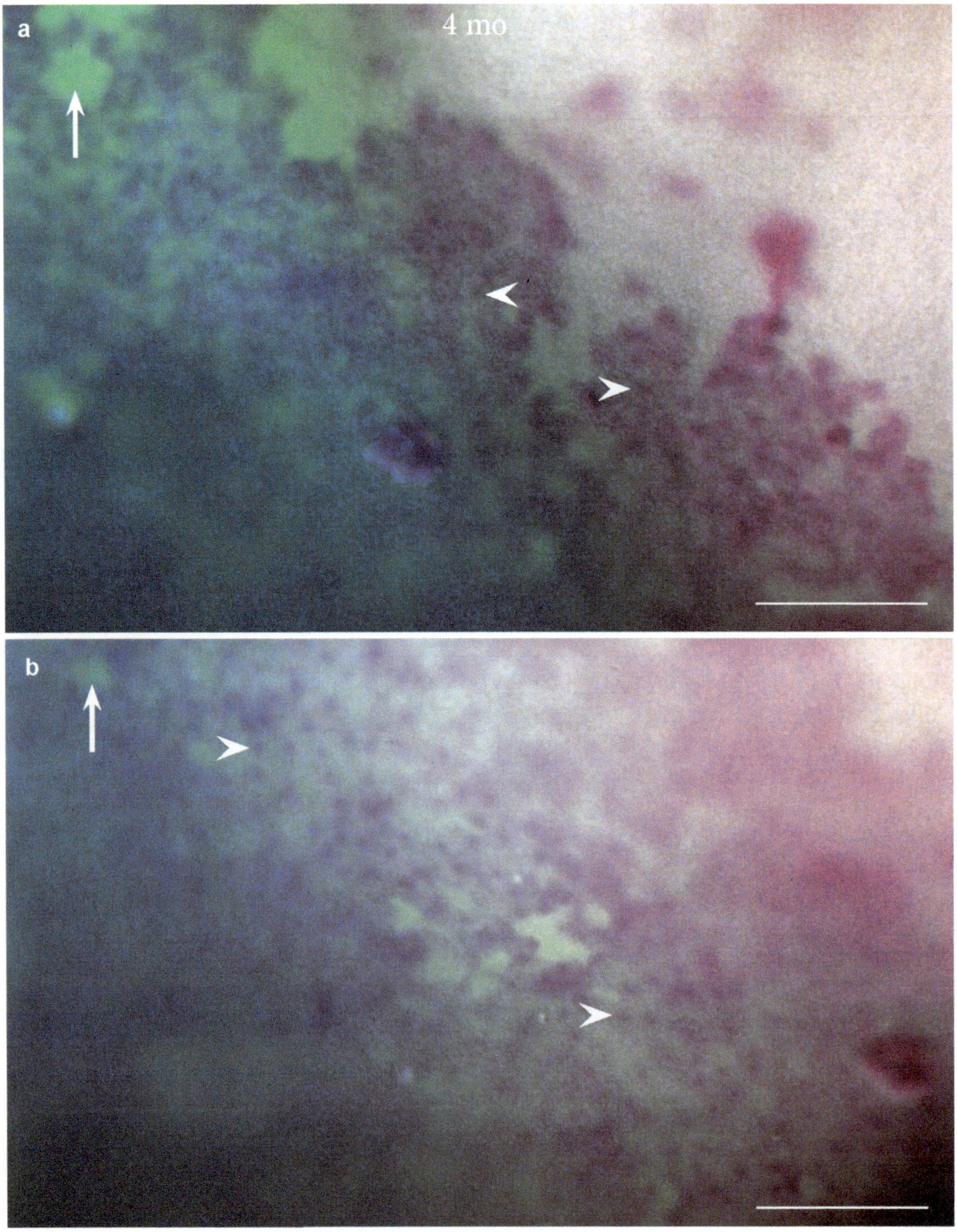

Fig. 5.26 These two areas show features commonly encountered in a severe KCS: confluent rose bengal staining of surface cells in which darkly stained dots (nuclei, *arrowheads*) are clearly discernible and in-between spaces (*arrows*) staining green with fluorescein diffusing into the tissues (cf. Chap. 2)

Case 4: 2 Years After Onset

Case Report

A 44-year-old malnourished man suffered a severe right-sided HZO with long-term sequelae such as corneal epitheliopathy, relapsing anterior uveitis, dilated pupil, and an absence of corneal sensitivity. Two years after onset, the right cornea showed large numbers of greyish surface cells; the left appeared normal (KCS tests: BUT not measurable/2, Schirmer 1 test 5/2; RBS 4/0)

The photographs of the right cornea were taken 2 years after HZO.

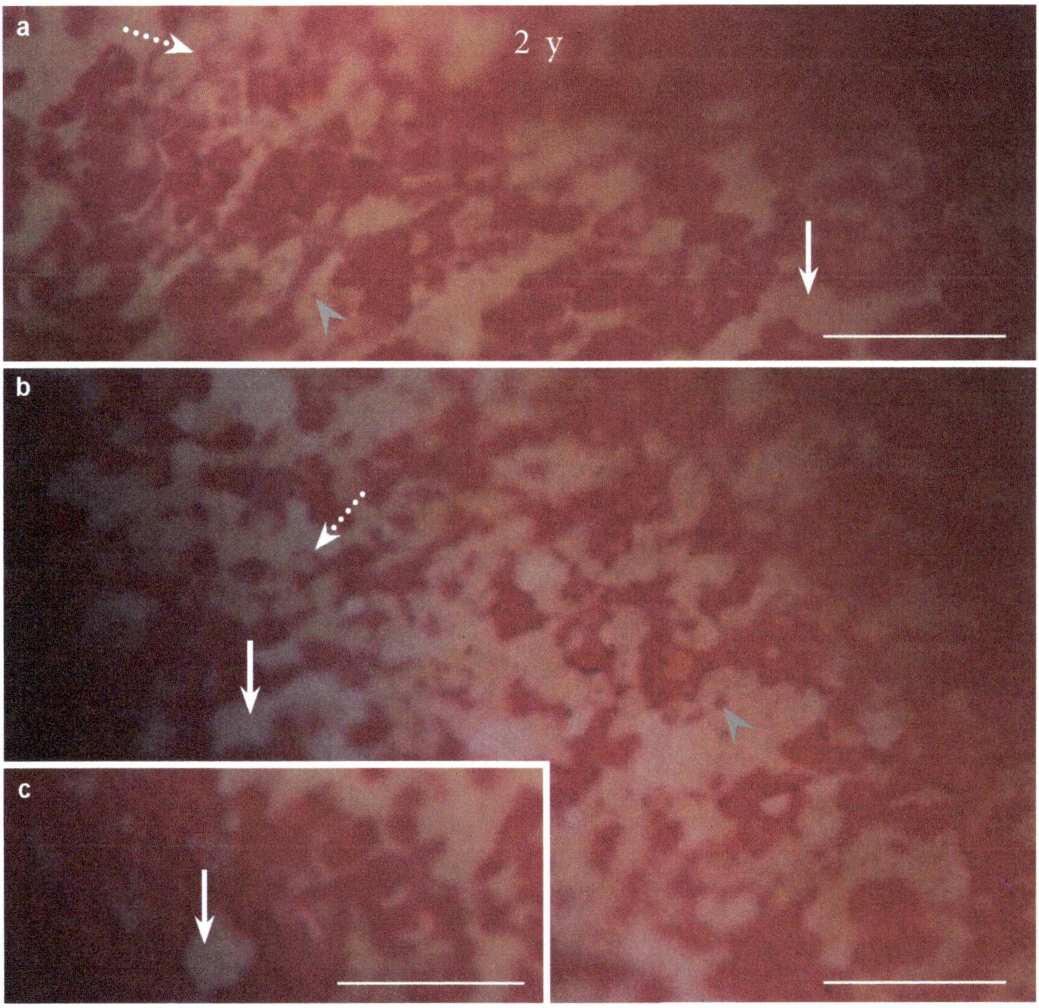

Fig. 5.27 (a–c) Areas of heavy rose bengal staining in which individual surface cells are difficult to distinguish. Visible are cell fragments (*arrowheads*), lines surrounding small spaces (*dotted arrows*), and clear in-between spaces (*plain arrows*). The hue of the staining varies between deeply red and yellowish, cf. Figs. 5.6 and 5.7). (Fluorescein and rose bengal)

Part II

Filamentary Keratopathy

About Filamentary Keratopathy

Filamentary keratopathy (also named filamentary keratitis) is not a disease per se but a clinical entity which owes its name to the presence of corneal appendices termed filaments. With the slit lamp, filaments appear as variously long and thick threads and/or vesicles attached to the corneal surface. Since first described by Leber in 1882, corneal filaments have been reported in a vast number of ocular surface diseases such as: KCS; infections (e.g., adenovirus, herpes simplex and vaccinia); trauma (abrasions, after short-wave diathermy, prolonged padding of an eye); oedematous states (recurrent erosions, contact lens wear); and some other conditions (keratoconus, neurotropic keratopathy, pemphigoid, erythema multiforme, advanced trachoma, keratitis of psoriasis, advanced glaucoma, superior limbic keratoconjunctivitis, chronic blepharospasm, aniridia, ocular albinism, surgery). In already irritated and painful eyes, filaments seem to aggravate the situation. Apparently, they may appear at any time, be located anywhere on the cornea and either disappear (spontaneously or with treatment) or persist for a long time despite treatment efforts.

Filamentary keratopathy is no rarity but it is not very common. In clinical practice, it is most often encountered in KCS, probably because KCS is such a common disease.

6 The Morphology and Dynamics of Filaments

A filament is a variously thick and variously long optically dense and light-reflecting *thread* attached at one or both ends to the surface. It may be naked or enveloped, entirely or in part, by *attached material* that shows two components: an *amorphous* (translucent) and a *granular* (optically dense and light-reflecting) one. In the majority of filaments both are discernible, mixed in various proportions; in some, particularly in the smaller ones, either only the amorphous or only the granular component can be discerned. Some filaments show a very dense light-reflecting nucleus in which no structures are discernible, and occasional ones seem enveloped by material that appears sticky.

The filaments show a rich variety of *shapes*. The simple ones appear as short thin threads with little material attached, small clumps or rounded structures attached by a short thread to the surface, or outstretched slender figures sometimes with a free protruding end. More complex filaments may appear as pearls on a string, show an attached long strand, double expansions, bulbous structures interconnected by variously thick threads or fused together, or quite bizarre configurations. Also the *sizes* vary. Roughly, the outstretched filaments measure between 60 μm and ≤ 3 mm in length and the rounded ones 50–450 μm in diameter.

The filaments *stain* both with fluorescein sodium and rose bengal. With *fluorescein* they appear yellow in retroillumination and green in focal illumination; in some, the green fluorescent hue may be difficult to elicit. With *rose bengal*, they show various shades of red.

The appearance of *surface attachments* varies with the sizes of the filaments. Thus, fine, thin threads are attached to diseased (stainable) surface cells; in larger filaments, the location in depth of the attachments is difficult to estimate but the underlying stroma appears clear. Their immediate surroundings show greyish surface cells staining with non-fluorescent fluorescein and/or rose bengal, some swollen cells and/or cystic spaces, and fine radiating lines. Green (fluorescent) staining with fluorescein, enlarging with time, indicates surface disruptions, either preexisting or caused by traction.

The *dynamics* of filaments imply *mechanisms* behind their varying appearances. Sequential photographs show their movements with blinks: they sweep the surface; flip up and down; some long ones fold and appear bulky before stretching again; others suddenly stretch and double their length; double attached threads stretch like a bow and relax forming a loop; some engage with each other; and some gather additional material while in others some parts disengage and disappear. Their *detachment* from the surface may leave a short protruding thread, a circular area of surface disturbance, or may result in a clean erosion. The individual filaments are probably short-lived.

Additional examples of morphology and dynamics of filamentary keratopathy are presented in connection with various surface conditions (Chap. 7).

H.M. Tabery, *Keratoconjunctivitis Sicca and Filamentary Keratopathy*,
DOI 10.1007/978-3-642-31028-7_6, © Springer-Verlag Berlin Heidelberg 2012

Prerequisites for Filament Formation

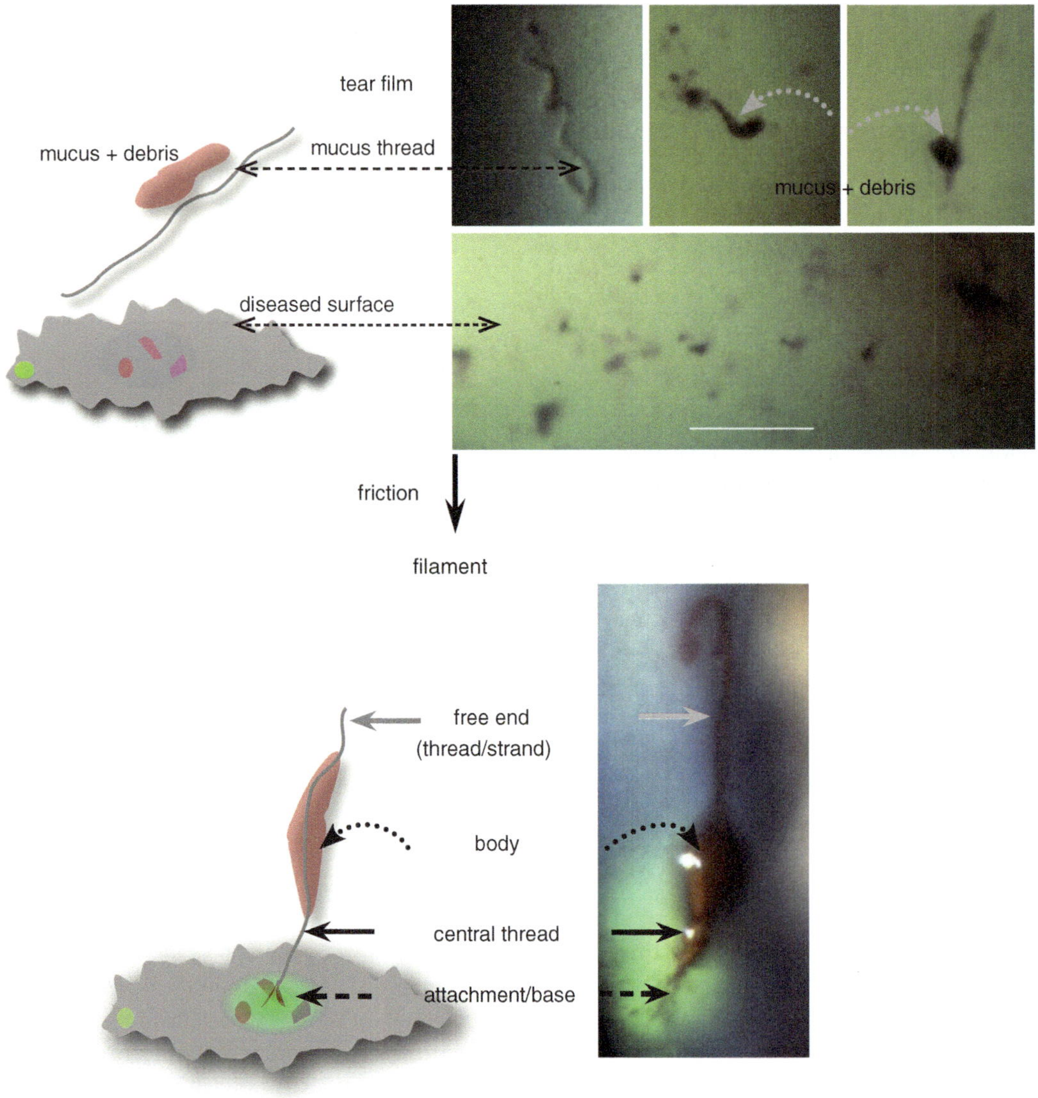

Fig. 6.1 Presumed mechanical *prerequisites for corneal filament formation* are (1) presence in the tear film of *material* (excess of mucus and cell debris) that can adhere to (2) *diseased surface*, and (3) *friction* between two surfaces (i.e., of the cornea and the tarsal conjunctiva). Variously thick and long threads, carrying or not carrying various amounts of material, attach at random at one or several points to the surface. Sweeping it with blinks several times each minute, they may engage with other filaments, coil, twist around themselves, gather additional material, or disrupt, or detach again. The perpetual motion results in a large variety of forms and sizes. The free end may be blunt or show a variously long protruding thread or strand

Prerequisites for Filament Formation (cont.)

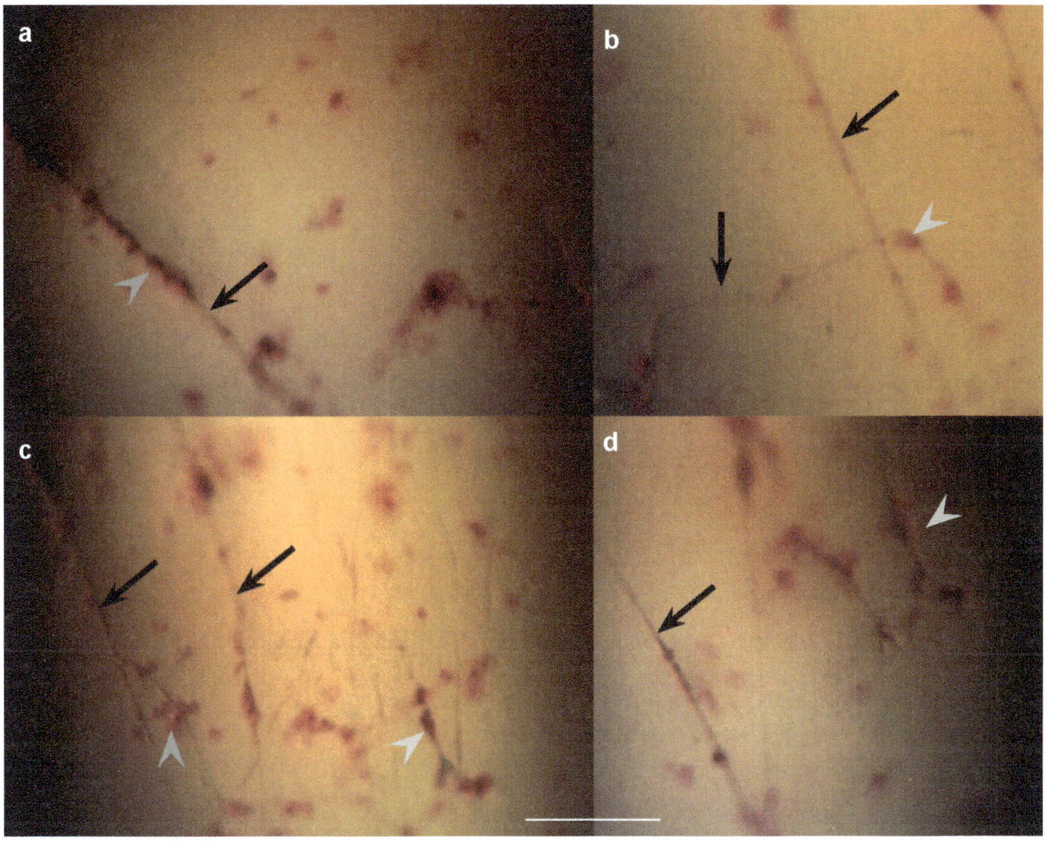

Fig. 6.2 a–d Variously thick and long mucus threads (*arrows*) rolling with blinks over the surface and gathering material (*arrowheads*)

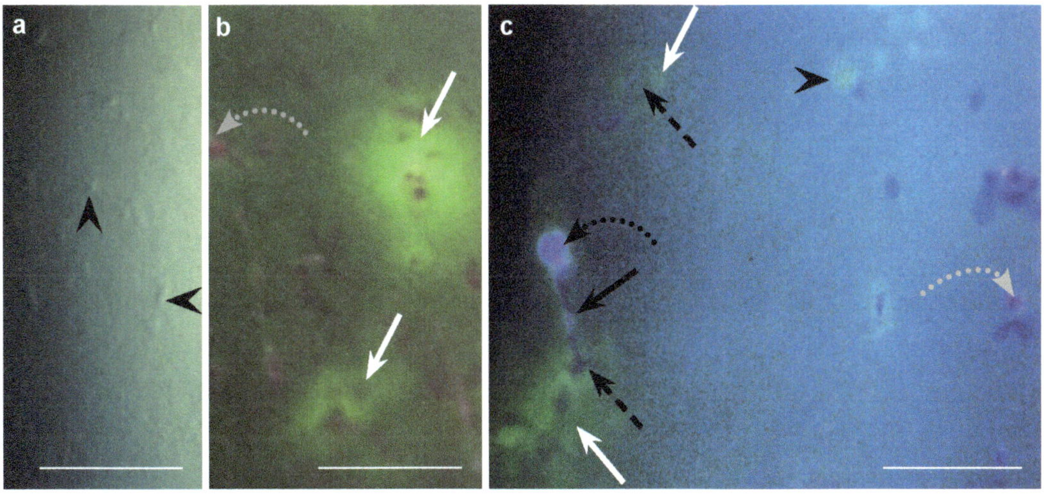

Fig. 6.3 (a, b) Examples of diseased surface: (a) oedematous epithelium showing cystic spaces (*arrowheads*); (b) green flecks indicating surface disruptions (*white arrows*), and rose bengal stained mucus (*bowed arrow*); (c) two small filaments attached (*dashed arrows*) to green stained areas (*white arrows*); the lower filament shows a central thread (*plain black arrow*) and a rounded body (*bowed black arrow*). The *bowed grey arrow* indicates mucus adhering to the surface and the *arrowhead* a cystic space (c Adapted from [3])

Filaments Before Staining

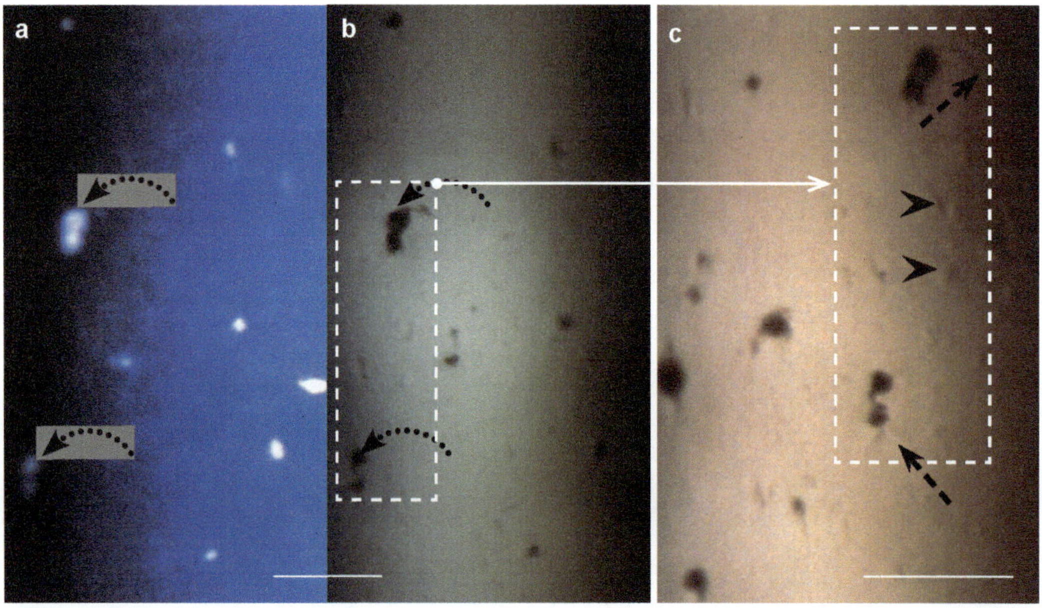

Fig. 6.4 (a, b) Small filaments with rounded bodies (*arrows*) which consist of material that is (a) light-reflecting (white) and (b) light-obstructing (dark). (The arrows are placed in corresponding locations.) The area in *frame* is shown at higher magnification in (c): the *arrows* indicate attachment points and the *arrowheads* cystic spaces

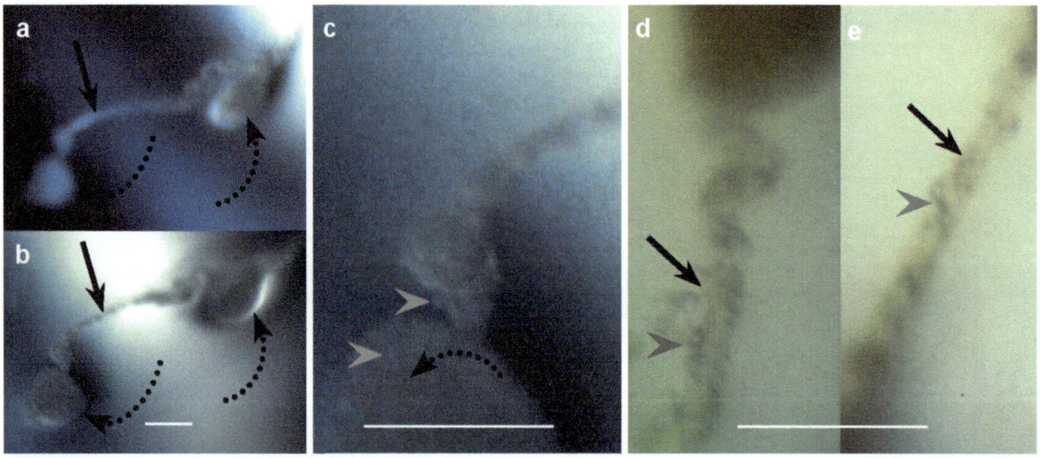

Fig. 6.5 A part of a large and complex filament; the *straight arrow* indicates a thick thread connecting two rounded bodies (*bowed arrows*). (a, b) show the light-reflecting and light-obstructing properties of the filament, and in (c–e) is visible a granular component (*arrowheads*) of the body (*bowed arrow*) and of the connecting thread (*straight arrows*)

Minifilaments; Staining with Fluorescein and Rose Bengal

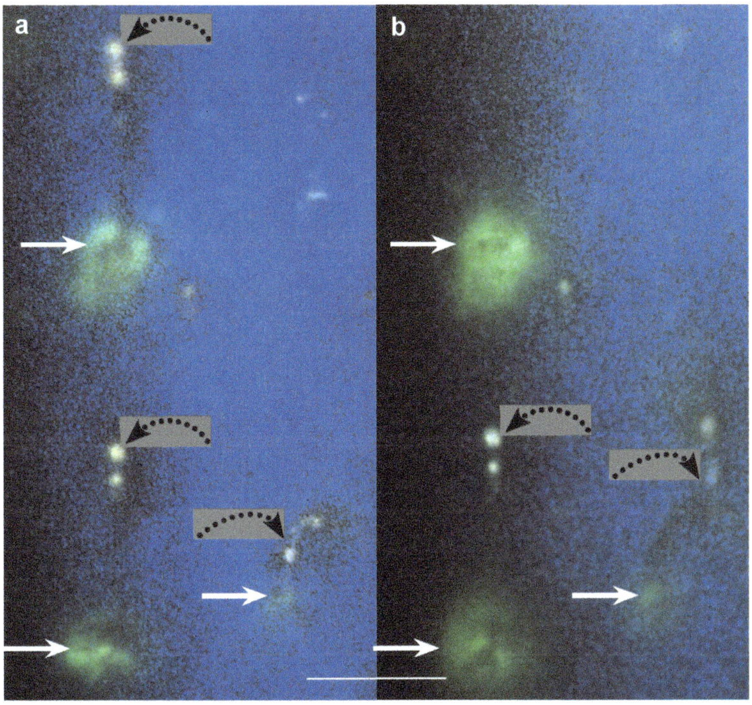

Fig. 6.6 (a, b) Three minifilaments (*bowed arrows*); they are strongly light-reflecting and no fluorescein staining is visible in them (cf. Fig. 6.7). Around their attachment points is visible fluorescein diffusion into the tissues (green flecks, *white arrows*). (b) The upper filament has disappeared between the photographs and the right lower one has stretched. (The white arrows are placed in corresponding locations)

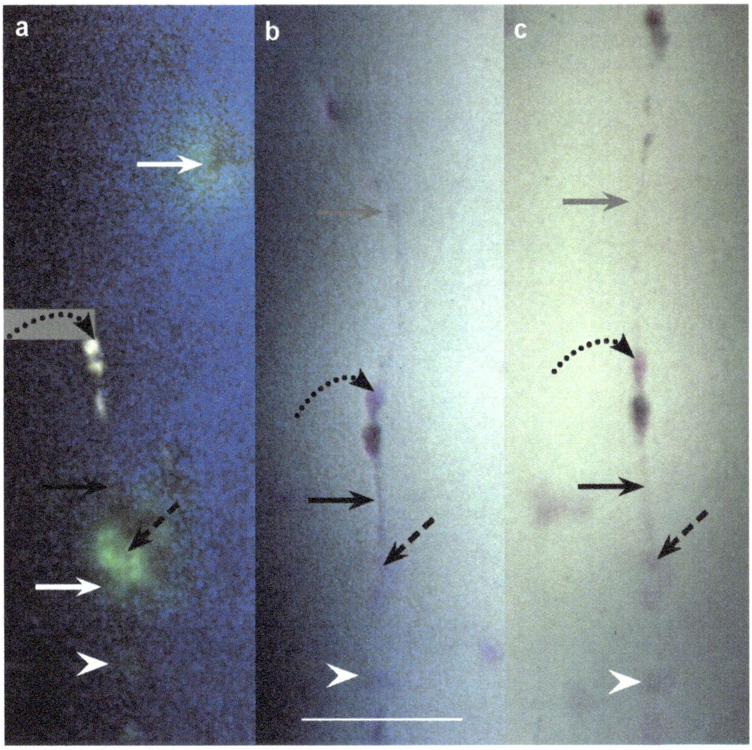

Fig. 6.7 (a) After the application of fluorescein is visible a minifilament (*bowed arrow*) attached (*dashed arrow*) to the lower one of the two green flecks (*white arrows*); the *black plain arrow* indicates its central thread. (b) The filament stains with rose bengal; the *grey arrow* indicates a continuation of the thread not visible in (a); (c) the thread is moving on a surface showing (a) green or (b, c) red stained surface cells (*arrowheads*). (The markers are placed in corresponding locations)

Minifilaments and Diseased Surface Cells

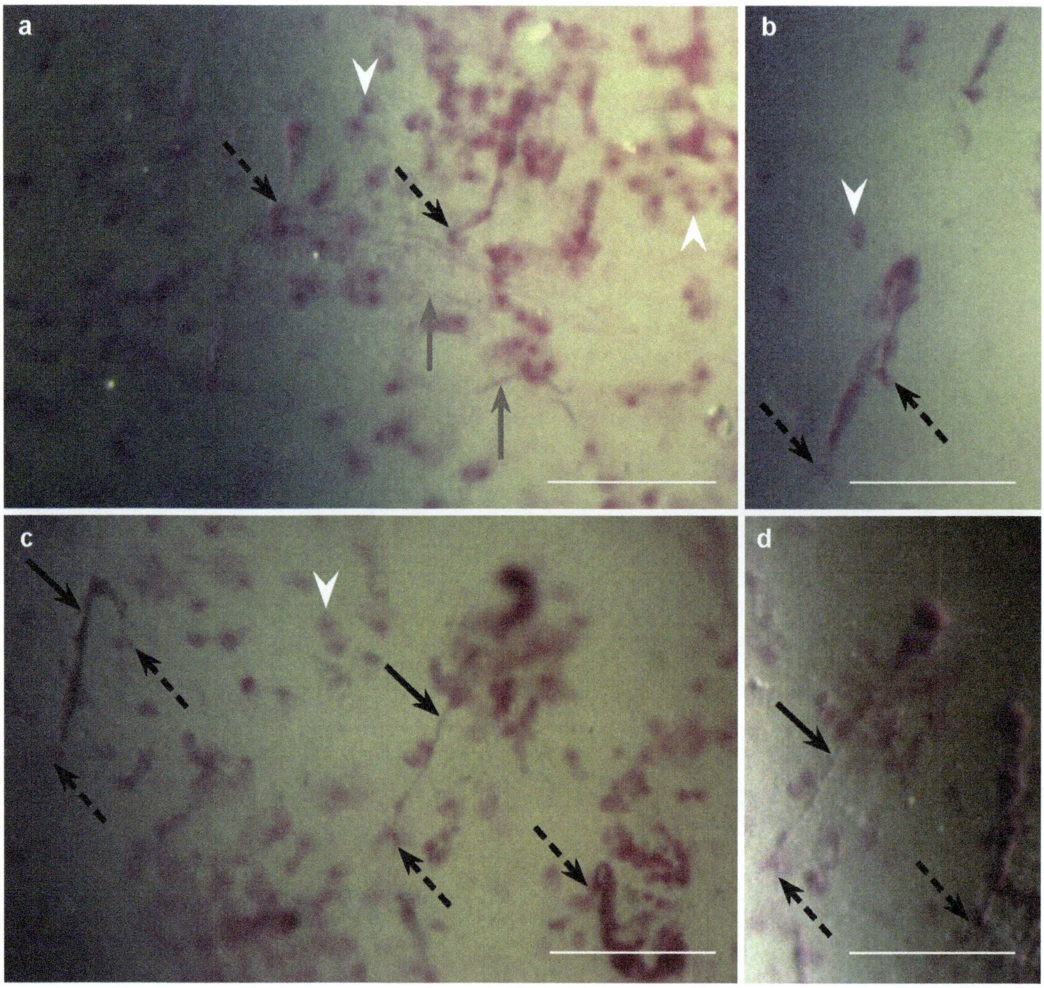

Fig. 6.8 (a–c) Many minifilaments stained red with rose bengal. Of their central threads (*plain black arrows*), some seem unstained. The attachment points (*dashed arrows*) often appear triangular or tent-like. A thread attached at both ends to the surface is visible in (c, left upper corner; cf. also Fig. 6.9). The *arrowheads* indicate rose bengal stained surface cells of which many contain a dark dot (nucleus). In (a) are additionally visible fine mucus threads on the surface (*grey arrows*) (c Adapted from [3])

Fig. 6.10 (a–h) A surface-attached (*dashed arrow*) thread (*plain arrow*) carrying a small amount of granular material. (b, e) show its light-reflecting property, (b, c, e) fluorescein diffusion into the tissues around its attachment (*white arrows*) and (f–h) rose bengal staining. The time sequence shows that it is attached only at one point; with blinks (c–e) the thread stretches possibly to its whole length and then (h) coils again. (The dashed arrows are placed in corresponding locations; c: blue filter)

Minifilaments and Their Dynamics

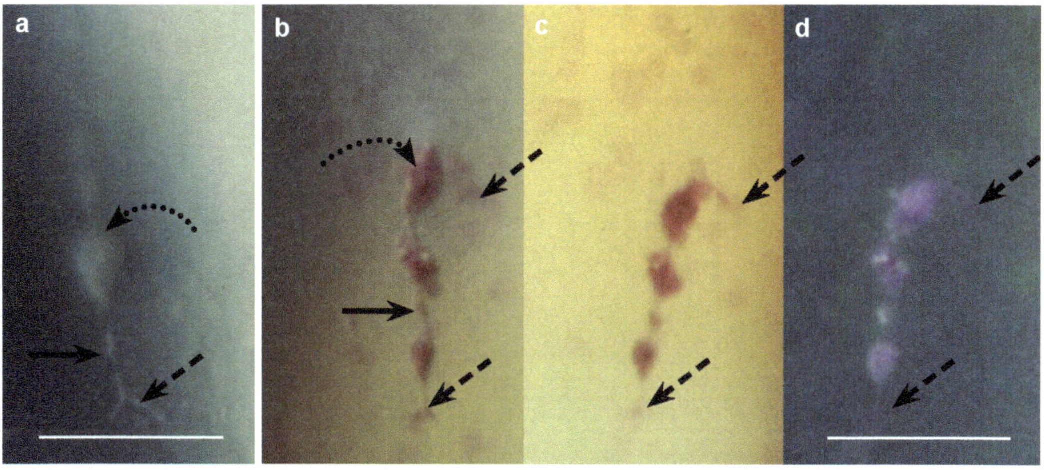

Fig. 6.9 (**a**) A small filament with a triangular attachment (*dashed arrow*), a short central thread (*plain arrow*) and a small body (*bowed arrow*). (**b–d**) Another filament in the same cornea, stained red with rose bengal; the thread (*plain arrow*), carrying small amounts of material (*bowed arrow*) like pearls on a string, is attached at both ends (dashed arrows) to the surface. The movements with blinks are limited. (The dashed arrows are placed in corresponding locations)

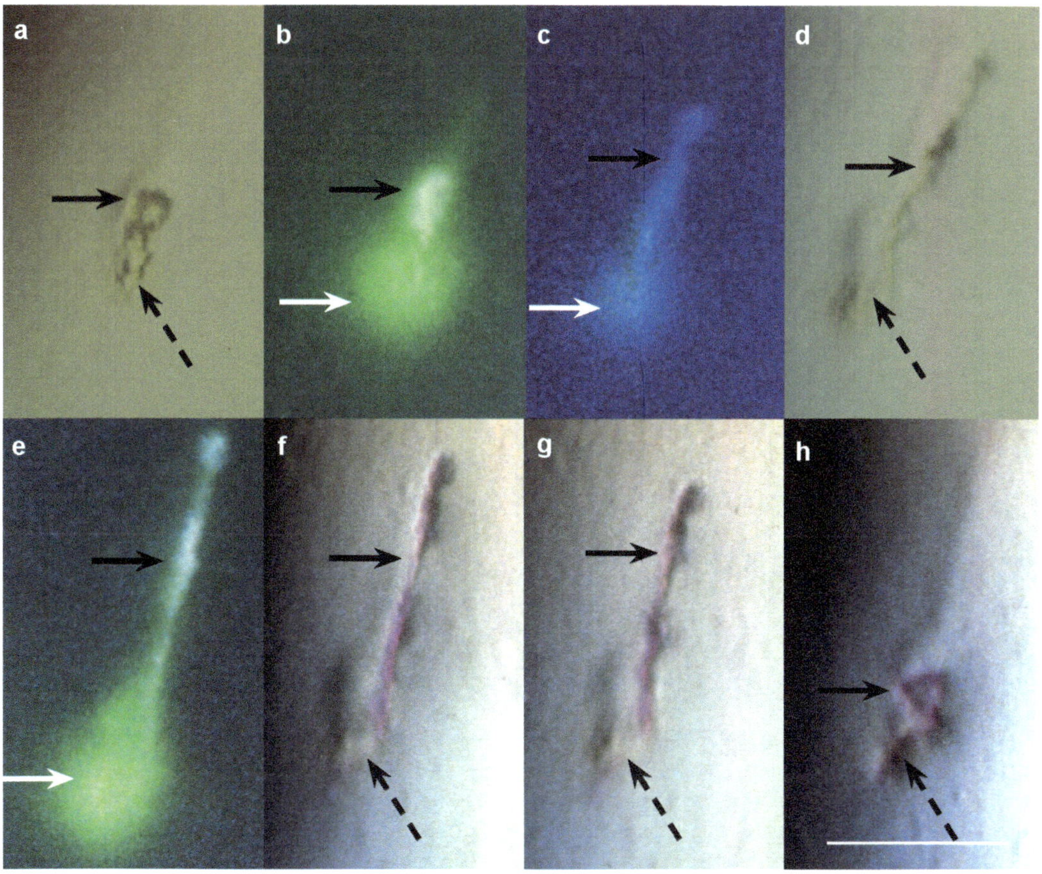

Long Threads and Filaments and Their Dynamics (1)

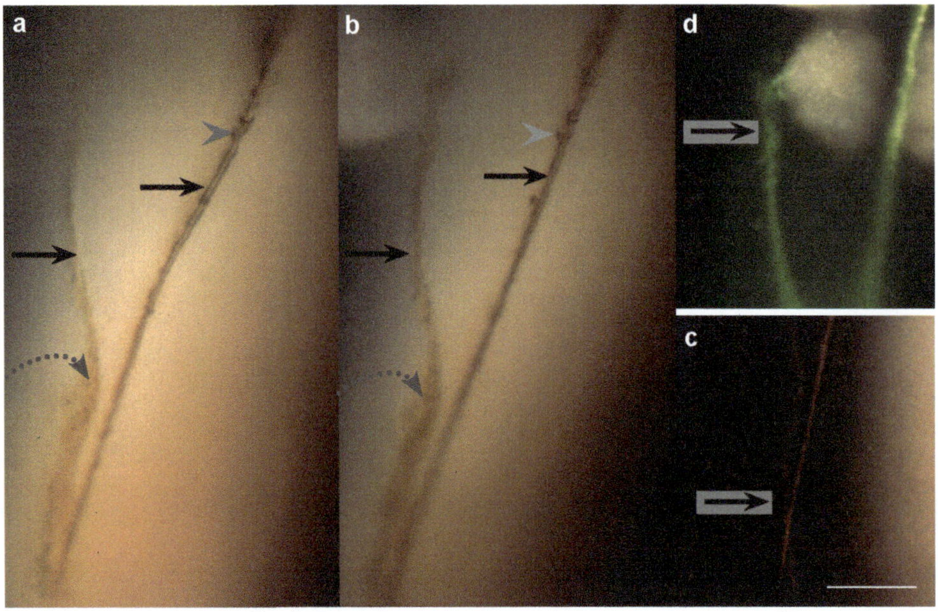

Fig. 6.11 (a–d) Two long threads (*straight arrows*) with a small amount of attached granular material (*arrowheads*); in (a), the lower part of the left one resembles a sheet (*bowed arrow*). (c) shows the lower part of the threads (*arrow*) and (d) their green fluorescein staining (upper part, *arrow*)

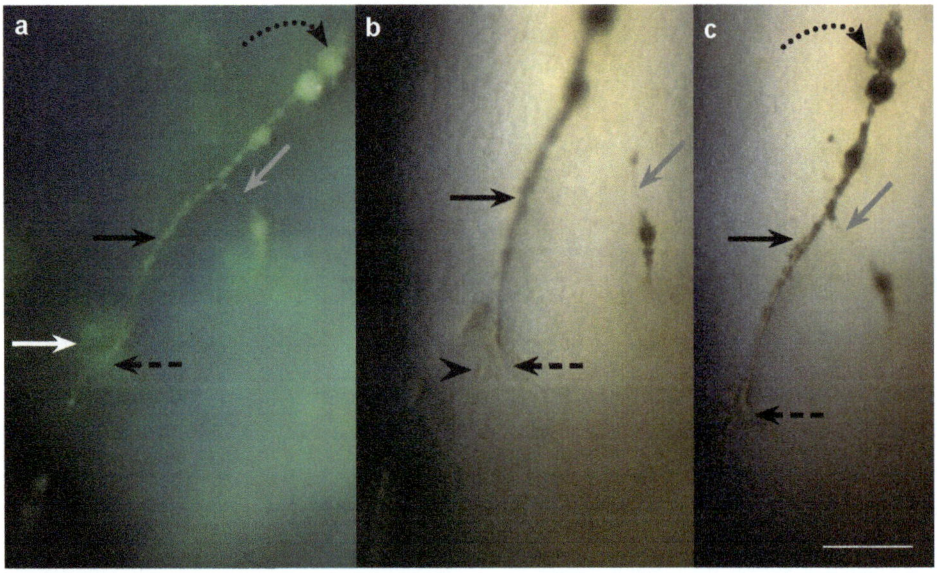

Fig. 6.12 (a–c) A long thread (*plain black arrows*) carrying small amounts of granular material and a small expansion at its free end (*bowed arrows*). Its attachment point (*dashed arrows*) shows (a) fluorescein diffusion into the tissues (*white arrow*) and (b) cystic changes (*arrowhead*). The *grey arrows* point to a free end of a small filament; an additional filament is visible in the left lower corner. The filaments move with blinks. (The dashed arrows are placed in corresponding locations)

Long Threads and Filaments and Their Dynamics (2)

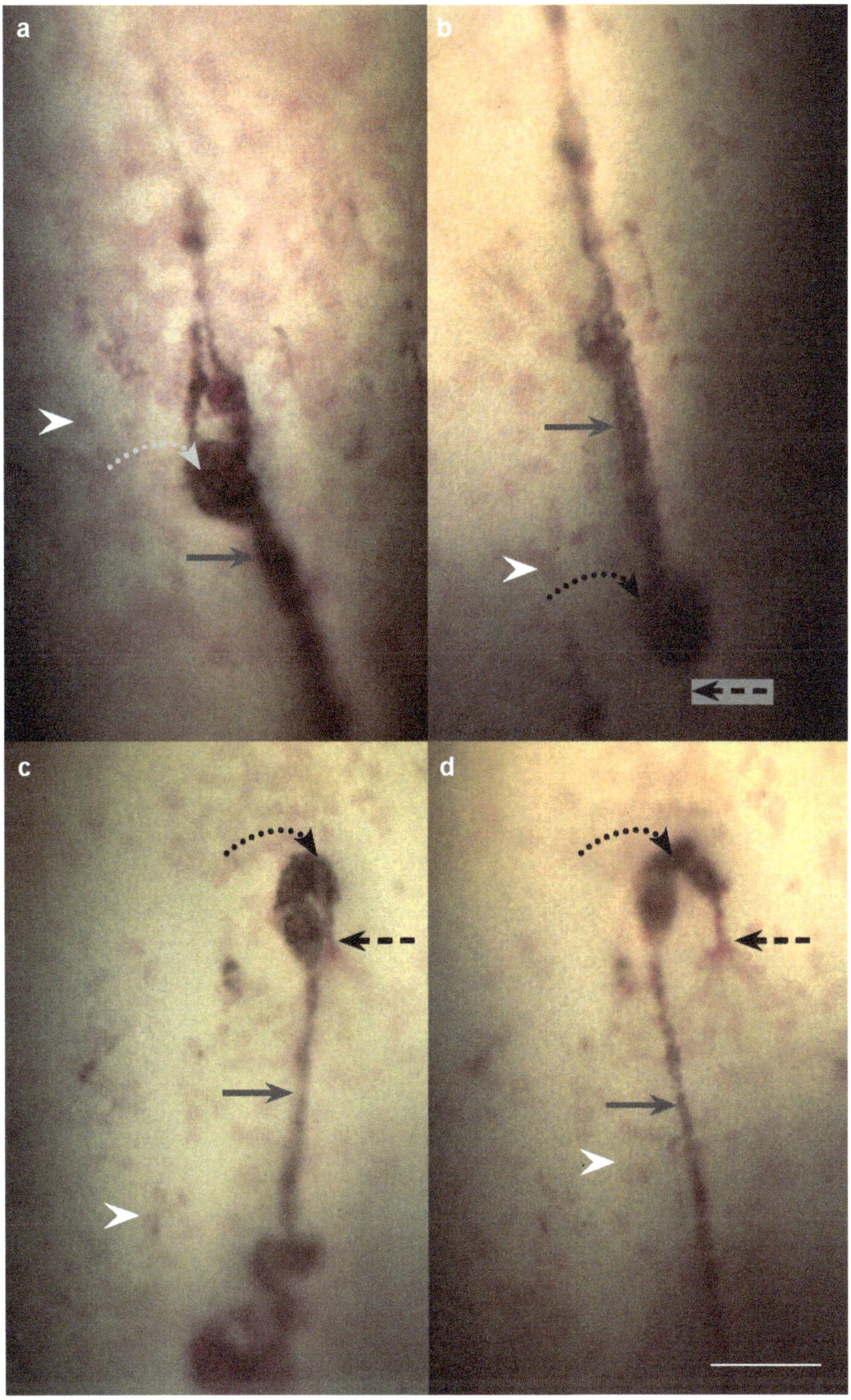

Fig. 6.13 Movements of a long filament with blinks. The *dashed arrows* indicate its attachment point, the *black bowed arrows* its body with a long attached thread (*plain arrows*) showing an expansion (a, *bowed arrow*). In (a, b), the filament is stretched upwards, in (c, d) the long thread points downwards. The surface shows heavy rose bengal cell staining (*arrowheads*). (The arrows in **c** and **d** are placed in corresponding locations)

Larger Rounded Filaments and Their Dynamics (1)

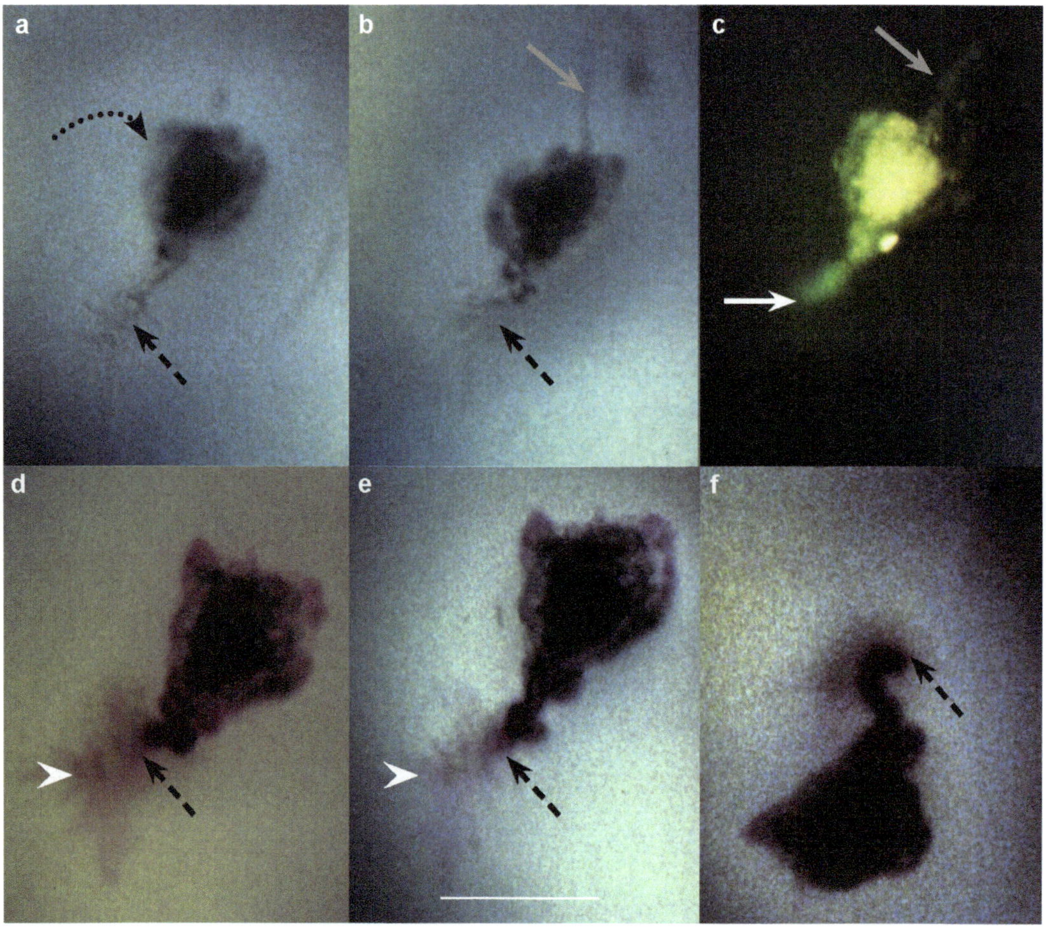

Fig. 6.14 An example of a medium-sized filament with a slightly irregular body (*bowed arrow*) showing (a, b, d, e) a compact and (c) strongly light-reflecting nucleus surrounded by less dense material staining (c) green with fluorescein and (d, e and f) red with rose bengal. The *dashed arrows* indicate the attachment point around which is visible (c) incipient fluorescein diffusion into the tissues (green, *white arrow*) and (d, e) rose bengal staining of surface cells (*arrowheads*). In (b, c) is additionally visible a protruding strand (*grey arrows*). In (f) the filament has flipped over and is pointing downwards. (The dashed arrows are placed in corresponding locations)

Fig. 6.16 A medium-sized filament (*bowed arrows*) moving around its attachment point (*dashed arrows*). In (a) the filament is pointing upwards, in (b) it is lying on the surface with its coiled central thread well visible (*plain arrow*) and in (c) it has flipped over and is pointing downwards. (The dashed arrows are placed in corresponding locations)

Larger Rounded Filaments and Their Dynamics (2)

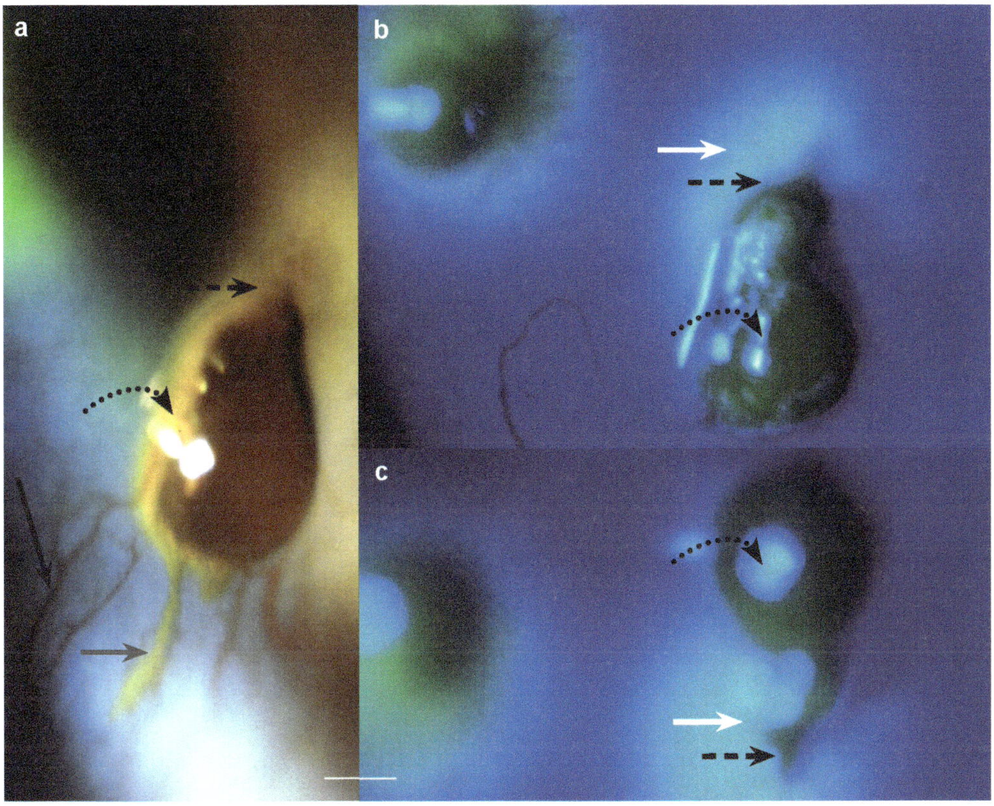

Fig. 6.15 A large, pear-shaped filament (*bowed arrows*) attached to the surface (*dashed arrows*) close to the lower limbus; the *grey arrow* in (a) indicates a protruding strand and the *long arrow* limbal vessels. (b, c) show fluorescein diffusion into the tissues around the attachment (*white arrows*). An additional filament is visible in the left upper corner. In (c), the filament has flipped over and is pointing upwards (b, c: blue filter; (b) Adapted from [4])

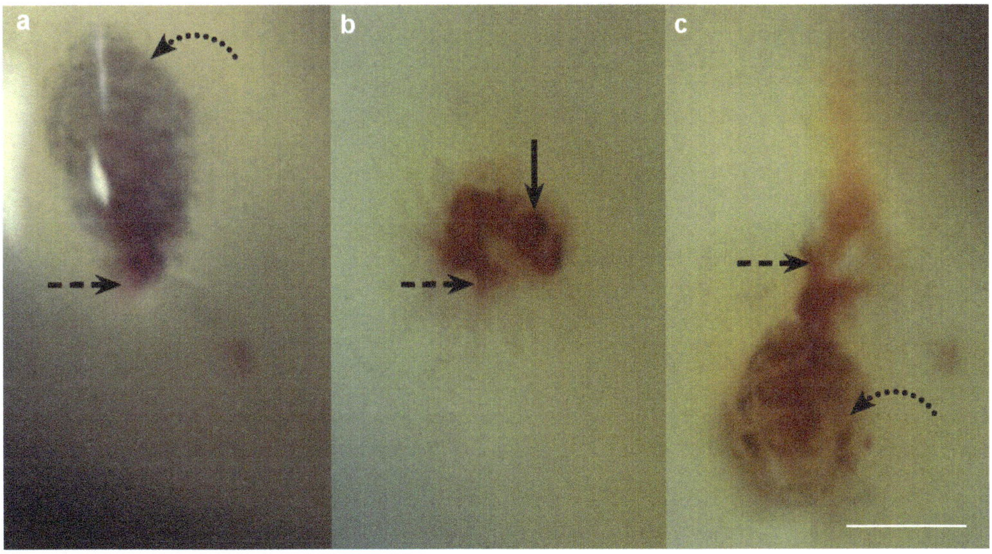

Changing Filament Appearance with Movements

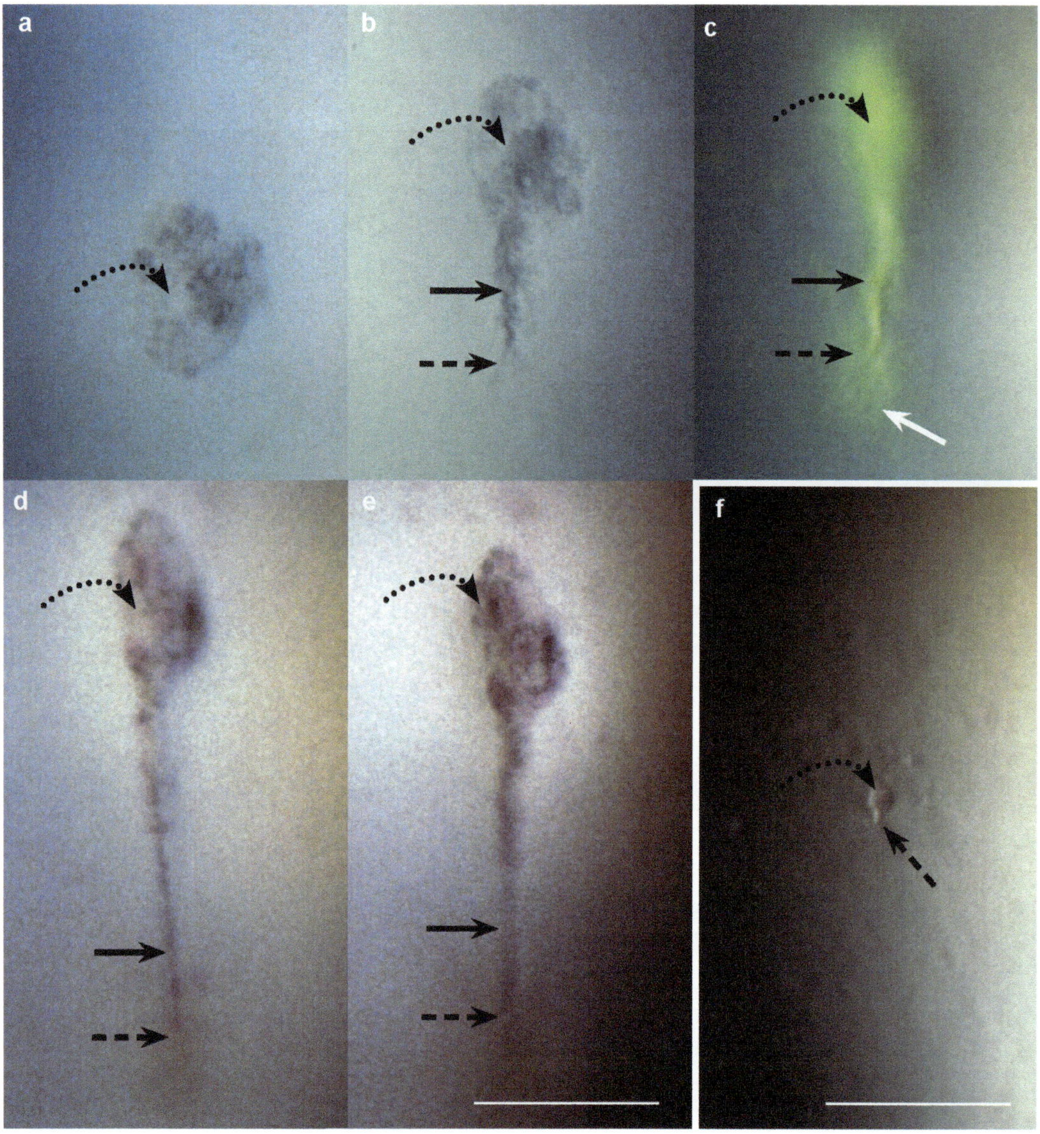

Fig. 6.17 (a) A lump of material (*arrow*) lying on the surface. (b) After a blink, it shows to be a filament (*bowed arrow*); the *dashed arrow* indicates its attachment and the *plain arrow* its central thread; (c) shows fluorescein staining of the filament and incipient fluorescein diffusion into the tissues around its attachment (*white arrow*); and in (d, e) is visible its granular appearance and the red hue of rose bengal. With blinks, the filament stretches and shortens. (The straight arrows are placed in corresponding locations.) (f) shows a very small filament (*bowed arrow*) captured in the same cornea; the *dashed arrow* indicates its attachment point

A Conjunctival Filament

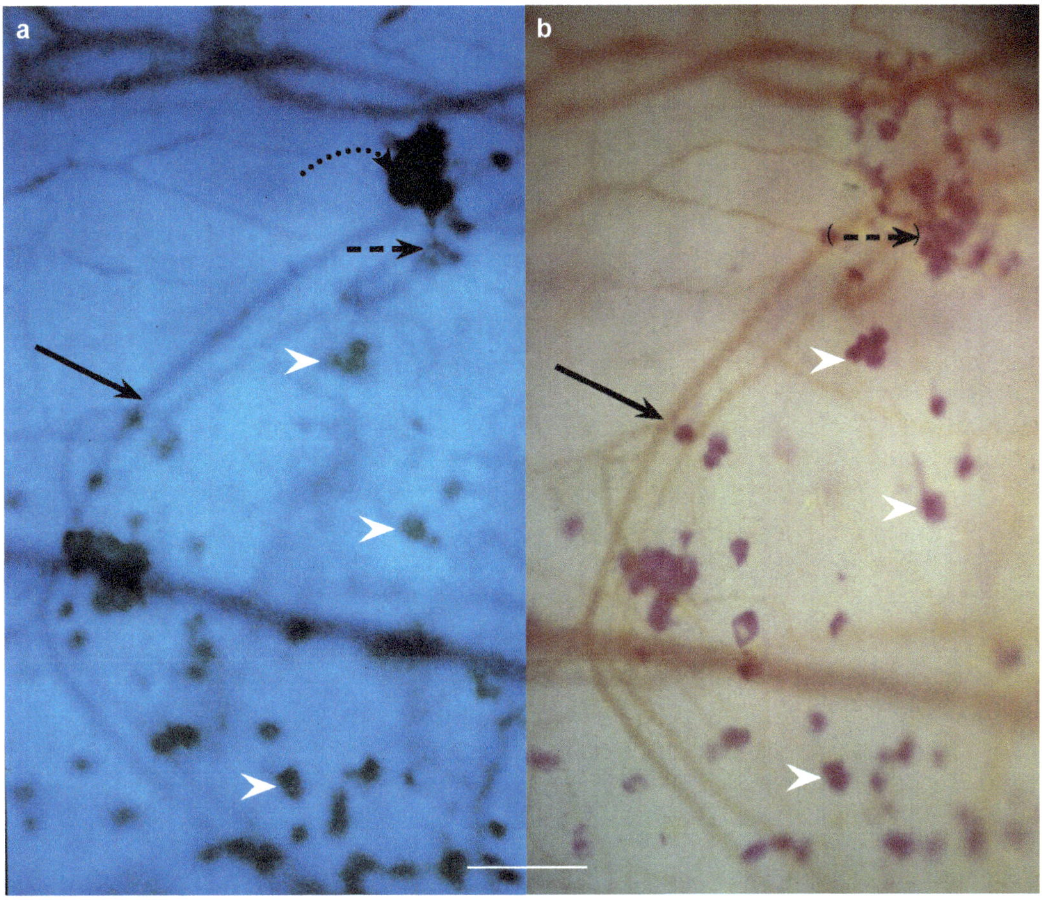

Fig. 6.18 A conjunctival filament. (a) shows the filament (*bowed arrow*) attached to the conjunctival surface (*dashed arrow*); the *arrowheads* indicate diseased surface cells stained with non-fluorescent fluorescein and the *long arrow* a conjunctival vessel (green filter). (b) After the application of rose bengal, the filament has disintegrated. Cells stained in (a) with non-fluorescent fluorescein stain (b) with rose bengal but the pattern is not exactly the same, partly because some diseased surface elements became displaced or disappeared between the photographs and partly because the conjunctiva itself is movable. (The markers are placed in corresponding locations)

Comment

Conjunctival filaments are extremely rare.

Surface Attachments of Larger Filaments

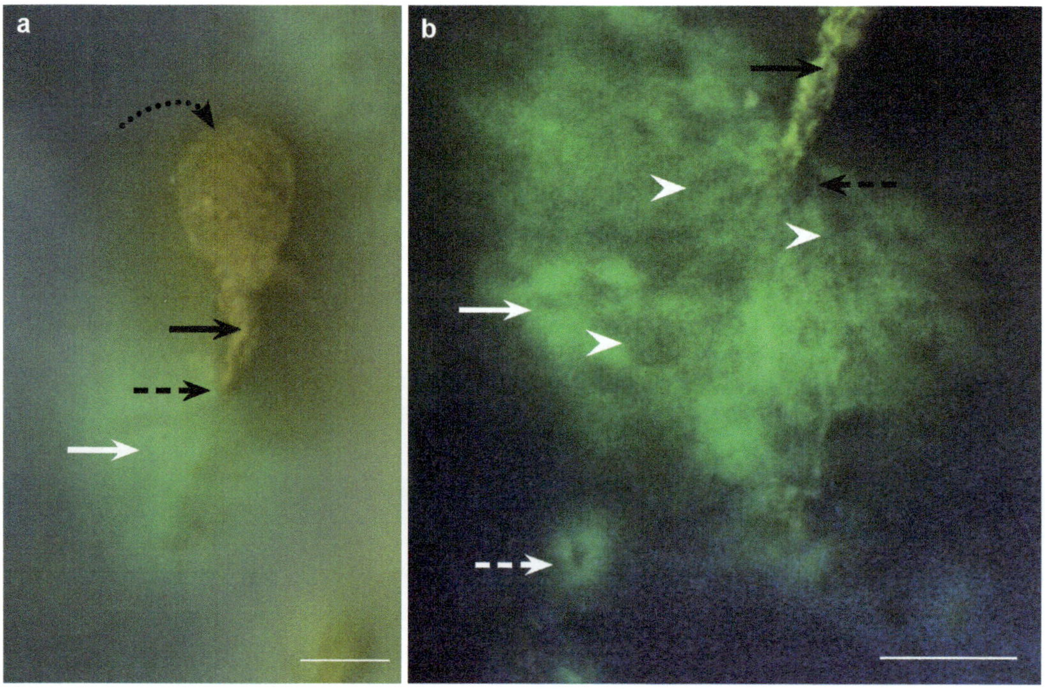

Fig. 6.19 Fluorescein diffusion into the tissues (green, *white arrows*) around attachment points (*dashed arrows*) of (a) a smaller (*bowed arrow*) and (b) a larger filament; the *plain black arrows* indicate central threads. In (b), the *arrowheads* point to surface cells stained with non-fluorescent fluorescein, and the *dashed white arrow* to a separate green fleck close to the filament base

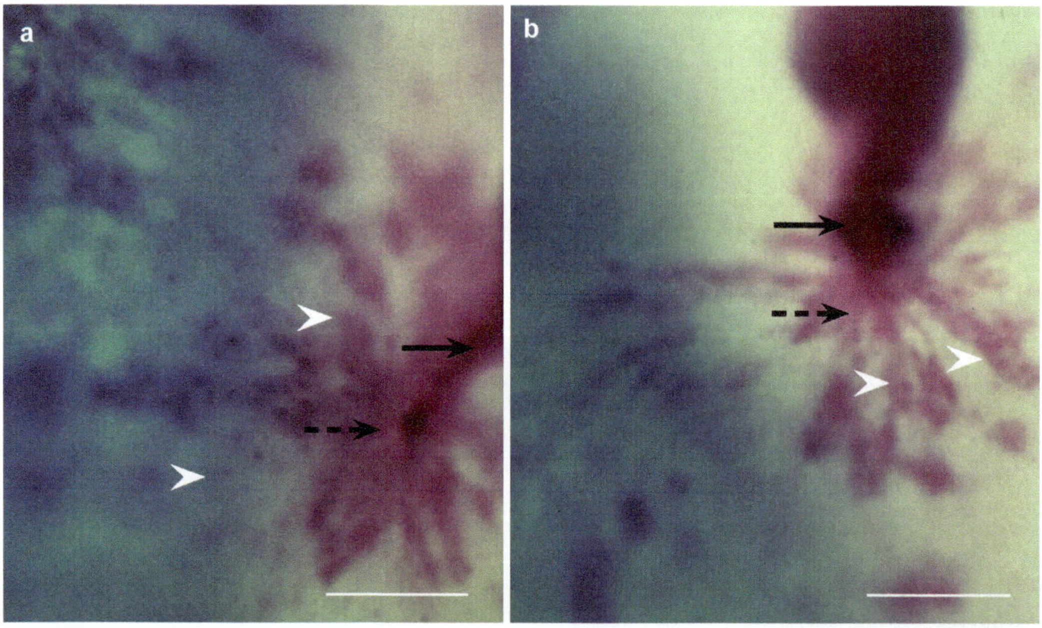

Fig. 6.20 (a, b) Rose bengal stained surface cells (*arrowheads*) seem to stream towards the attachment points (*dashed arrows*); the *plain arrows* indicate the filaments' central threads

Surface Detachments of Larger Filaments

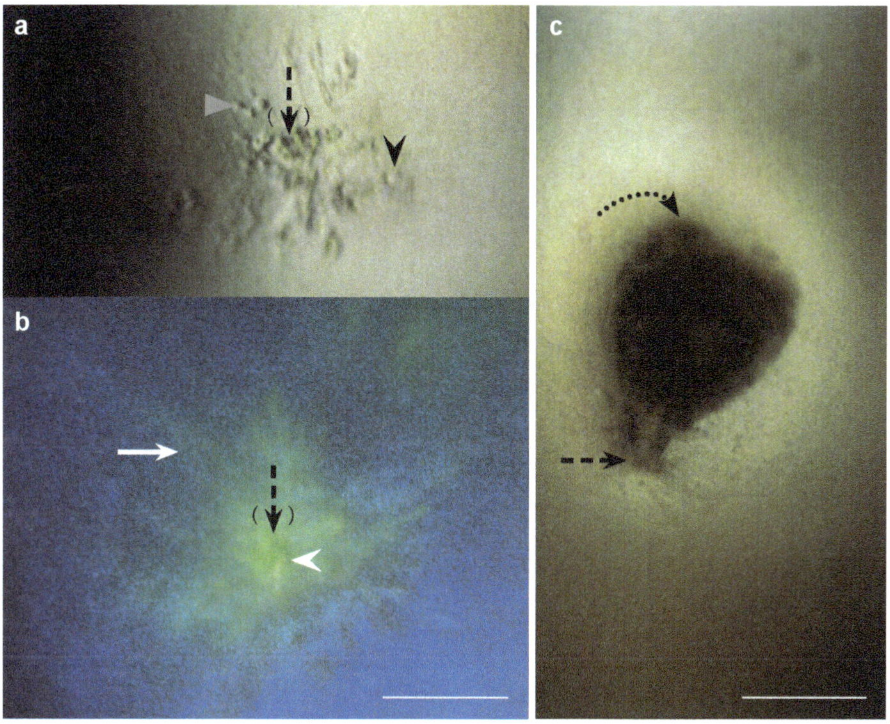

Fig. 6.21 (a, b) After a filament detachment (*dashed arrows*) the surface shows (a) rounded bodies (*grey arrowhead*) and cystic spaces (*black arrowhead*), and (b) non-fluorescent (*arrowhead*) and fluorescent (*white arrow*) fluorescein staining showing a streaming pattern towards the centre (cf. Fig. 6.20). (c) A rounded filament (*bowed arrow*) present close to the area shown in (a, b); the dashed arrow indicates its attachment point

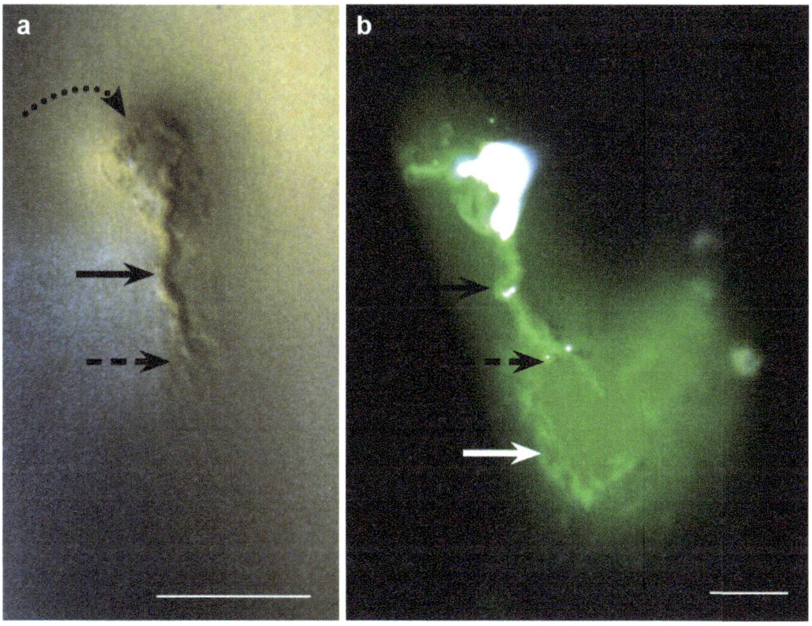

Fig. 6.22 (**a**) A filament (*bowed arrow*) with a partly coiled central thread (*plain arrow*); the *dashed arrow* indicates its attachment point. In (b) is visible a surface erosion (*white arrow*) at the base of a similar filament in the same cornea, occurring spontaneously during the examination. The *plain black arrow* indicates its central thread and the *dashed arrow* its attachment (cf. also Fig. 7.46)

7 Case Reports

This chapter demonstrates filaments occurring in some of the various conditions reported in the literature. Three of the patients (Cases 1, 2 and 4) had KCS (in primary Sjögren's syndrome). Case 1 shows variously large filaments, and their dynamics, observed during a 3-month period. At the same time, it demonstrates a rare diagnostic pitfall; a long period of time that may elapse between symptom onset and diagnosis of underlying disease; a disappearance of symptoms but not of findings; and no deterioration of the surface condition during 14 years in a patient declining treatment.

Case 2 demonstrates filaments coming and going during 5 years in conjunction with pronounced KCS surface changes including mucus adherence to the surface; in this patient, treated mainly with lubricating eye drops, the surface condition remained unchanged during the observation period of 5 years. Case 4 shows the dynamics of a very large filament against a background of KCS surface changes.

In Cases 3 and 5 are shown two rarely captured phenomena, in Case 3 filaments surrounded by a distinct clear layer of which the interpretation remains open and in Case 5 a long strand leaving surface imprints visualising a sticky property of a mucus component.

In Cases 6–12, filaments developed in conditions per se not rare but only rarely accompanied by filamentary keratopathy, and Case 13 shows a very long filament just avulsed from the epithelium.

And what is a pseudofilament? A firmly attached bit of a nylon thread, protruding and sweeping the surface and, similarly to mucus threads, gathering material.

H.M. Tabery, *Keratoconjunctivitis Sicca and Filamentary Keratopathy*,
DOI 10.1007/978-3-642-31028-7_7, © Springer-Verlag Berlin Heidelberg 2012

Case 1: A Diagnostic Mystery Resolved

Case Report

A 42-year-old man working with material containing glass fibres presented with foreign body sensation in the right eye. The eye was injected, and the corneal epithelium showed punctate fluorescein staining and a few fibre-like formations. The left eye was white. The (presumed) fibres were removed, and he was treated with antibiotic ointment for a couple of days. The symptoms persisted and an addition of cortisone eye drops had no effect. One month after onset both eyes were irritated and injected, and surface staining was suggestive of KCS; the right cornea showed several larger and smaller filaments and the left cornea a few small ones. The patient had no other symptoms except for recurrent facial erythema possibly due to acne rosacea. He was treated with lubricating eye drops and for a couple of months also with tetracycline p.o. The effect of treatment was uncertain. The symptoms slowly regressed but the findings were basically the same; at follow-up visits, both corneae showed small filaments. About a year after onset, the findings were consistent with KCS except for the Schirmer 1 test (25/21, and 20/20 six months later), but after a further year (2 years after symptom onset) the findings fulfilled the diagnostic criteria (BUT 5/5, Schirmer 1 test 1/3, RBS 7/7); the patient was referred for investigation and diagnosed with primary Sjögren's syndrome. During the following year, he did not use any eye drops because symptom-free, and the findings remained more or less unchanged with only small filaments coming and going. The patient was last seen 14 years after onset.

The photographs of the right cornea were taken 4 weeks, 5 weeks, 3 months and 14 years after symptom onset.

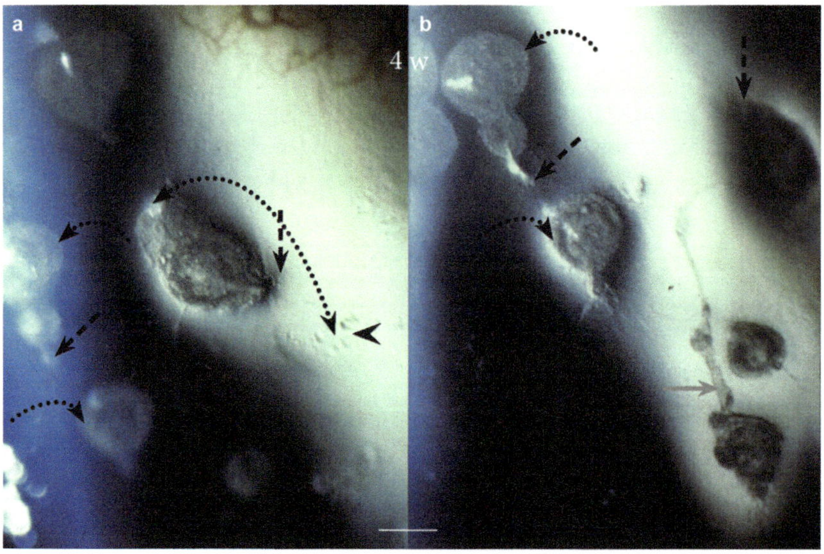

Fig. 7.1 (**a**, **b**) Several rounded filaments close to the upper limbus. The *dashed arrows* indicating attachment points and the *bowed arrows* indicating filament bodies are placed in corresponding locations. In (**a**) the filament in the centre seems to consist of two bodies of which the left one has detached from the surface (*double arrow*); the *arrowhead* points to a few cystic spaces where it might have been attached (cf. Fig. 6.21). In (**b**) the same filament (right upper corner) has flipped over and is pointing downwards; the *grey arrow* indicates a long mucus strand attached to the body of a filament located in the right lower corner (Adapted from [4])

Case 1: A Diagnostic Mystery Resolved (cont.)

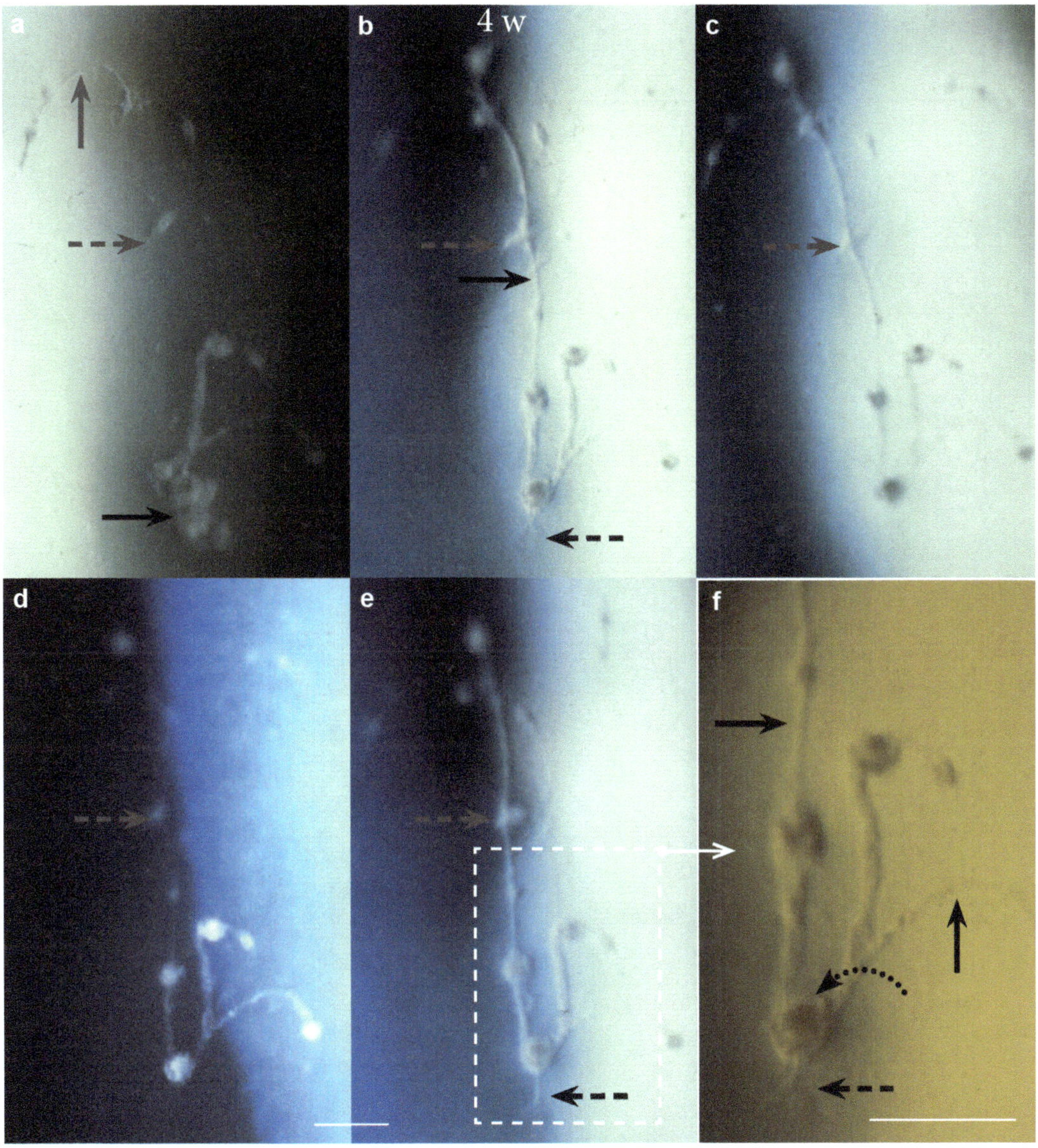

Fig. 7.2 (a–e) Sequential photographs of a complex filament: in (a) is visible a thread (*black plain arrow*), lying coiled on the surface, and two adjoining threads showing bulbous enlargements; a double-attached filament (*grey plain arrow*); and a small filament (*grey dashed arrow*, for orientation placed in the same location in all photographs). (b) With blinks, the thread (*black plain arrow*) stretches and the attachment point (*dashed arrow*) becomes visible; the adjoining structures remain more or less in place (throughout). (c–e) The thread remains stretched. (d) shows the light-reflecting property of the threads and their bulbous enlargements (or 'bodies'). The lower part of the filament indicated by *frame* in (e) is shown at higher magnification in (f): the *dashed arrow* indicates its attachment point, the *plain arrows* mucus threads and the *bowed arrow* one of its bulbous enlargements (f Adapted from [4])

Case 1: A Diagnostic Mystery Resolved (cont.)

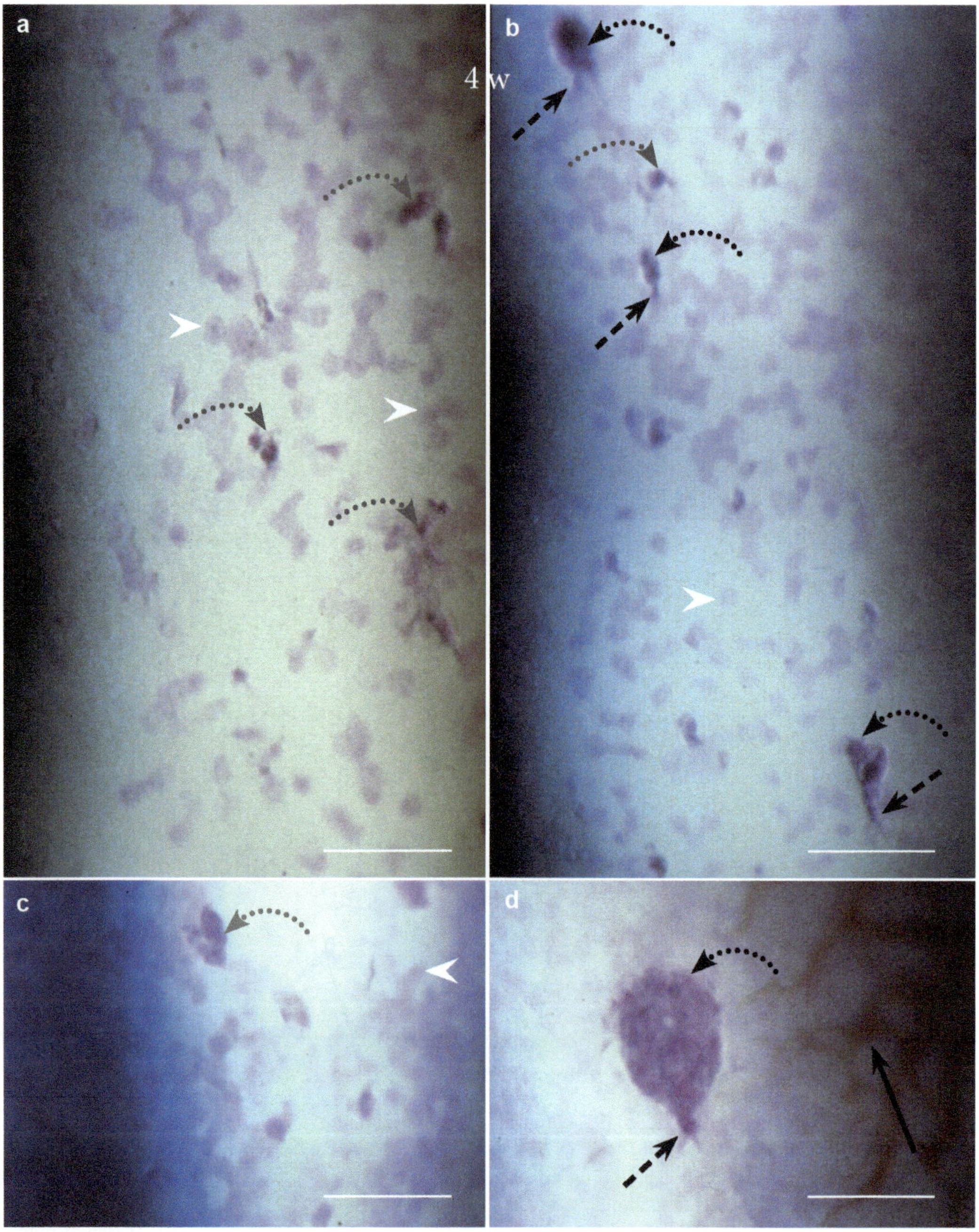

Fig. 7.3 (a–c) With rose bengal, these areas show many red stained surface cells (*white arrowheads*), attached surface debris and/or mucus (*bowed grey arrows*) and small filaments (*bowed black arrows*); the *dashed arrows* indicate attachment points. (d) The body of this filament (*bowed arrow*) appears granular; the *dashed arrow* indicates its attachment point and the *plain arrow* points to limbal vessels. No densely stained dots within the stained cells (nuclei) were captured at this occasion. Cf. Fig. 7.4

Case 1: A Diagnostic Mystery Resolved (cont.)

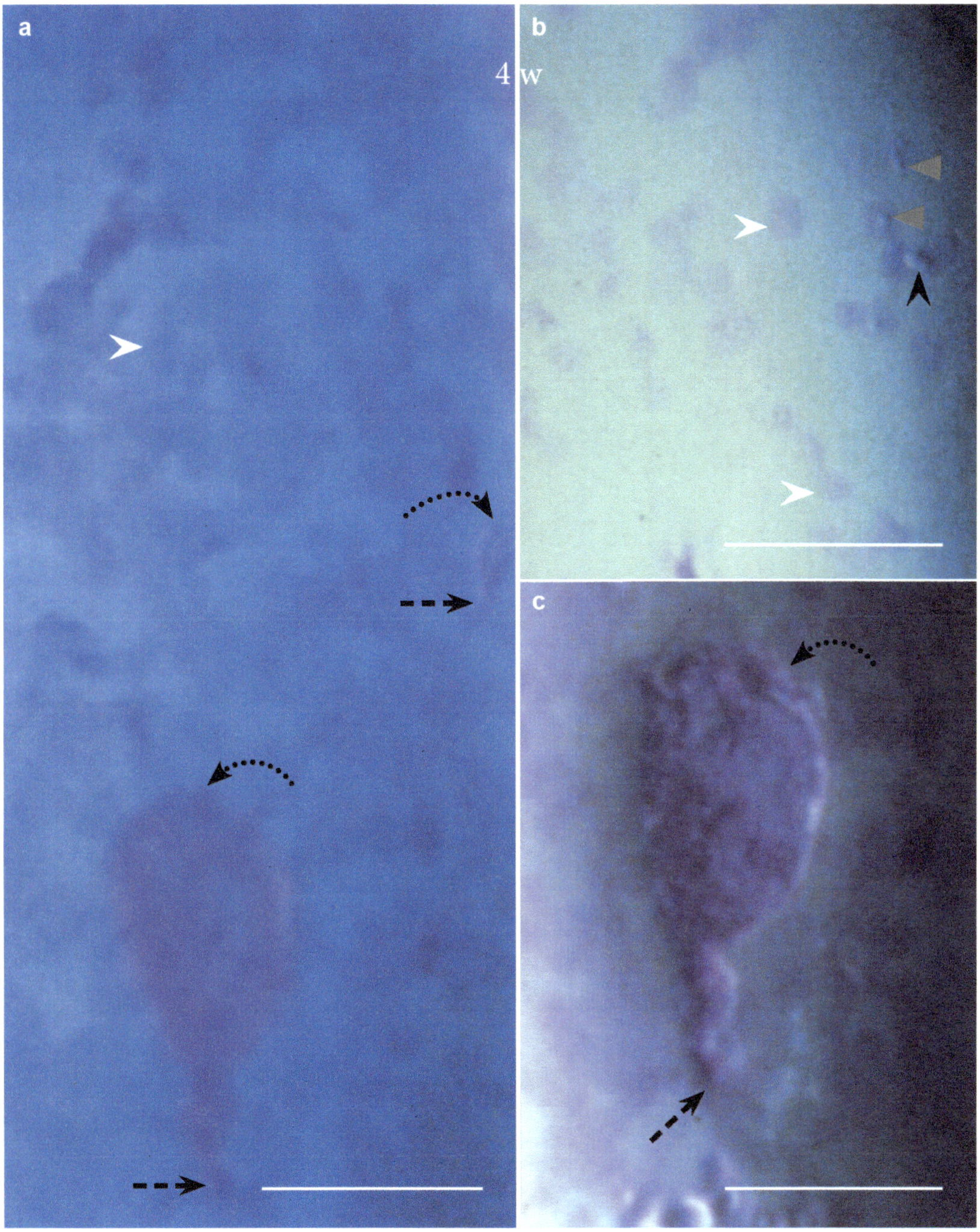

Fig. 7.4 (a) One larger and one small filament (*bowed arrows*) with attachment points indicated by *straight arrows*; the background shows many rose bengal stained surface cells (*white arrowhead*). (b) Rose bengal stained surface cells (*white arrowheads*), a larger cystic space (*black arrowhead*) and small cystic spaces or rounded bodies (*grey arrowheads*). (c) shows a filament (body indicated by *bowed arrow,* attachment by *straight arrow*) seen against a background showing many rose bengal stained surface cells; the surface of the filament appears granular

Case 1: A Diagnostic Mystery Resolved (cont.)

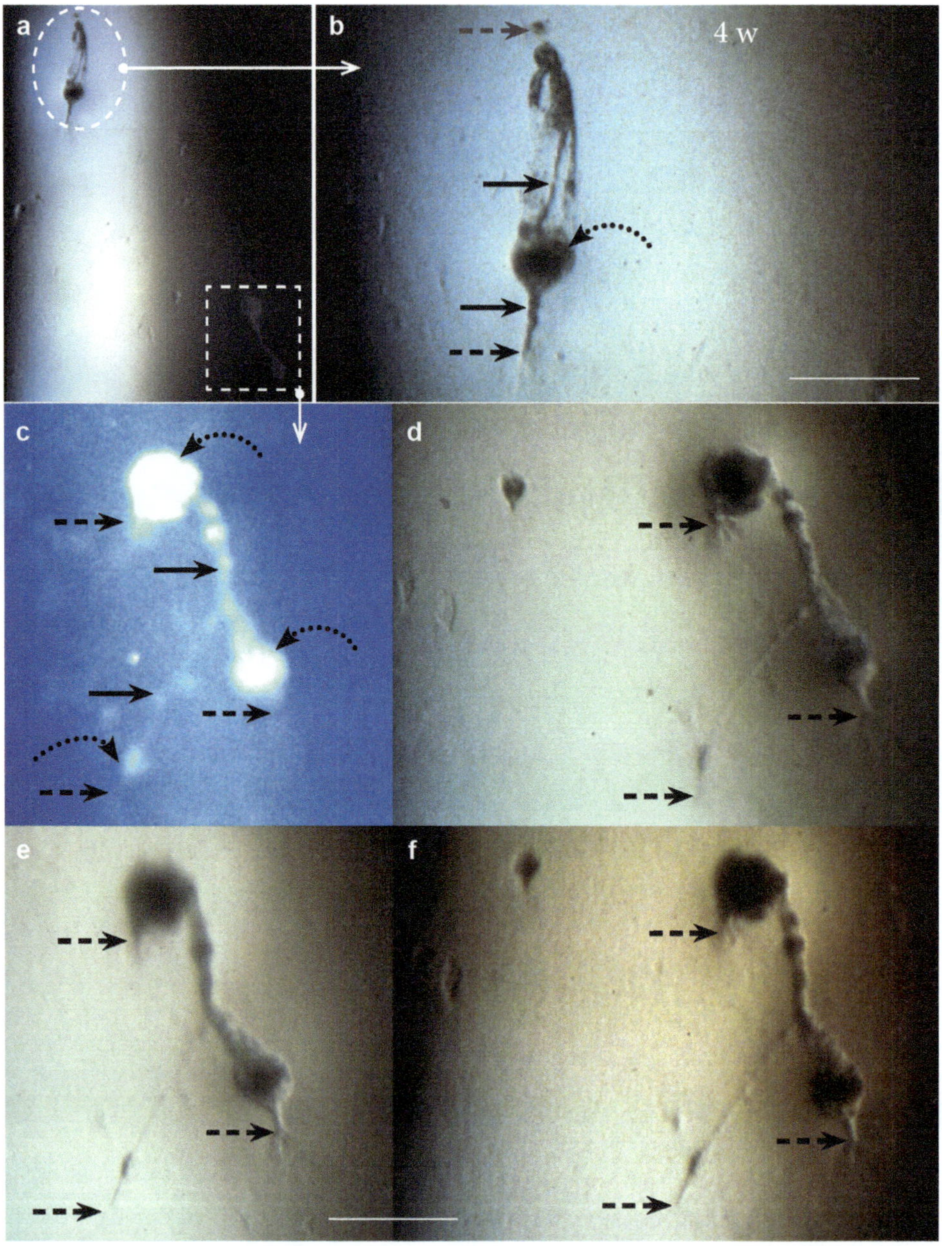

Fig. 7.5 (a) Survey. (b) The filament indicated by *oval frame* in (a) shows an attachment point (*dashed arrow*), a central thread (*plain arrows*) and a bulbous expansion (*bowed arrow*); the filament's upper end may just have detached from the surface (*grey arrow*). (c–f) The filament in *rectangular frame* in (a): (c) It has 3 attachment points (*dashed arrows*), 3 bulbous expansions ('bodies', *bowed arrows*) and 2 interconnecting threads (*plain arrows*); it is strongly light reflecting. (d–i) show in time sequence its slight movements with blinks in relation to the attachment points (*arrows*). (g–i) As in Fig. 7.5c–f, this 'tripple' filament shows only slight movements in relation to the attachment points (*arrows*). (j) After staining with rose bengal, the lower thread has ruptured and is lying coiled (*grey arrow*) on the surface. (k) Rose bengal stained surface cells (*arrowhead*) close to the upper bulbous expansion (*arrow*). (l) shows the lower bulbous expansion (*black arrow*), the coiled mucus thread on the surface (*grey arrow*) and rose bengal stained surface cells (*arrowhead*) (b Adapted from [4])

Case 1: A Diagnostic Mystery Resolved (cont.)

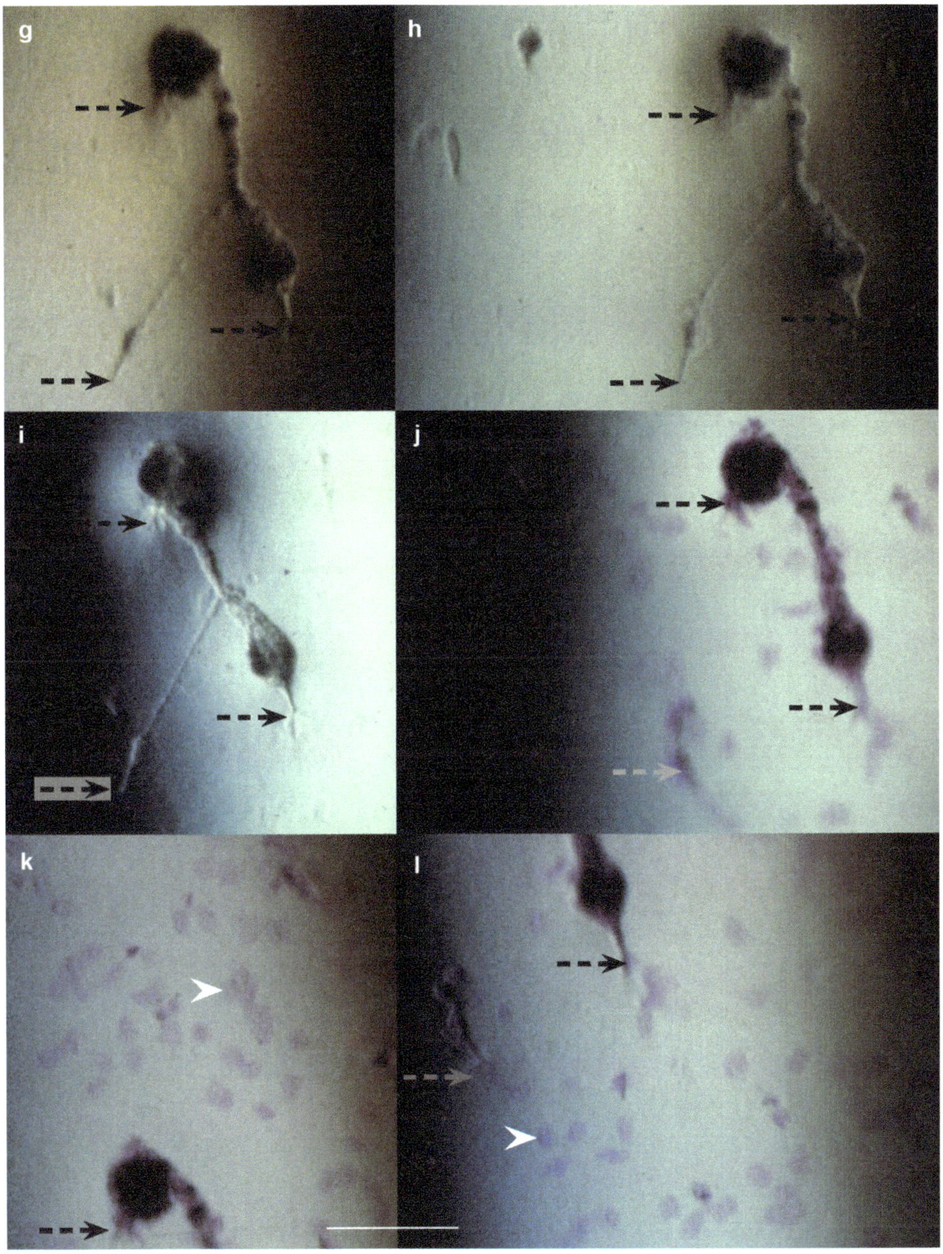

Fig. 7.5 (continued)

Case 1: A Diagnostic Mystery Resolved (cont.)

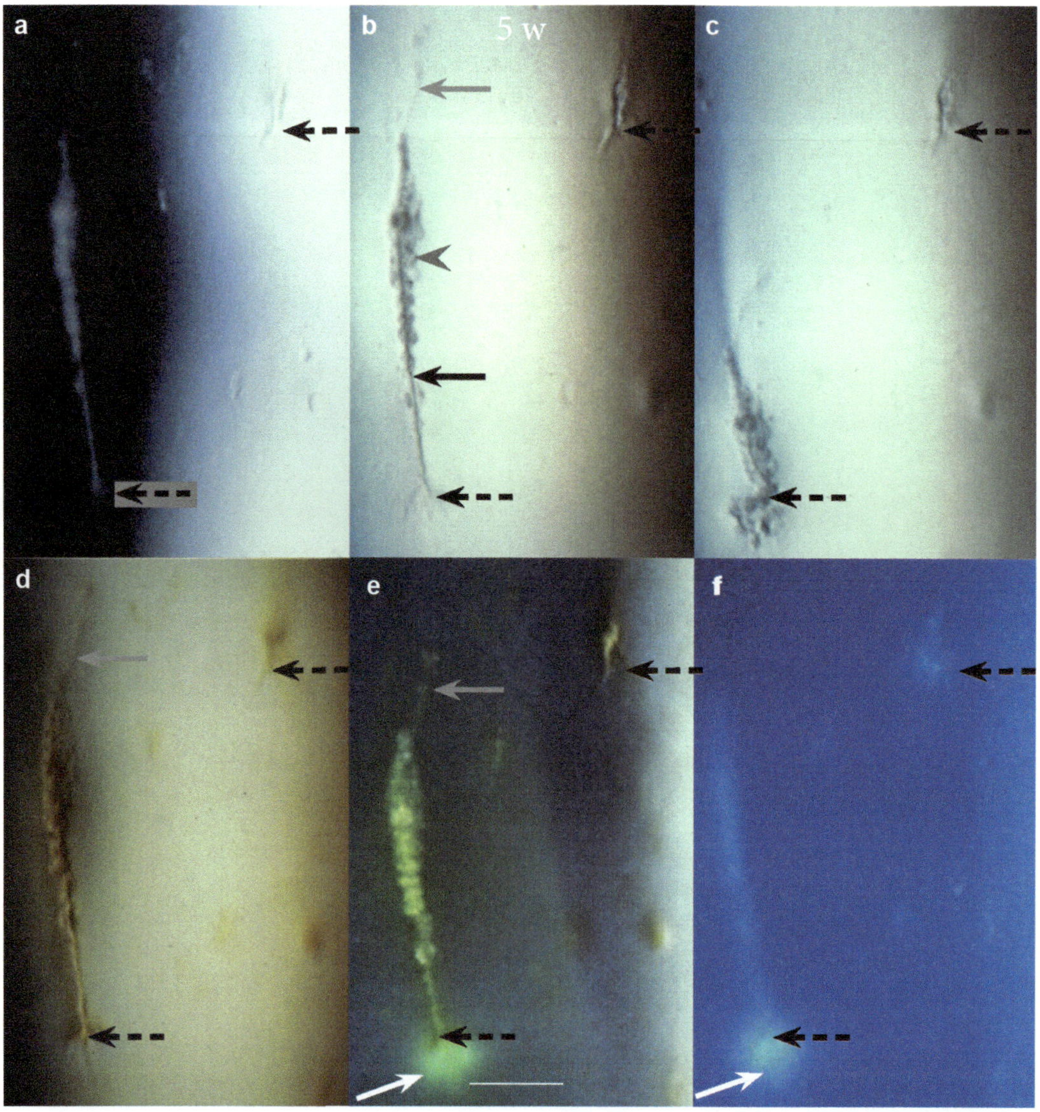

Fig. 7.6 Two of several filaments present on the right cornea. In all photographs, the *dashed arrows* indicate their attachment points. The long filament (a) is light-reflecting; (b) shows a well visible central thread (*plain black arrow*), a strand (*grey arrow*) protruding from its free end and granularity (*grey arrowhead*); (c) moves with blinks; (d) stains yellow with fluorescein. In (e, f) is visible green fluorescence of the filament and around the attachment point (*white arrow*). (The markers are placed in corresponding locations; blue filter used in (f).) Figure 7.7 shows the dynamics of the same filament stained red with rose bengal (Adapted from [4])

Case 1: A Diagnostic Mystery Resolved (cont.)

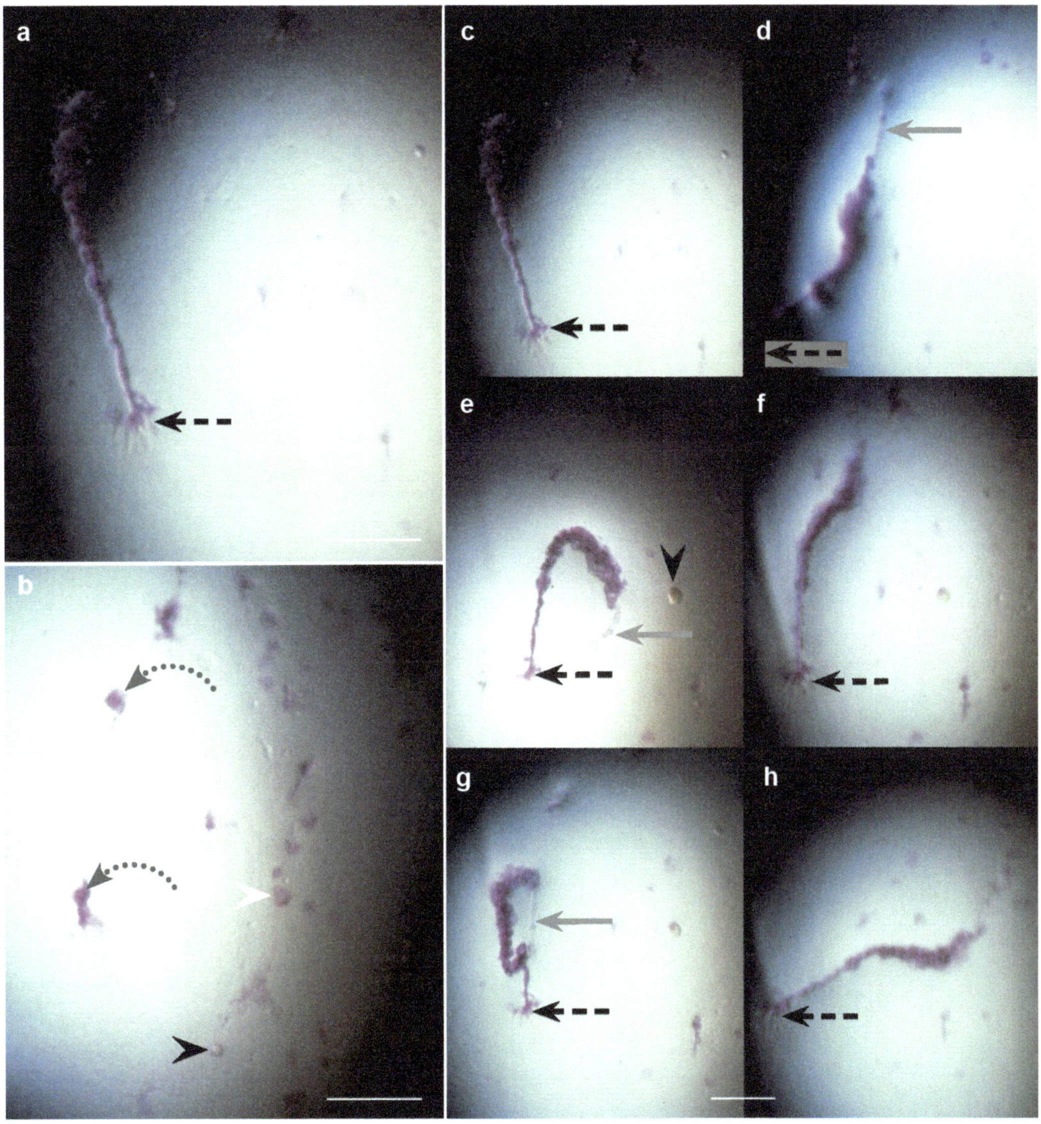

Fig. 7.7 (a) The same filament as in Fig. 7.6, stained with rose bengal. The *dashed arrow* indicates its attachment point. (b) Surface cells (*white arrowhead*) and mucus (*bowed arrows*) stained red with rose bengal; the *black arrowhead* indicates a cystic space. (c–h) show the filament's sweeping movements with blinks. The *dashed arrows* indicate its attachment, the *grey arrows* the strand protruding from its upper end and the *arrowhead* in (e) a cystic space (Adapted from [4])

Case 1: A Diagnostic Mystery Resolved (cont.)

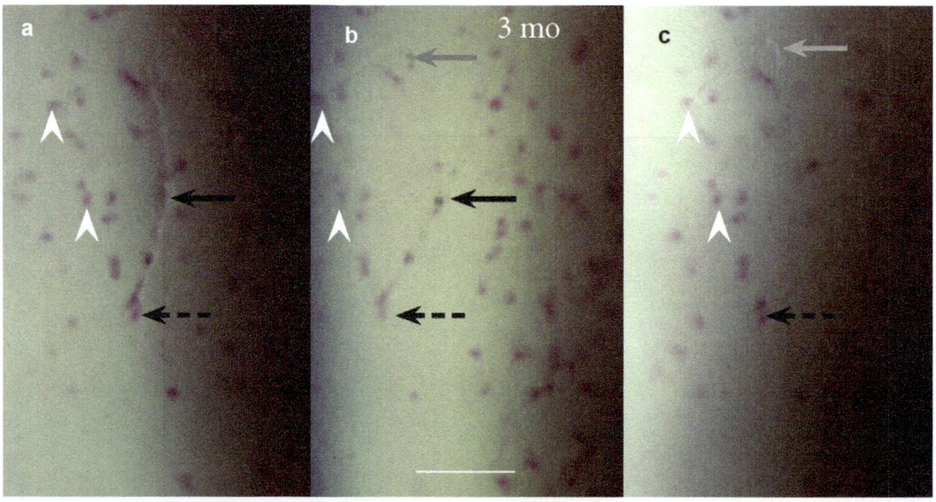

Fig. 7.8 Three consecutive photographs showing (**a**, **b**) a mucus thread (*plain arrows*) attached to the surface (*dashed arrows*) and rose bengal stained surface cells (*arrowheads*). The *grey arrow* in (**b**) points to a new mucus thread that in (**c**) is still present while the original thread has disappeared. (The markers are placed in corresponding locations)

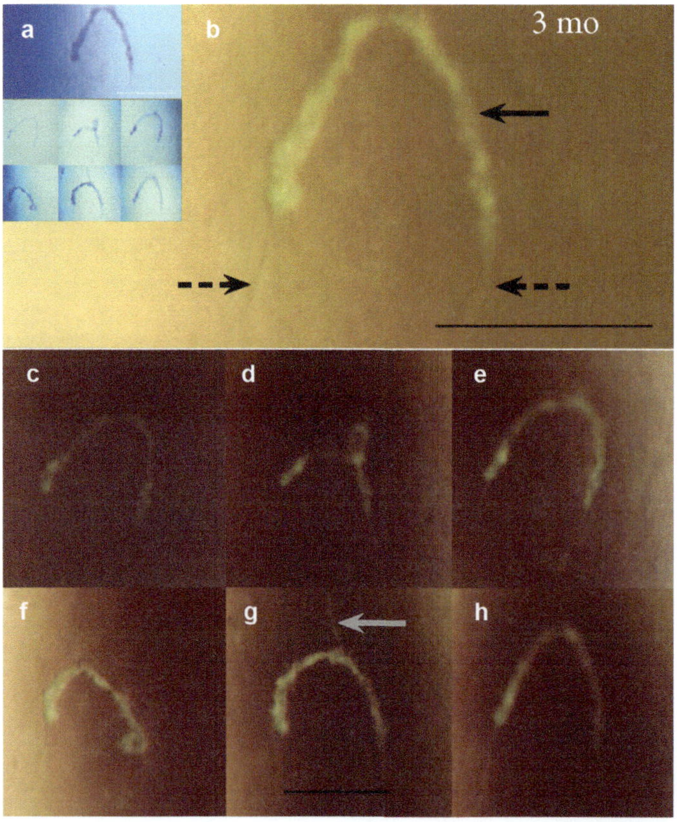

Fig. 7.9 A double-attached thread carrying a small amount of material. (**a**) shows at low magnification the original photographs; in (**b**–**h**) the colours are inverted. (**b**) The thread (*plain arrow*) is attached at two points (*dashed arrows*) to the surface. With blinks, it (**c**) stretches upwards like a bow, (**d**) forms a loop, (**e**) stretches again, (**f**) partly coils, (**g**) shows an attached thin strand (*arrow*) and (**h**) stretches upward

Case 1: A Diagnostic Mystery Resolved (cont.)

Fourteen years after onset, the patient's test values could not be worse (BUT 0/0, Schirmer 1 test 0/0, RBS 9/9), and both corneae showed greyish epithelial flecks staining green with fluorescein and a few small filaments. He declined treatment because symptom-free.

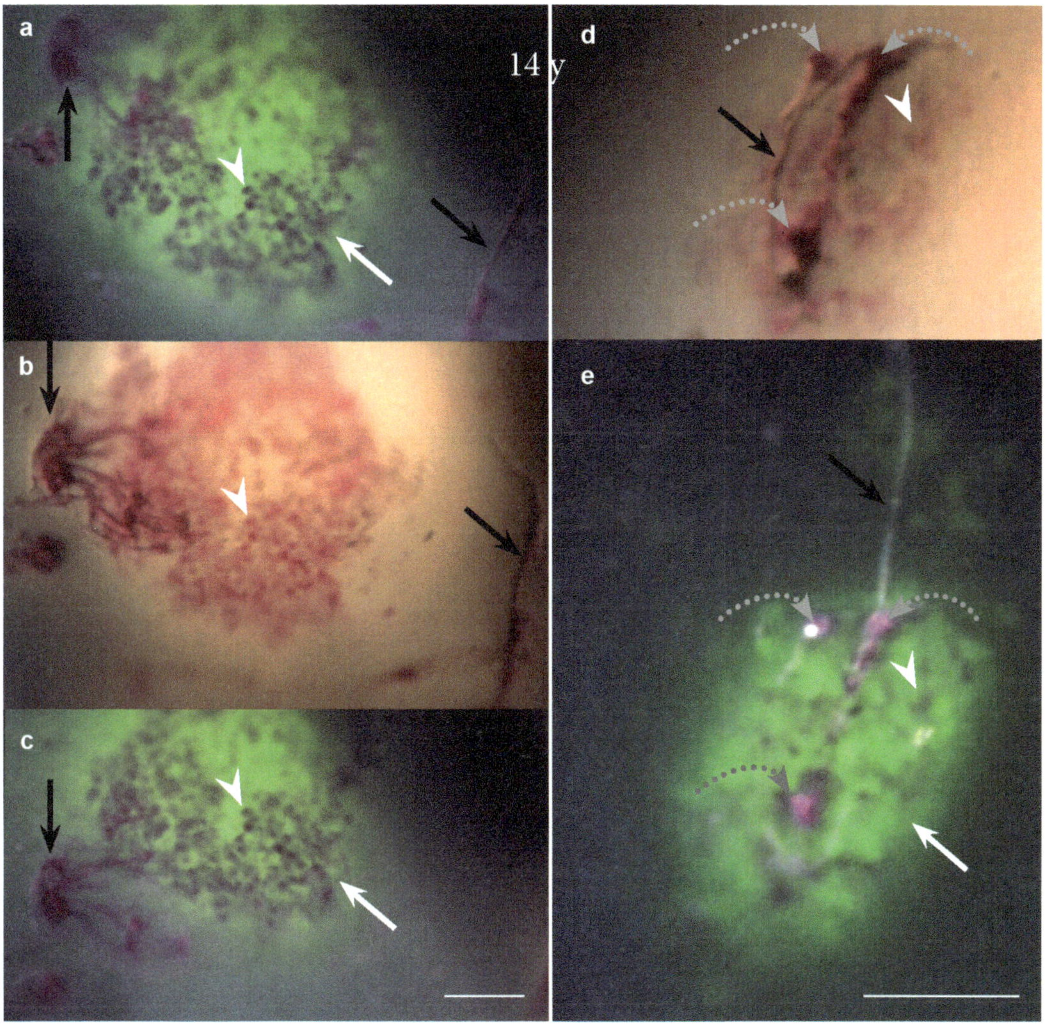

Fig. 7.10 (a–c) A fleck showing rose bengal stained surface cells (*arrowheads*) and (a, c) fluorescein diffusion into the tissues (green, *white arrows*). The *black arrows* indicate mucus moving on the surface. (The arrowheads are placed in corresponding locations). (d, e) Another fleck showing green fluorescein staining (e, *white arrow*), rose bengal stained surface cells (*arrowheads*), lumps of mucus adhering to the surface (*bowed arrows*) and a mucus thread (*straight black arrow*), which in (d) is lying upon the fleck and in (e) is pointing upwards. (The bowed arrows and the arrowheads are placed in corresponding locations)

Case 2: Filaments in a Severe KCS

Case Report

A 52-year-old woman with primary Sjögren's syndrome and agamoglobulinemia-A. Dry eye symptoms started about 14 years before her first visit to the Eye Clinic. At presentation, the BUT was 4/4, Schirmer 1 test 13/13 and RBS 9/9; the eyes were white but both corneae showed large filaments. She was treated with lubricating eye drops.

The photographs of the left eye were taken at presentation and then yearly for 4 years.

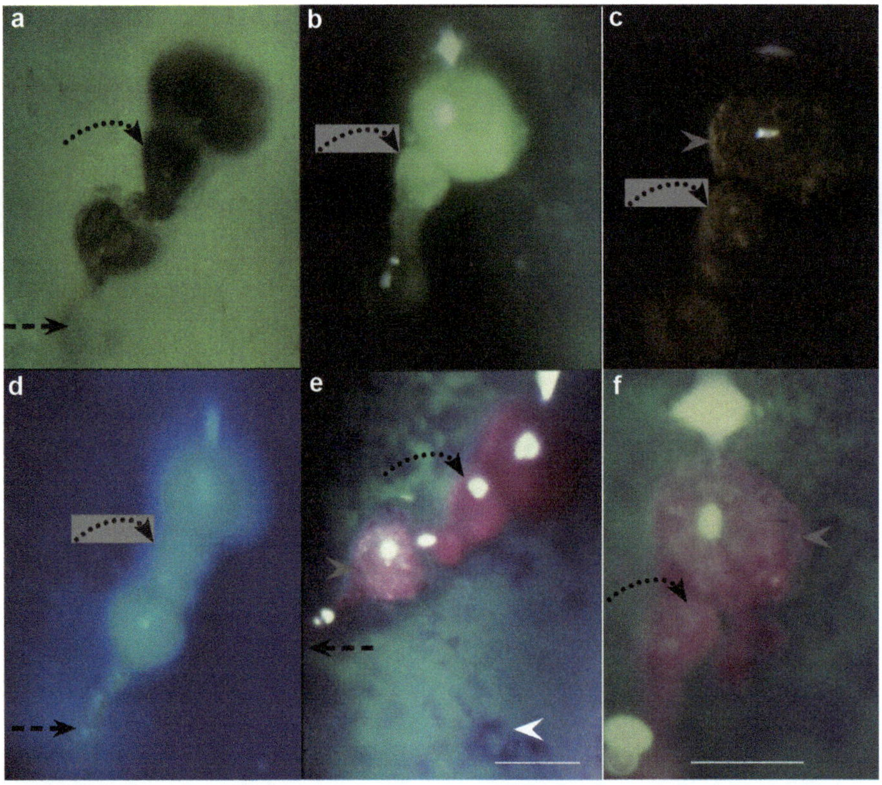

Fig. 7.11 A large filament (*bowed arrows*). The *dashed arrows* indicate its attachment point and the *white arrowhead* in (e) surface cells stained with rose bengal. The contents of the filament are (a) dense, and (b, d) light-reflecting; the surface appears smooth, the discernible contents granular (c, e and f, *grey arrowheads*). (e, f) The filament stains with rose bengal; the green background is caused by fluorescein diffusion into the tissues (d: blue filter)

Fig. 7.13 Five additional filaments. In all photographs, *dashed arrows* indicate their attachment points, *plain arrows* central threads, black *bowed arrows* their bodies and *white arrowheads* stained surface cells. (a, b) This filament shows (a) granularity of contents (*arrowhead*) and (b) a translucent surrounding layer (*white bowed arrowhead*). In (c), the attachment of the central thread is in focus; its location in depth within the epithelium cannot be estimated. In (d, e) are visible rose bengal stained surface cells *(arrowheads)* streaming towards the attachment points

Case 2: Filaments in a Severe KCS (cont.)

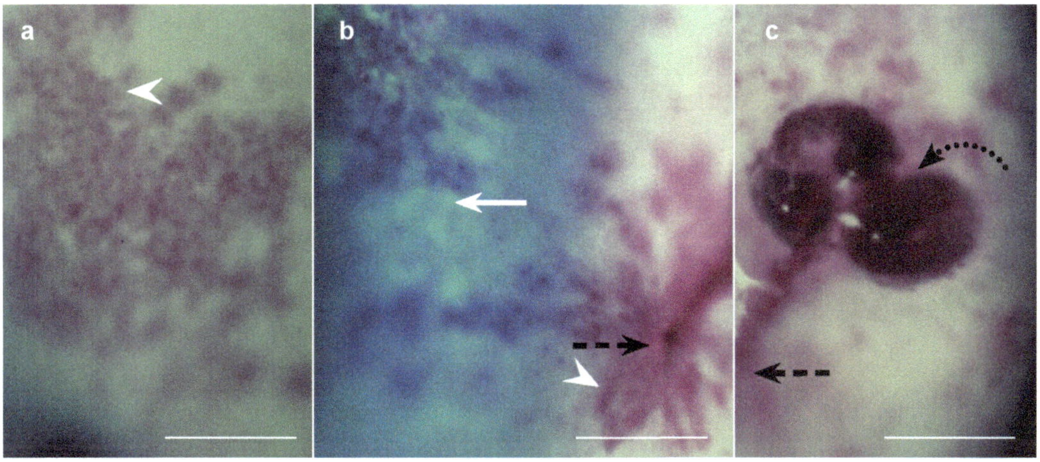

Fig. 7.12 In (a) are visible many rose bengal stained cells containing dark dots (nuclei, *arrowhead*); in (b) an attachment of a filament (*dashed arrow*), rose bengal stained cells (*arrowhead*) streaming towards it and fluorescein diffusion into the tissues (green, *white arrow*); and in (c) another filament (*bowed arrow*). The *dashed arrow* points to its attachment

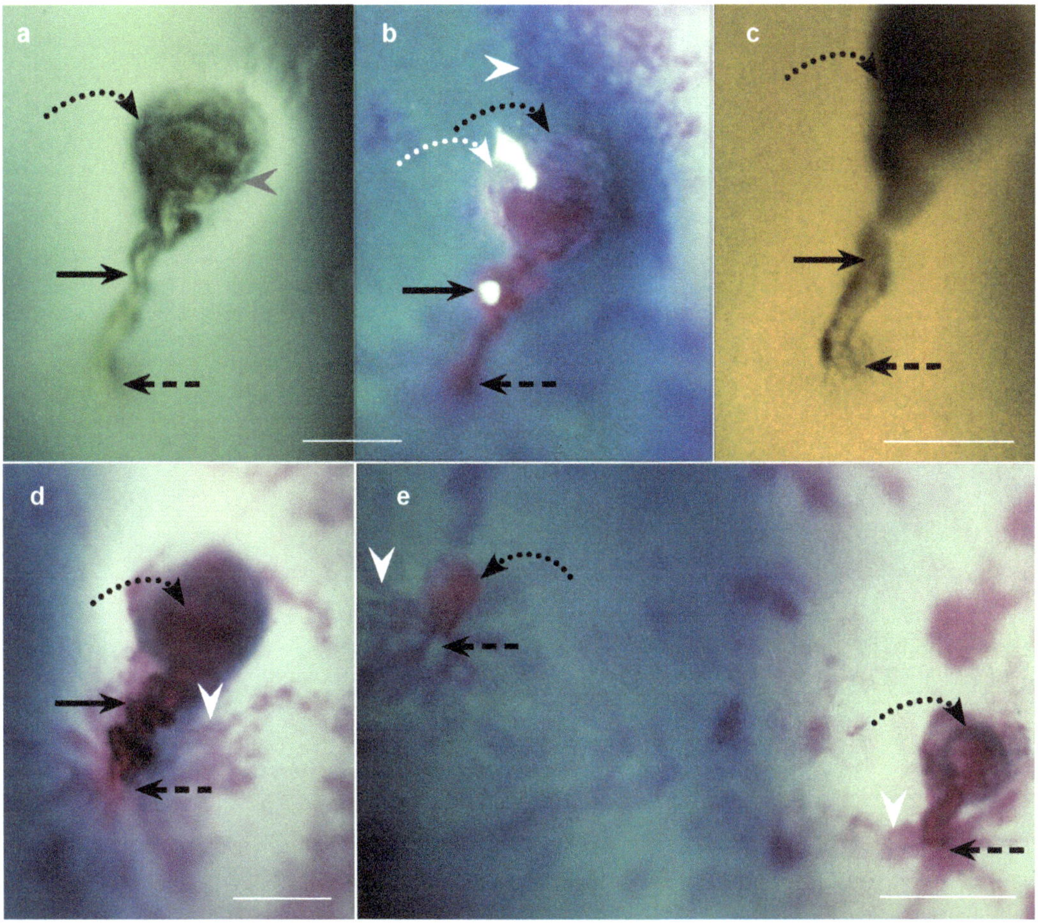

Case 2: Filaments in a Severe KCS (cont.)

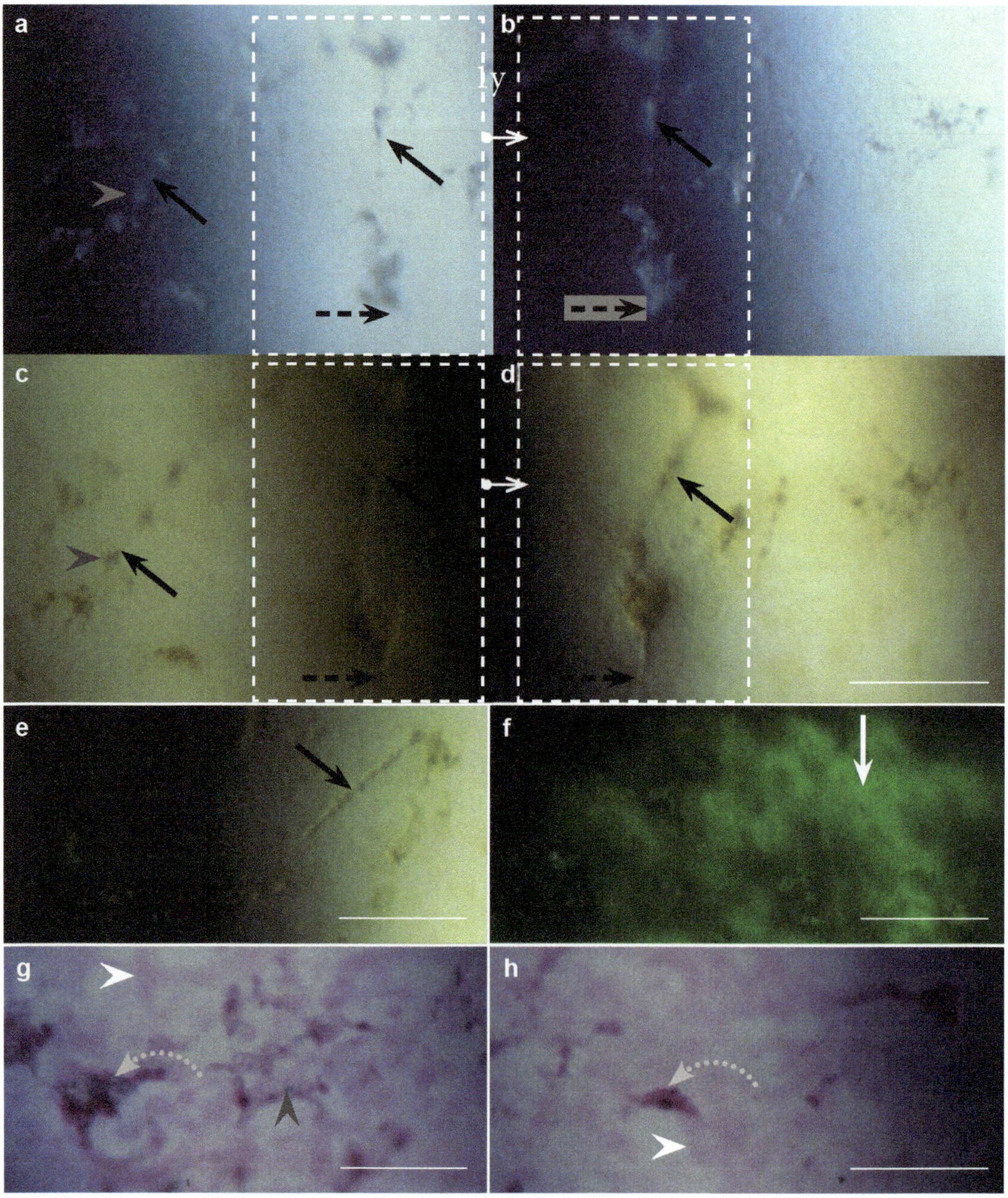

Fig. 7.14 (**a–d**) Mucus threads (*plain arrows*) with attached debris (*arrowheads*) and a small filament attached (*dashed arrow*) to the surface; the structures show only minimal movements with blinks. (The *frames* indicate the same area and the markers are placed in corresponding locations.) (**e**) shows another mucus thread on the surface (*arrow*), (**f**) fluorescein diffusion into the tissues (green, *arrow*), (**g**, **h**) rose bengal staining of surface cells (*white arrowheads*), cell debris/fragments (g, *grey arrowhead*) and pieces of mucus (*bowed arrows*)

One year after presentation, both eyes were irritated, mildly injected and showed smaller and larger filaments; the left cornea was more involved. BUT was 3/4, Schirmer 1 test 4/11, RBS 8/8.

Case 2: Filaments in a Severe KCS (cont.)

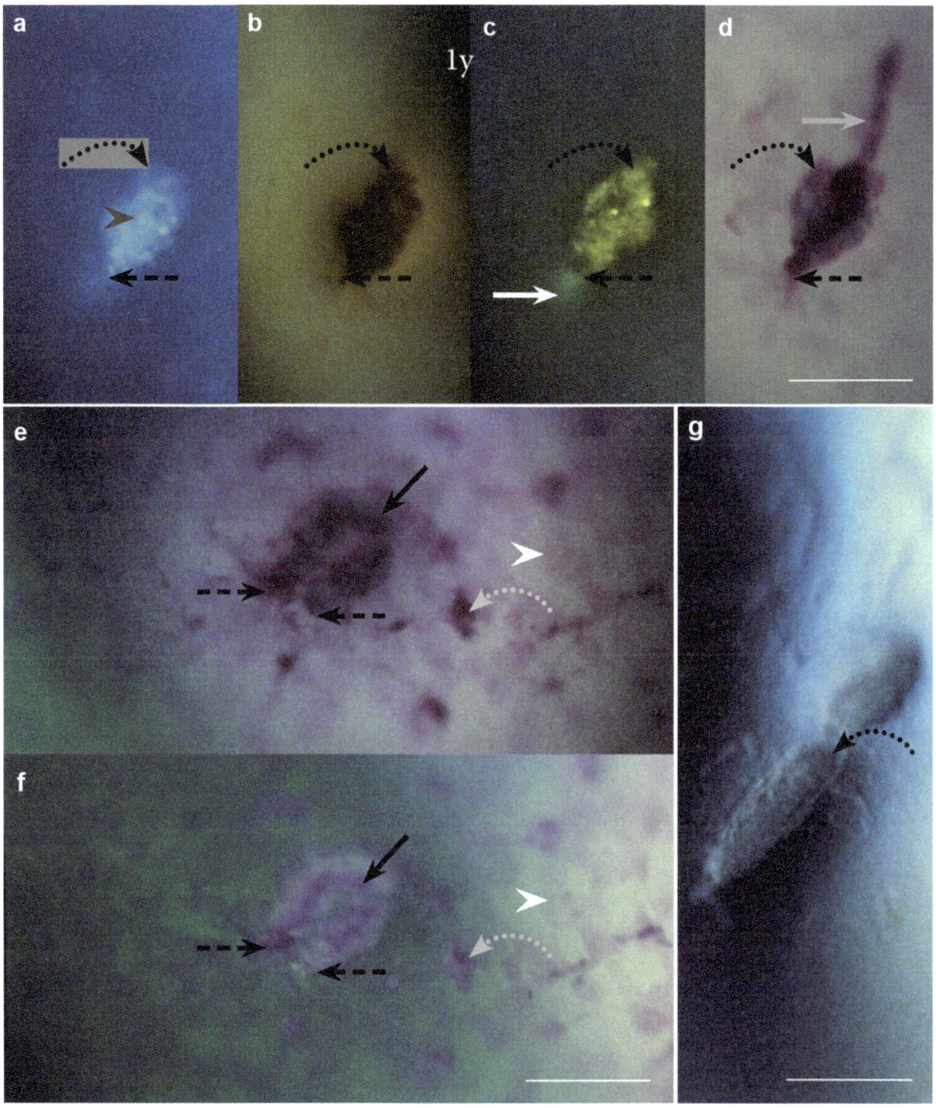

Fig. 7.15 (a–d) A filament (*bowed arrows*) with attachment point indicated by *dashed arrows*. In (a) is visible its light-reflecting property and granularity (*arrowhead*), in (b) its density, in (c) incipient fluorescein diffusion into the tissues around its attachment point (green, *white arrow*). In (d), after rose bengal staining, has appeared a strand (*grey arrow*) at the filament's free end. (e, f) This filament seems to consist of a central thread (*plain arrows*) enveloped by mucus and cell debris and attached at both ends (*dashed arrows*) to the surface showing rose bengal stained surface cells (*arrowheads*), lumps of mucus (*bowed arrows*), and fluorescein diffusion into the tissues (green). (The markers are placed in corresponding locations.) (g) shows a part of another filament (*arrow*) captured at the same occasion

Case 2: Filaments in a Severe KCS (cont.)

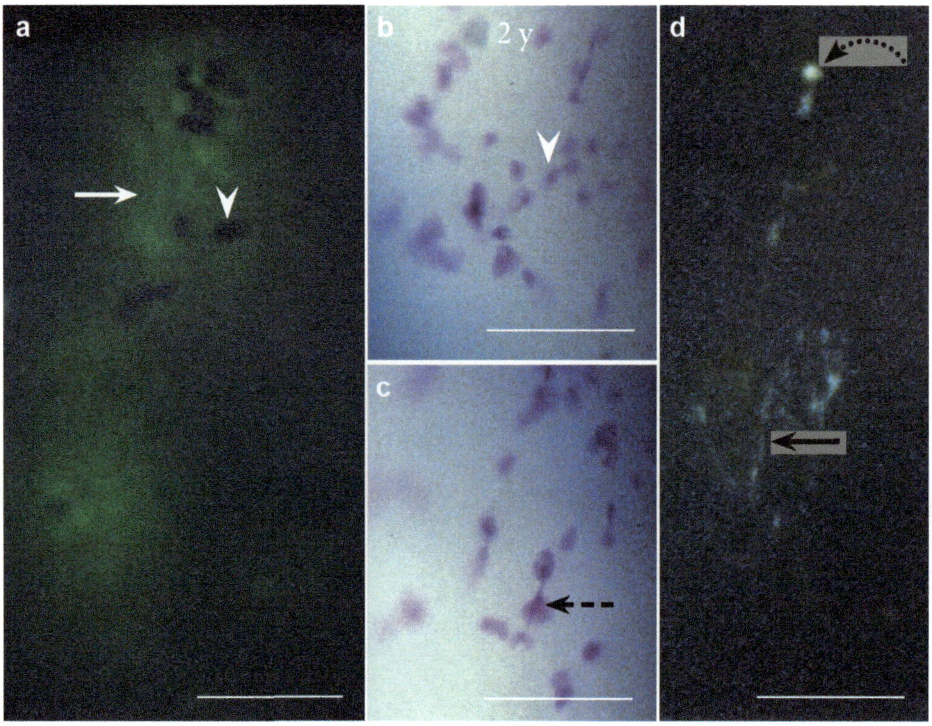

Fig. 7.16 (a) shows green flecks (*arrow*) and rose bengal stained surface cells (*arrowhead*). (b) Some of the stained cells contain a darker dot (nucleus, *arrowhead*). (c) The *dashed arrow* points to a structure with tent-like form suggestive of attachment point of a minifilament. (d) Light-reflecting mucus threads (*straight arrow*) on the surface and a minifilament (*bowed arrow*)

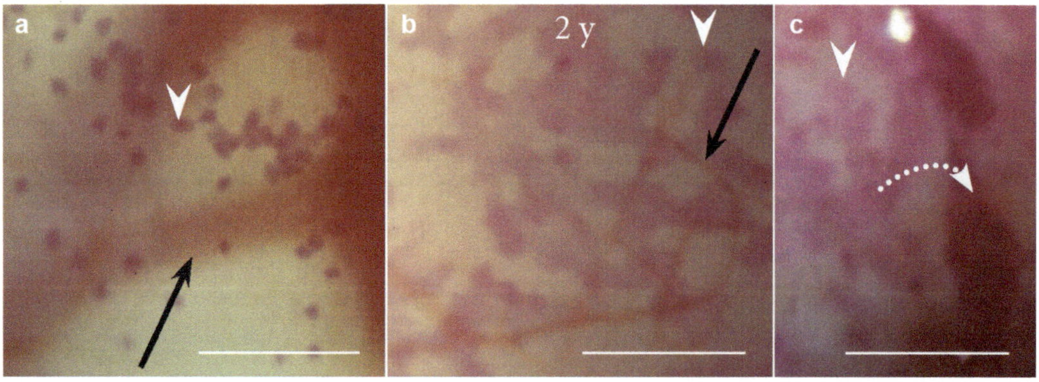

Fig. 7.17 The nasal conjunctiva shows (a) small and (b, c) larger cells staining with rose bengal (*arrowheads*). (c) A piece of mucus (*bowed arrow*) is lying on the surface. The *straight arrows* indicate conjunctival vessels

Two years after presentation the patient, treated with lubricating eye drops and topical acetylcysteine, had little symptoms. The left cornea showed a few small filaments; none were present on the right one. The BUT was 3/2, Schirmer 1 test 8/0 and RBS 8/8.

Case 2: Filaments in a Severe KCS (cont.)

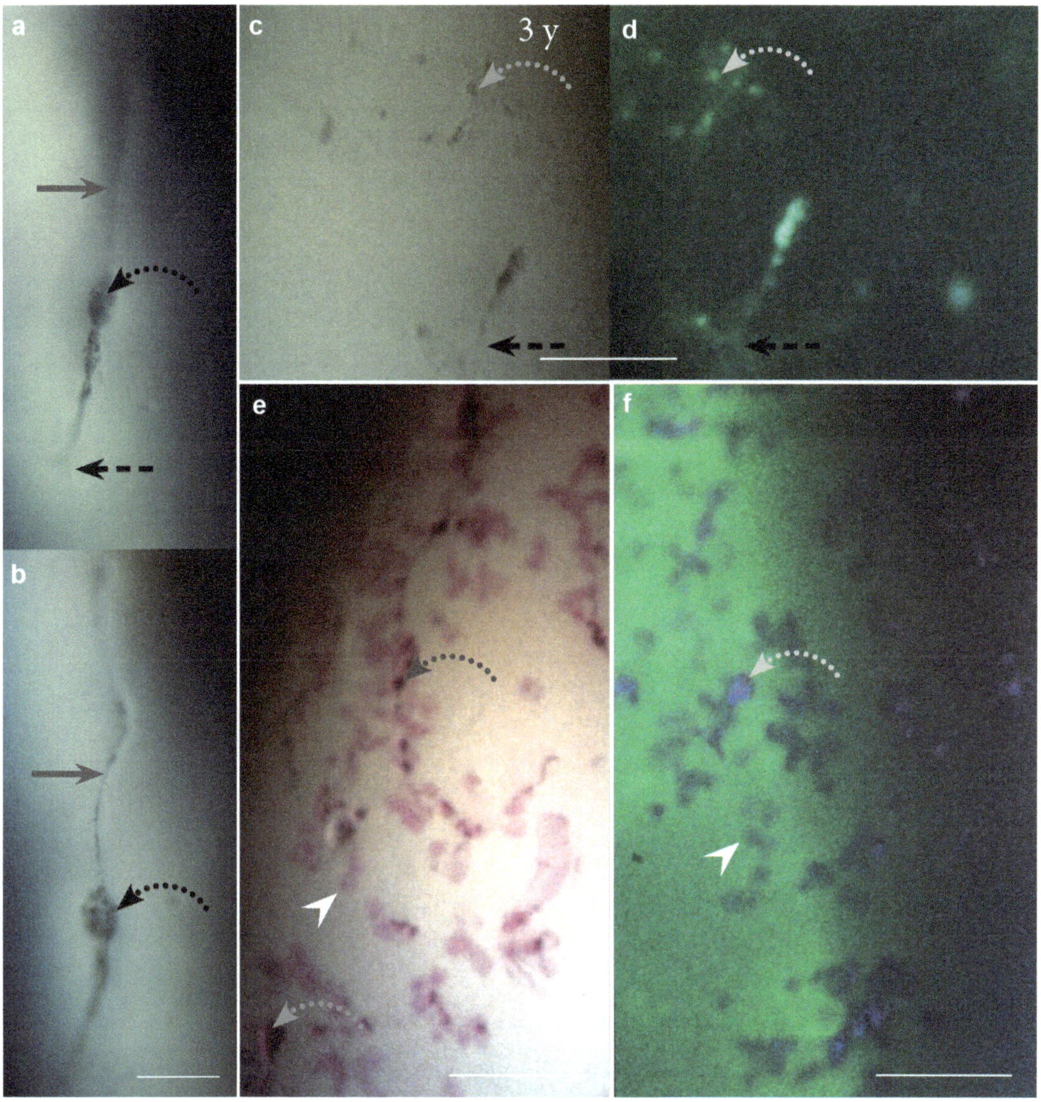

Fig. 7.18 (a, b) A filament (*bowed arrow*) with a protruding strand (*grey arrow*) sweeping the surface. The *dashed arrow* indicates the filament's attachment point. (c, d) A small filament with attachment indicated by *dashed arrows*, and mucus adhering to the surface (*bowed arrows*); in (d) is visible the light-reflecting property of the mucus. (The arrows are placed in corresponding locations.) (e, f) show rose bengal staining of surface cells (*arrowheads*) and pieces of mucus adhering to the surface (*arrows*); the green background in (f) reveals fluorescein diffusion into the tissues. (Not the same areas)

Three years after presentation, the symptoms and treatment were unchanged. Both eyes were white; the left cornea showed only a few small filaments. The BUT was 0/0, Schirmer 1 test 1/1 and RBS 8/9.

Case 2: Filaments in a Severe KCS (cont.)

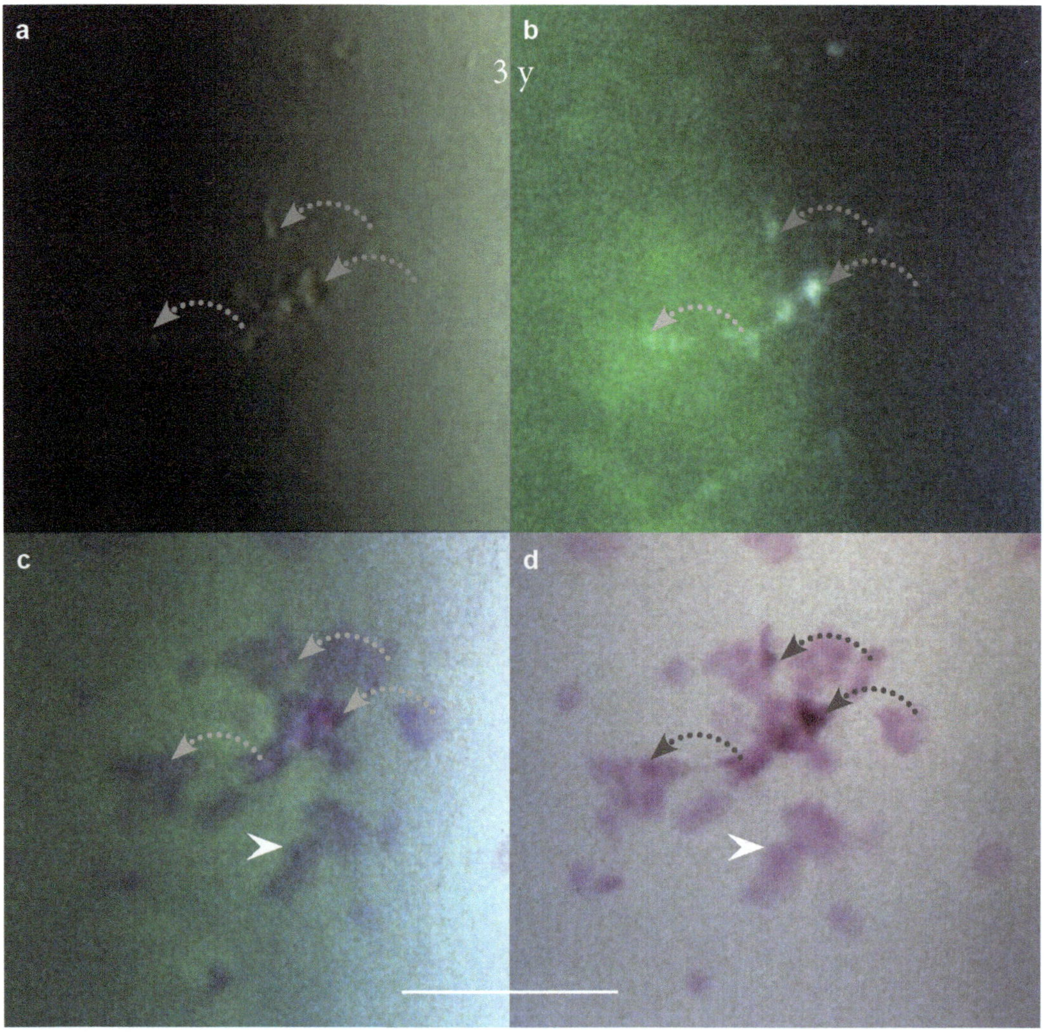

Fig. 7.19 This area shows mucus (*arrows*) adhering to the surface. (**a**) Before staining, the mucus is discernible as small lumps; (**b**) immediately after the application of fluorescein, the light-reflecting mucus appears white in the green stained tear film; (**c**, **d**) rose bengal reveals adherence of the mucus to red stained surface cells (*arrowheads*). (The markers are placed in corresponding locations)

Case 2: Filaments in a Severe KCS (cont.)

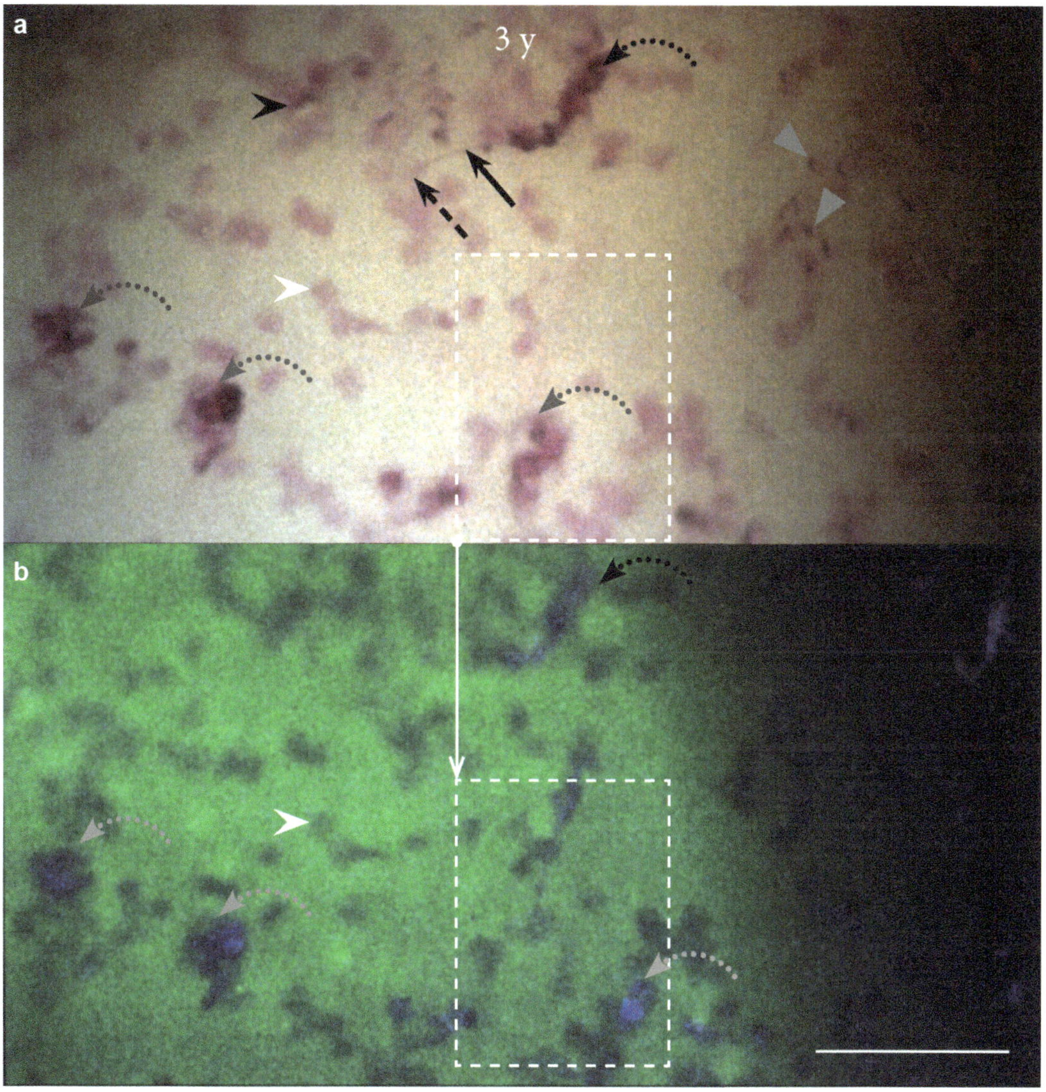

Fig. 7.20 (a, b) Another area showing mucus on the surface (*grey bowed arrows*) and rose bengal stained surface cells (*white arrowheads*). The piece of mucus indicated by *black bowed arrow* might represent a small filament attached (*dashed arrow*) to the surface by a thin thread (*plain arrow*); the *grey arrowheads* in (a) indicate rounded bodies. (b) After a couple of blinks, some of the mucus (*grey bowed arrows*) has remained in place but some has changed position (in *frame*, cf. (a)). The green background is caused by fluorescein diffusion into the tissues. (The bowed arrows and the white arrowheads are placed in corresponding locations; a Adapted from [4])

Case 2: Filaments in a Severe KCS (cont.)

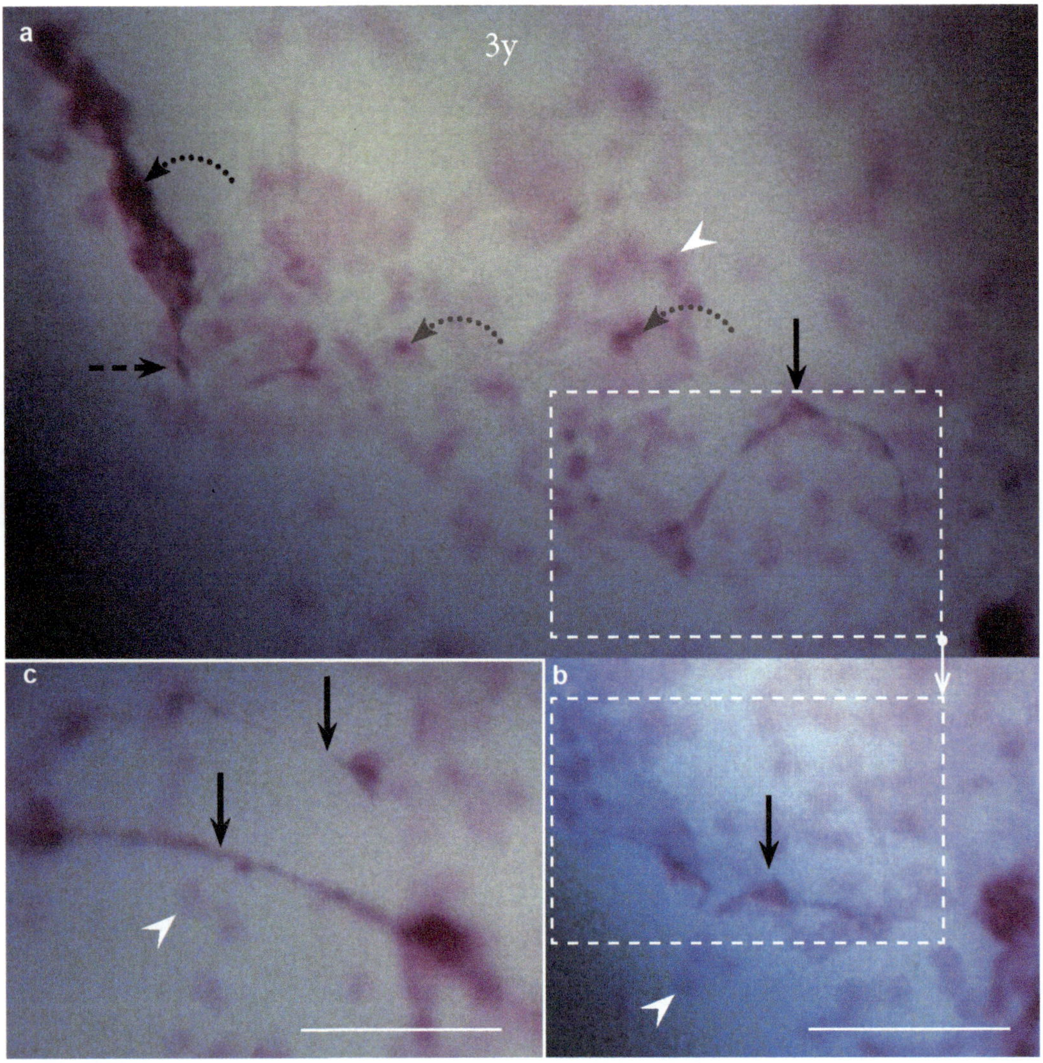

Fig. 7.21 (a) A filament (*bowed black arrow*) with surface attachment indicated by *dashed arrow*, rose bengal stained surface cells (*arrowhead*), and a mucus thread (*plain arrow*) attached to the surface at both ends and stretched like a bow; (b) after a blink, it has ruptured and is now lying on the surface (*arrow*); the *frames* indicate the same area. (c) shows mucus threads (*arrows*) and rose bengal stained surface cells (*arrowhead*)

Case 2: Filaments in a Severe KCS (cont.)

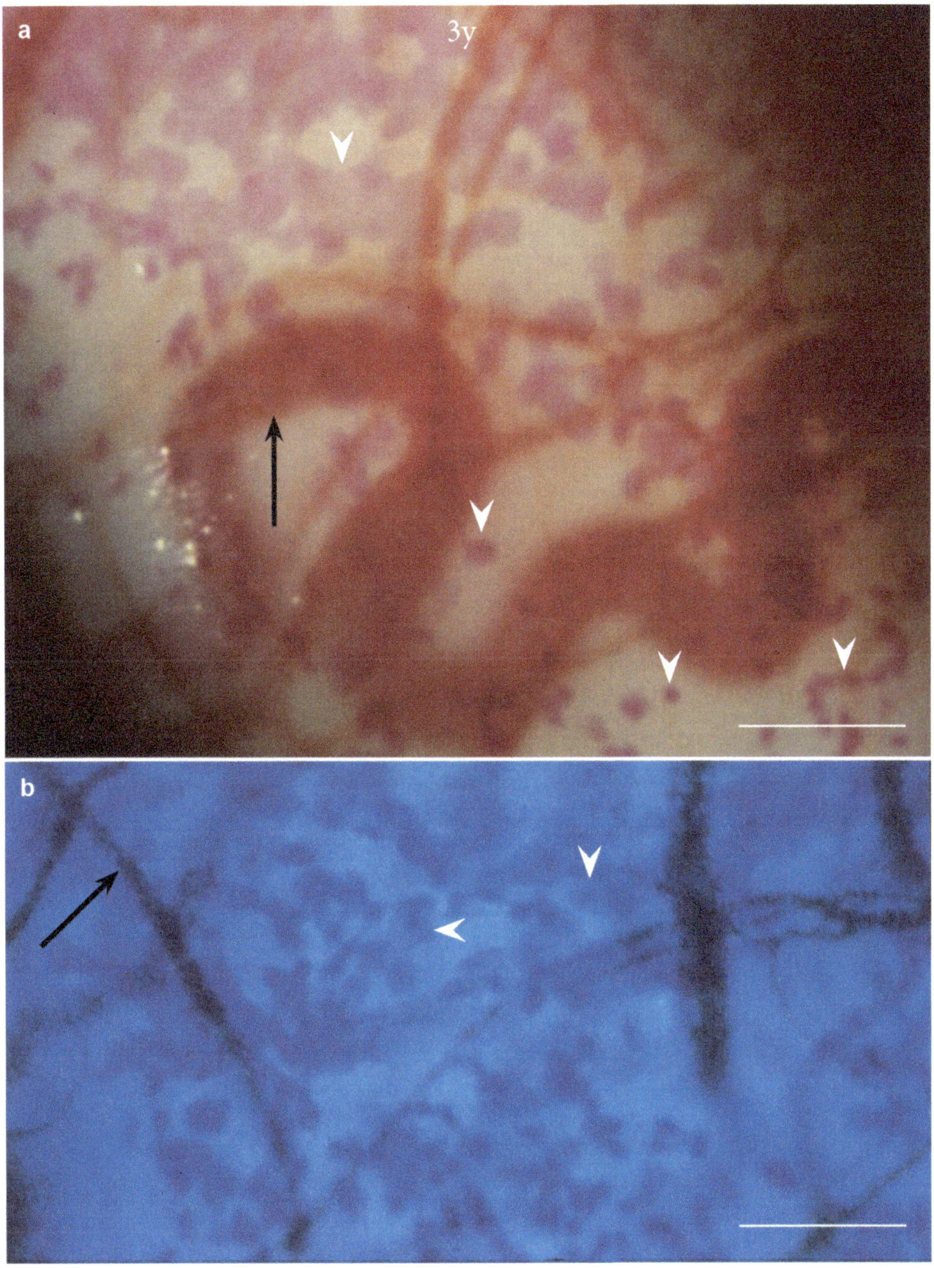

Fig. 7.22 The nasal conjunctiva shows many larger and smaller surface cells staining with rose bengal (*arrowheads*). The *arrows* indicate conjunctival vessels (b: green filter)

Case 2: Filaments in a Severe KCS (cont.)

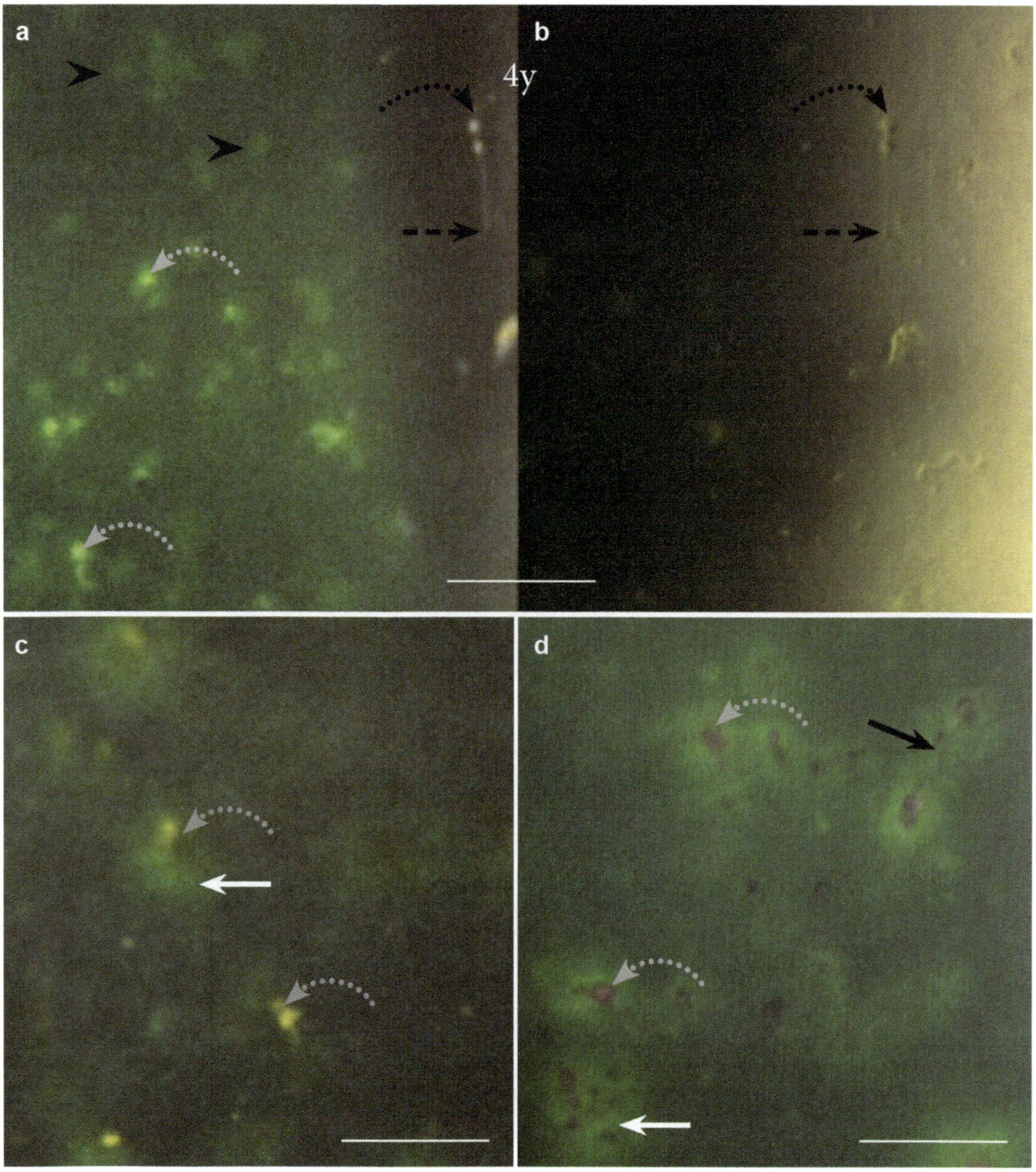

Fig. 7.23 (a, b) This area shows a minifilament (*bowed black arrows)* with attachment point indicated by *dashed arrows*; small pieces of surface-attached mucus (yellowish dots, *bowed grey arrows*); and green cystic spaces (*arrowheads*). (The black arrows are placed in corresponding locations.) (c, d) Two different areas showing small pieces of mucus (*bowed arrows*) appearing yellow with fluorescein and brightly red with rose bengal. The *white arrows* indicate green flecks caused by fluorescein diffusion into the tissues and the *black arrow* in (d) a mucus thread

Four years after presentation, the patient had as little symptoms as before. She had stopped acetylcysteine drops about a month before and was using only lubricating eye drops. The eyes were white and both corneae showed many small filaments. The BUT was 0/0, Schirmer 1 test 1/1 and RBS 8/8.

Case 2: Filaments in a Severe KCS (cont.)

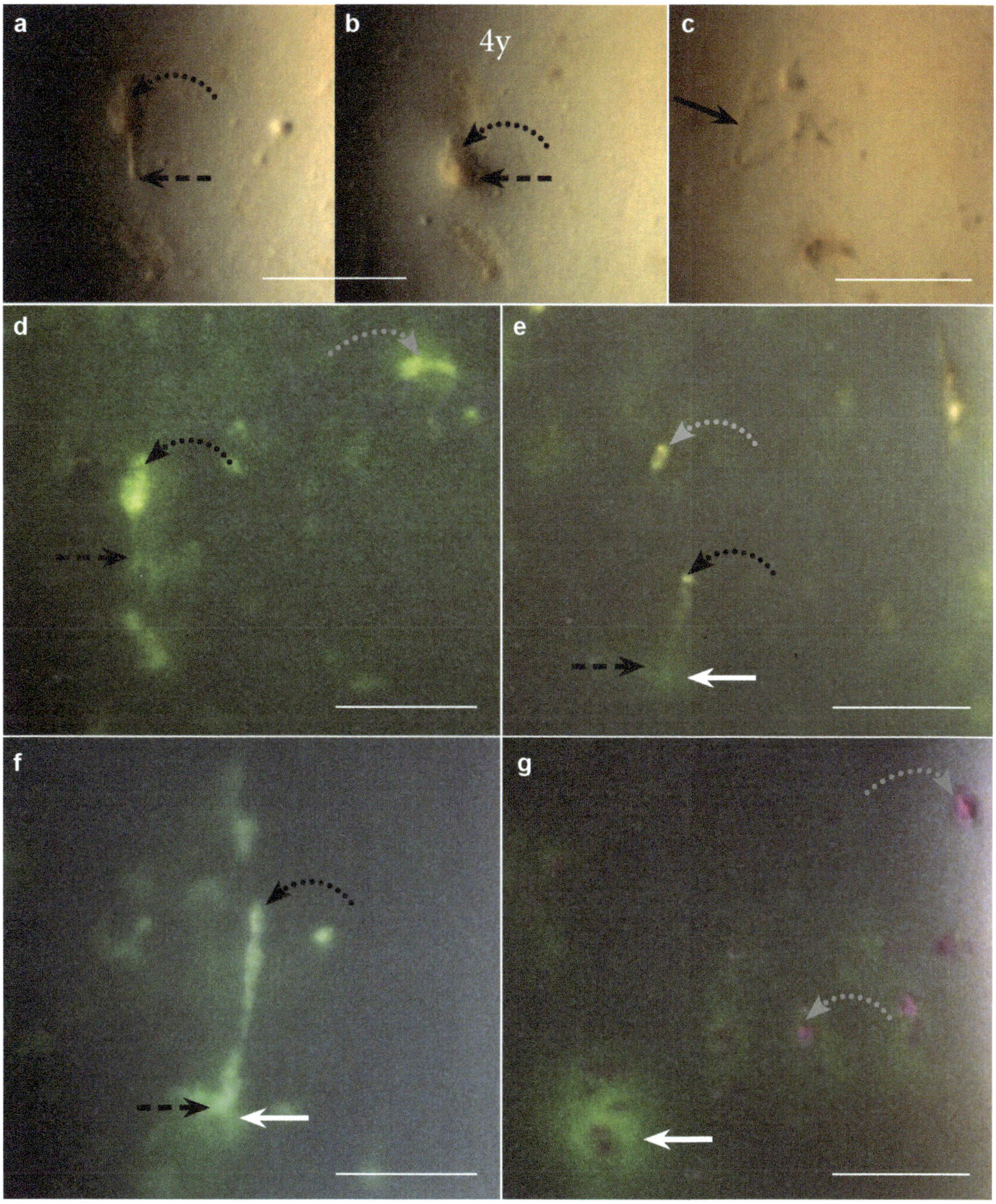

Fig. 7.24 (a, b) A small filament (*bowed arrows*), (a) stretched and (b) crumpled, overlying its attachment point (*dashed arrows*). (c) shows a mucus thread on the surface (*arrow*). (d–f) Four different areas showing minifilaments (*black bowed arrows*), fluorescein diffusion into the tissues (*white arrows*) around their attachment points (*dashed arrows*) and pieces of mucus on the surface (*grey bowed arrows*). In (g) are visible rose bengal stained pieces of mucus on the surface (*bowed arrows*) and green flecks (*white arrow*) caused by fluorescein diffusion into the tissues

Case 2: Filaments in a Severe KCS (cont.)

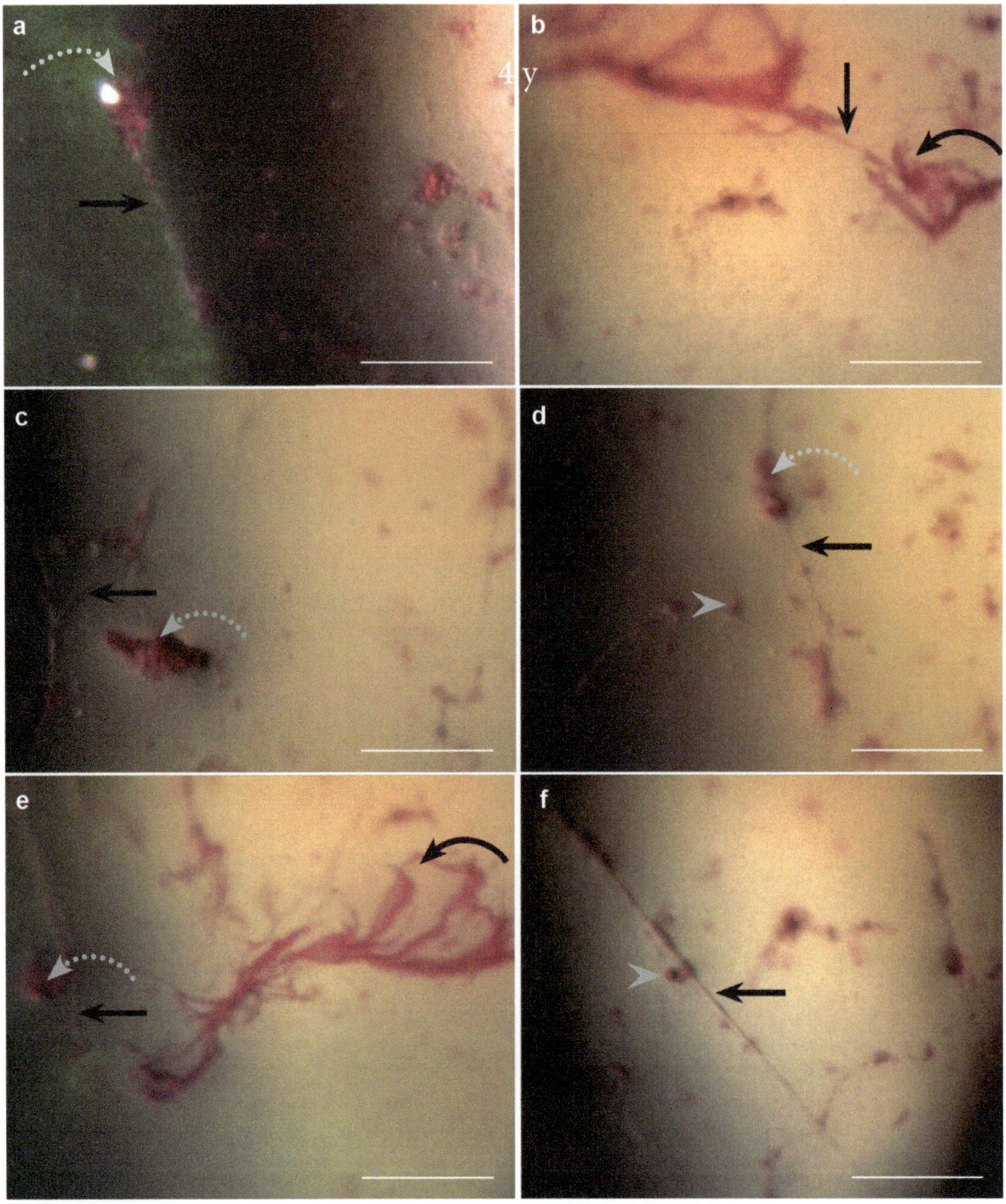

Fig. 7.25 (a–f) Mucus threads (*straight arrows*), crumpled mucus sheets (*black bowed arrows*), lumps of mucus and cell debris (*grey bowed arrows*) and cell debris (*arrowheads*) on the surface or in the precorneal tear film

Addendum

After a further year, when last seen, the situation was unchanged. The patient had little symptoms, was using only lubricating eye drops, and both corneae showed the same changes as the preceding year. The BUT was 0/0, Schirmer 1 test 0/0 and RBS 8/8.

Case 3: Filaments After Marginal Infiltrates

Case Report

A 73-year-old woman with rheumatoid arthritis was referred to the Eye Clinic because of irritation and redness of the right eye. The eye was injected and showed marginal infiltrations at the upper and lower corneal limbus, which healed with topical steroid. After that the cornea showed several filaments both at the upper and lower limbus; all disappeared within 4 weeks.

The photographs of the right cornea were taken at presentation and a week later.

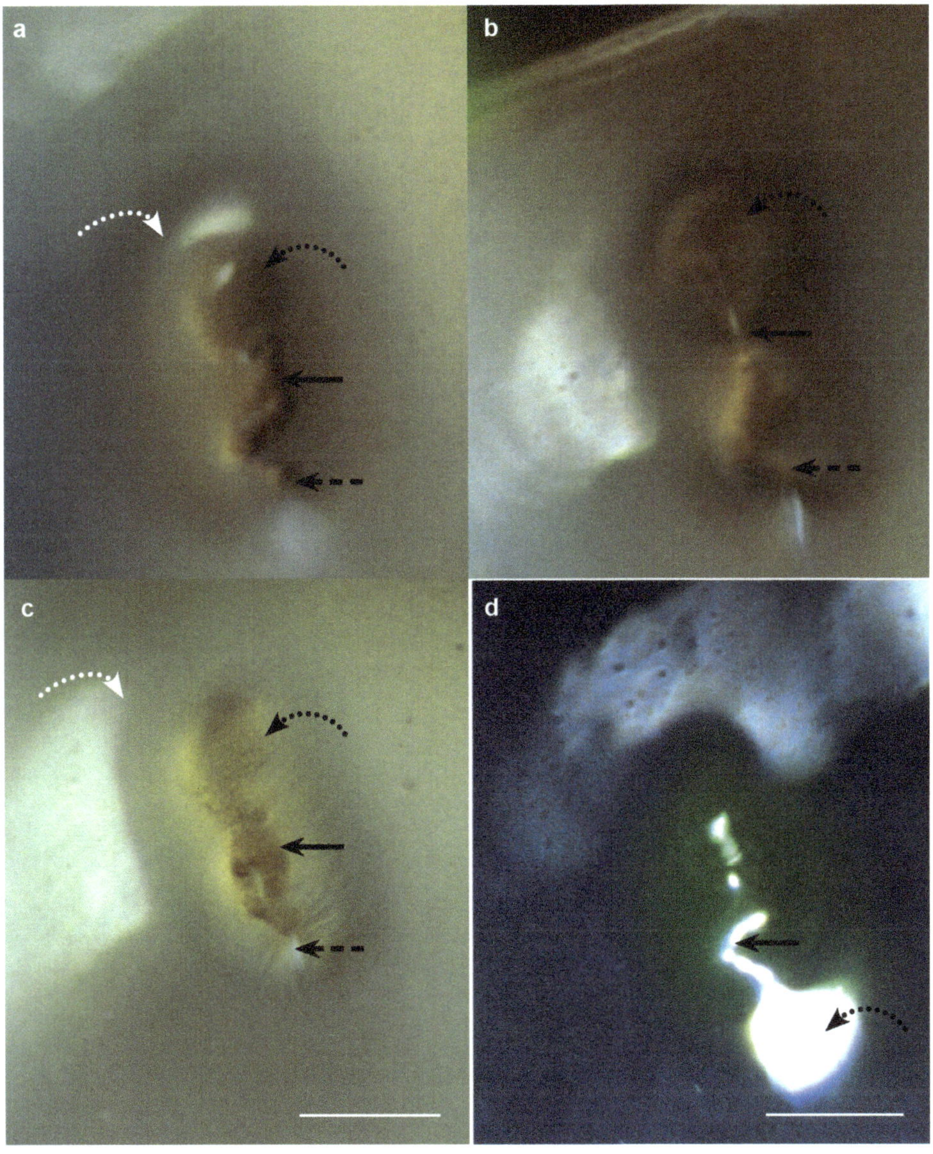

Fig. 7.26 (a–c) A filament close to the upper limbus. The *dashed arrows* indicate its attachment point, the black *bowed arrows* its body and the *plain arrows* its central thread; the light reflections (*white bowed arrows*) imply a surrounding homogenous layer, cf. Figs. 7.27 and 7.28 (overleaf). (d) has captured the strong light-reflecting property of filaments (a different filament, pointing downwards; cf. Fig. 7.5c)

Case 3: Filaments After Marginal Infiltrates (cont.)

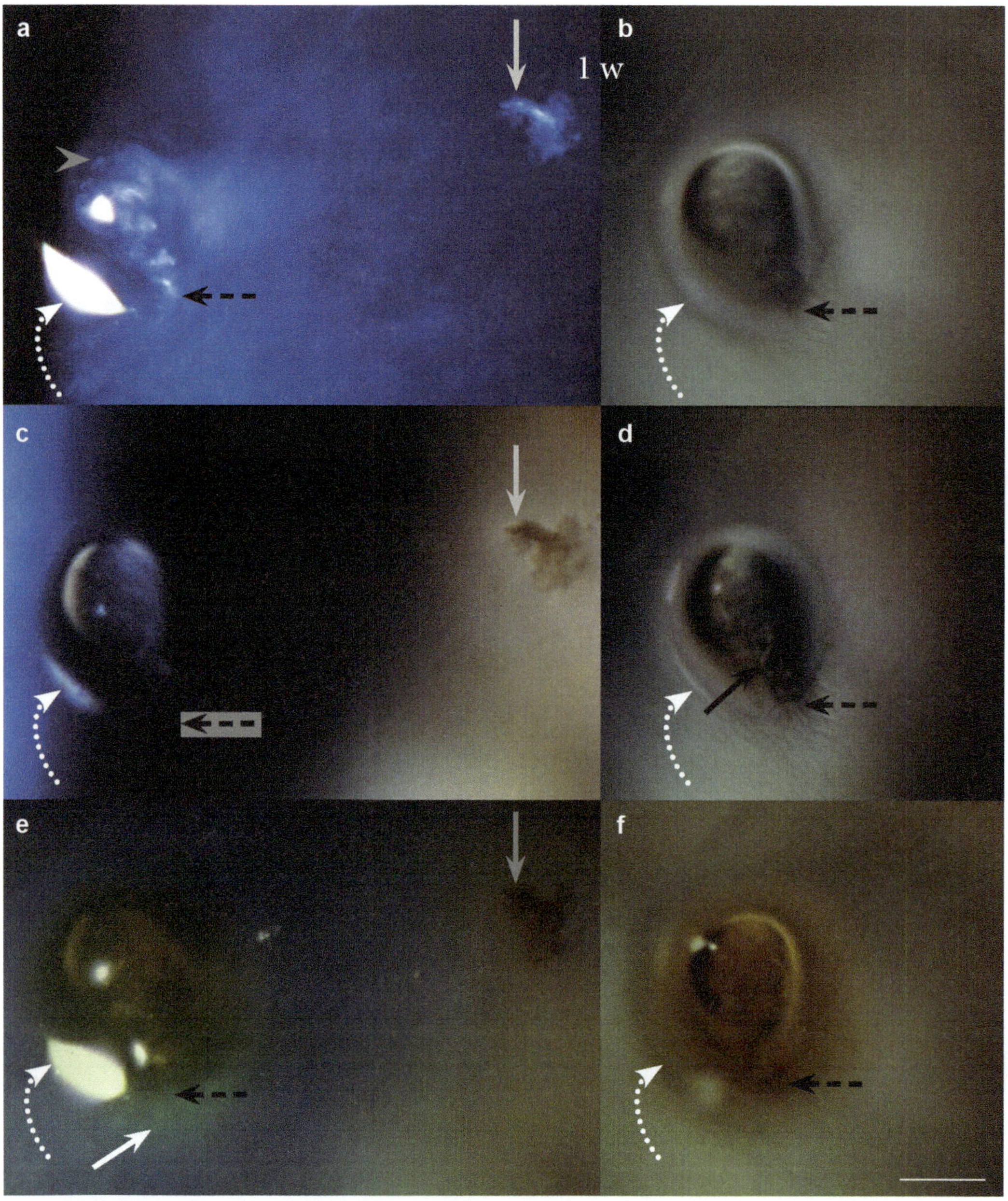

Fig. 7.27 The temporal upper part of the cornea shows a rounded filament (*black dashed arrows*) surrounded by a clear layer (*bowed arrows*), visible as such (b, d and f) or implied by light reflected from it (a, c and e); the filament contains very little discernible cell debris (a, *arrowhead*); the *plain arrow* in (d) indicates the filament's central thread. (e, f) After the application of fluorescein the filament's dull brownish hue contrasts with the vivid green one revealing fluorescein penetration into the tissues (e, *white arrow*) around the attachment point (cf. Figs. 7.38 and 7.46). (a, c and e) additionally show a short protruding thread (*grey arrows*), suggestive of remains of a torn-off filament; the thread and its surroundings are (a) light-reflecting and (e) stain yellow with fluorescein. (The black dashed arrows are placed in the same locations in all photographs)

Case 3: Filaments After Marginal Infiltrates (cont.)

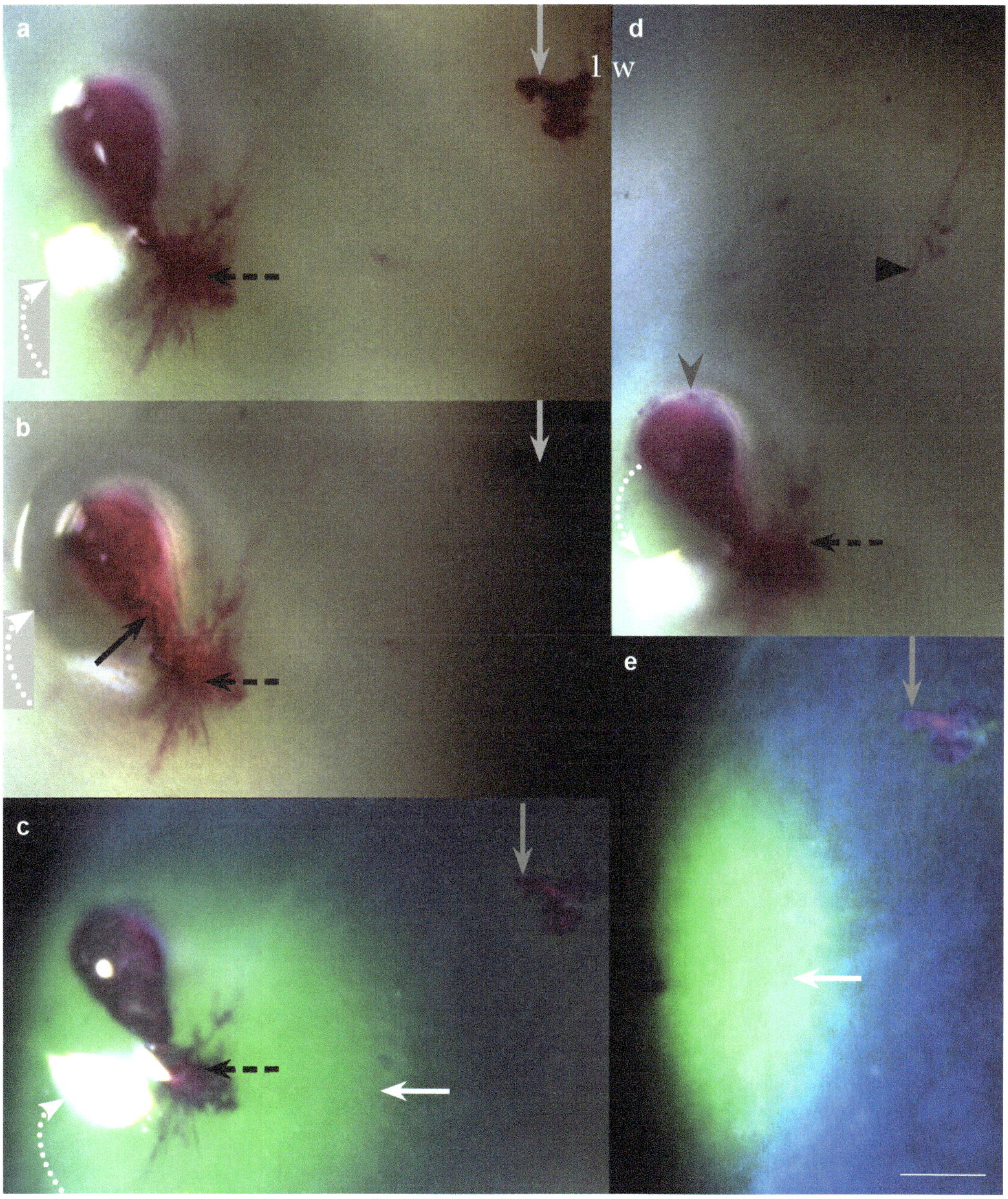

Fig. 7.28 The same filament as in Fig. 7.27. (a–c) With rose bengal, the filament, the surface surrounding its attachment (*dashed arrows)* and the protruding thread with its surroundings *(grey arrows*) stain red but the layer surrounding the filament (*bowed arrows*) is clear. The *plain arrow* in (b) indicates the filament's central thread. (c) The green staining (*white arrow*) has enlarged (cf. Fig. 7.27e). In (d) the *grey arrowhead* indicates cell debris attached to the filament (cf. Fig. 7.27a) and the *black arrowhead* a line, possibly an imprint of a long thread (visible also in (a) and (b); cf. also Figs. 7.37 and 7.38). (e) The extensive green staining (*white arrow*) surrounding the filament's attachment contrasts with the minimal one around the attachment of the thread (*plain arrow*). (a–d) Except for the attachment, there is almost none red staining of surface cells. (The black dashed arrows are placed in the same locations in all photographs; b Adapted from [4])

Case 4: Giant Filaments in KCS

Case Report

A 44-year-old woman with primary Sjögren's syndrome and dry eye symptoms for 8 years, treated with lubricating eye drops. At presentation, both conjunctivae were slightly injected and both corneae showed large filaments at the lower limbus. Test values: BUT 1/1, Schirmer 1 test 1/1, RBS 7/7.

The photographs of the right cornea were taken at presentation.

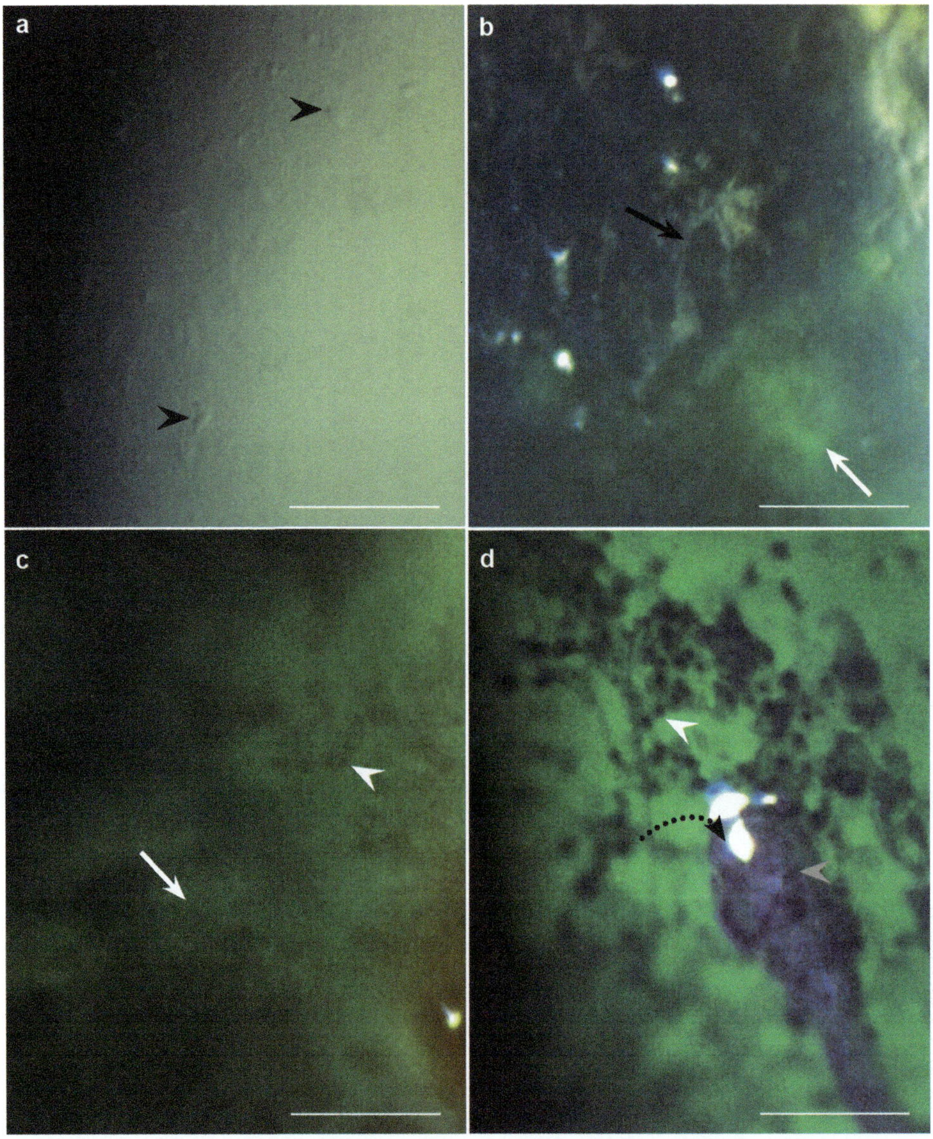

Fig. 7.29 (**a**) Cystic spaces *(arrowheads)*; (**b**) mucus threads (*black arrow*) and incipient fluorescein diffusion into the tissues (green, *white arrow*); (**c**) fluorescein diffusion (green, *arrow*) and cells stained with non-fluorescent fluorescein (*arrowhead*); (**d**) shows the upper part of a filament (*arrow*) containing cell debris (*grey arrowhead*), and rose bengal stained cells containing dark dots (nuclei, *white arrowhead*)

Case 4: Giant Filaments in KCS (cont.)

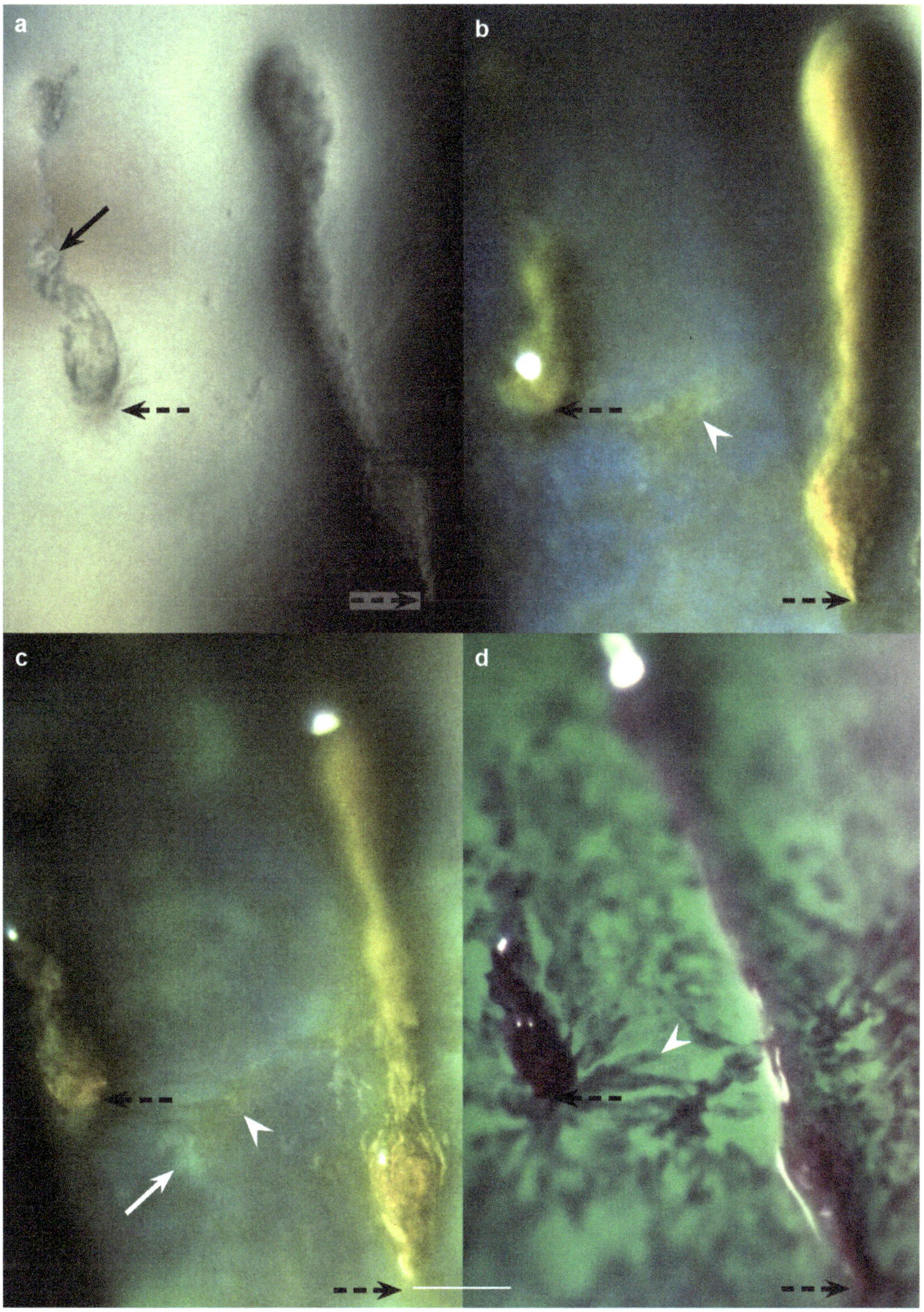

Fig. 7.30 Two filaments (a) before staining, (b) shortly after the application of fluorescein, (c) a little later, and (d) with addition of rose bengal. The *dashed arrows* indicate attachment points, the *arrowheads* stained surface cells, the *black arrow* in (a) a partly coiled central thread and the *white arrow* in (c) fluorescein diffusion into the tissues. (The dashed arrows are placed in corresponding locations)

Case 4: Giant Filaments in KCS (cont.)

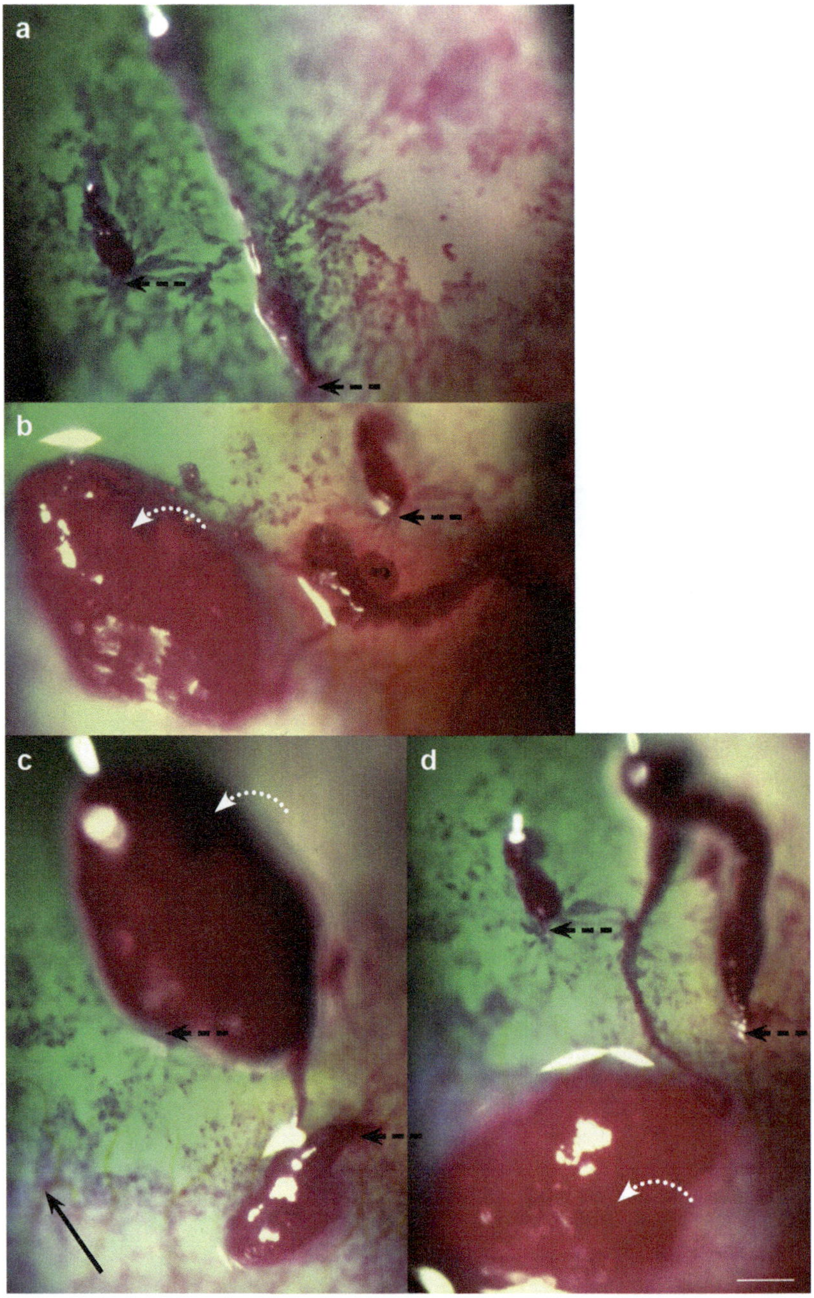

Fig. 7.31 Sequential photographs of the two filaments shown in Fig. 7.30. The filaments are located close to the lower limbus and move upon a surface showing green staining caused by fluorescein diffusion into the tissues and red rose bengal staining of surface cells. The *dashed arrows* indicating the filaments' attachment points are placed in the same locations in all photographs. (**a**) After a blink, both filaments are stretched upwards; (**b**) after a further blink appears a large lump of red stained mucus (*bowed arrow*) which (**c** and **d**) is attached to the right filament and moves up and down with blinks (*bowed arrows*); the *long black arrow* in (**c**) points to a limbal vessel. (**e**) The right filament has folded upon itself, the red mucus lump is still attached to it but (**f**) disappears after another blink, and the long thread of the filament stretches upwards just to (**g**) compress again; attached to its upper end is a small lump (*bowed arrowheads* in **f** and **g**) that is no longer visible in (**h**)

Case 4: Giant Filaments in KCS (cont.)

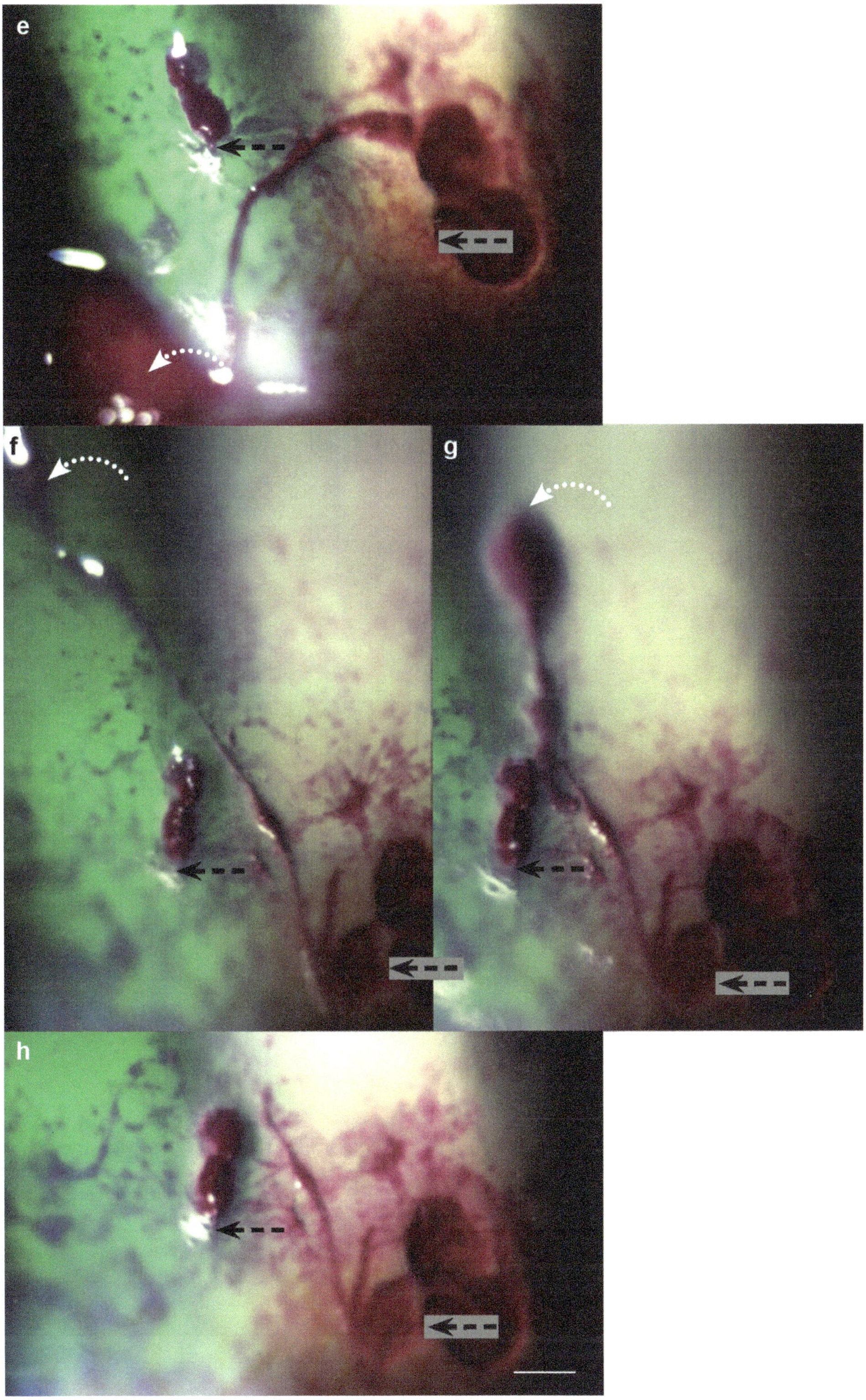

Fig. 7.31 (continued)

Case 5: Filaments After Herpes Zoster Ophthalmicus

Case Report

An 81-year-old man with left-sided HZO 6 months previously presented with a red and painful left eye; the duration of symptoms was about a week. The eye was injected and showed corneal epithelial oedema, several filaments, and anterior uveitis with keratic precipitates. The symptoms subsided rapidly with topical steroid and mydriatics. The filaments disappeared within a week. During the follow-up was found impaired corneal sensibility.

The photographs of the left cornea were taken at presentation (referred to as day 1) and on days 2, 5 and 8.

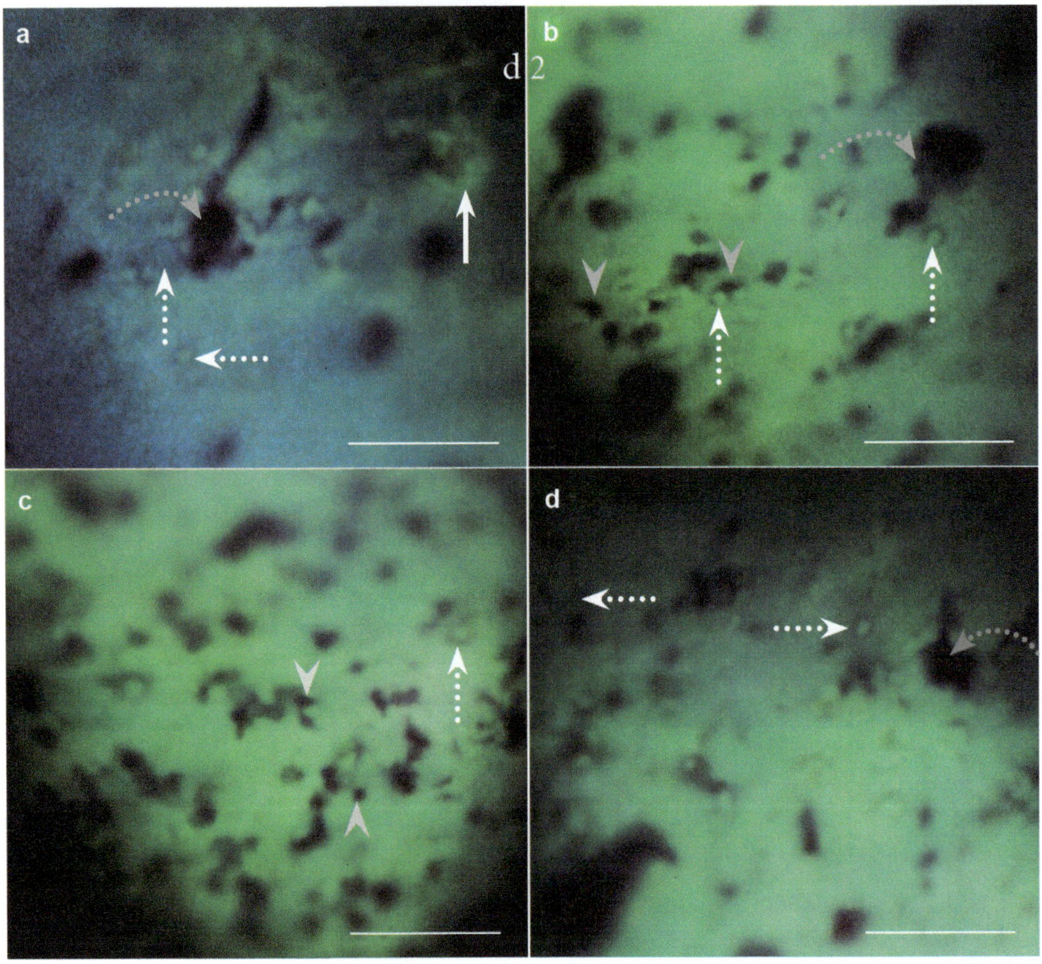

Fig. 7.32 (a–d) Deranged epithelium showing many cell fragments (*arrowheads*), lines surrounding small spots (*doted arrows*), and larger rose bengal stained patches (*bowed arrows*). The *plain white arrow* in (a) indicates incipient fluorescein diffusion into the tissues (green). In the subsequent photographs (b–d), the green staining has increased (cf. Figs. 5.2, 5.3, 5.12 and 5.23). A filament captured at the same occasion is shown in Fig. 7.36 (overleaf)

Case 5: Filaments After Herpes Zoster Ophthalmicus (cont.)

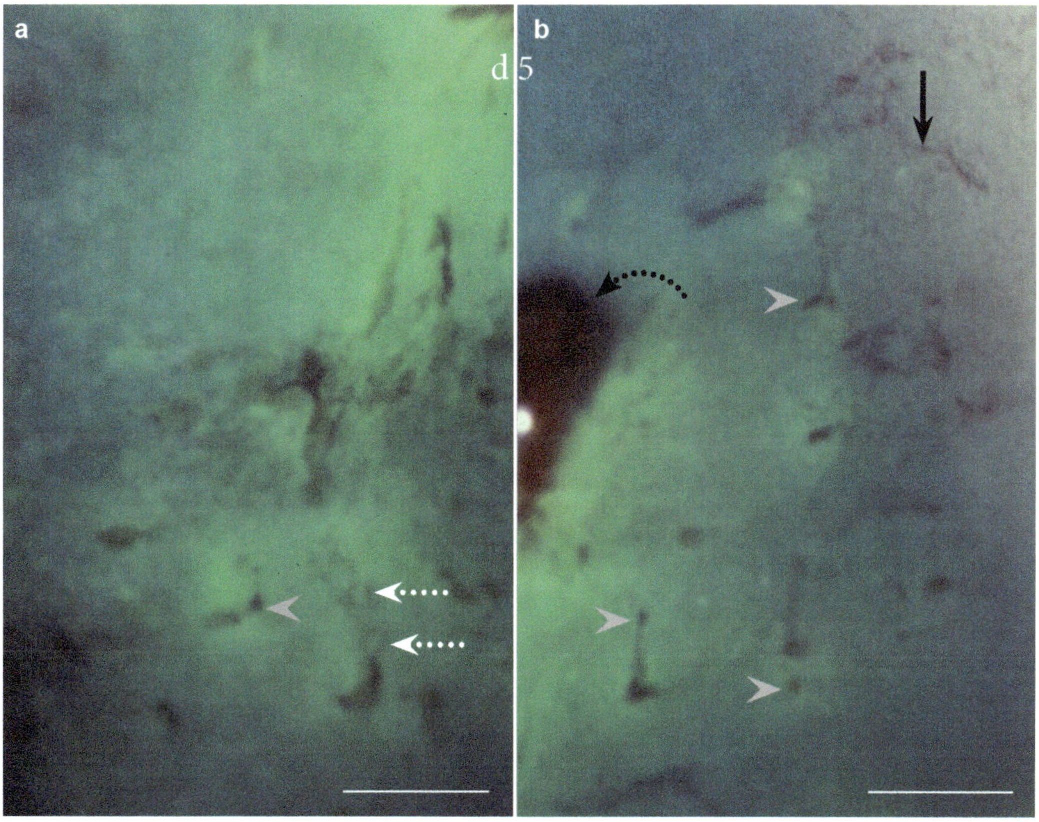

Fig. 7.33 Cell fragments (*arrowheads*), lines surrounding small spaces (*dotted arrows*), a mucus thread (a, *straight arrow*), and green staining revealing fluorescein diffusion into the tissues. The *bowed arrow* in (b) indicates a part of a filament shown in Figs. 7.37 and 7.38

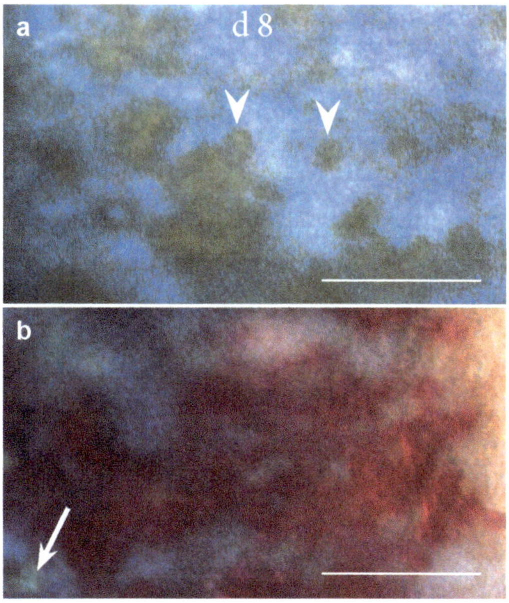

Fig. 7.34 The lower part of the cornea shows (a) surface cells staining brown with non-fluorescent fluorescein (*arrowheads*) and (b) a heavy, confluent rose bengal staining in which individual cells cannot be discerned (cf. Fig. 5.4). The *arrow* indicates incipient fluorescein diffusion into the tissues. At this occasion filaments were no longer present

Case 5: Filaments After Herpes Zoster Ophthalmicus (cont.)

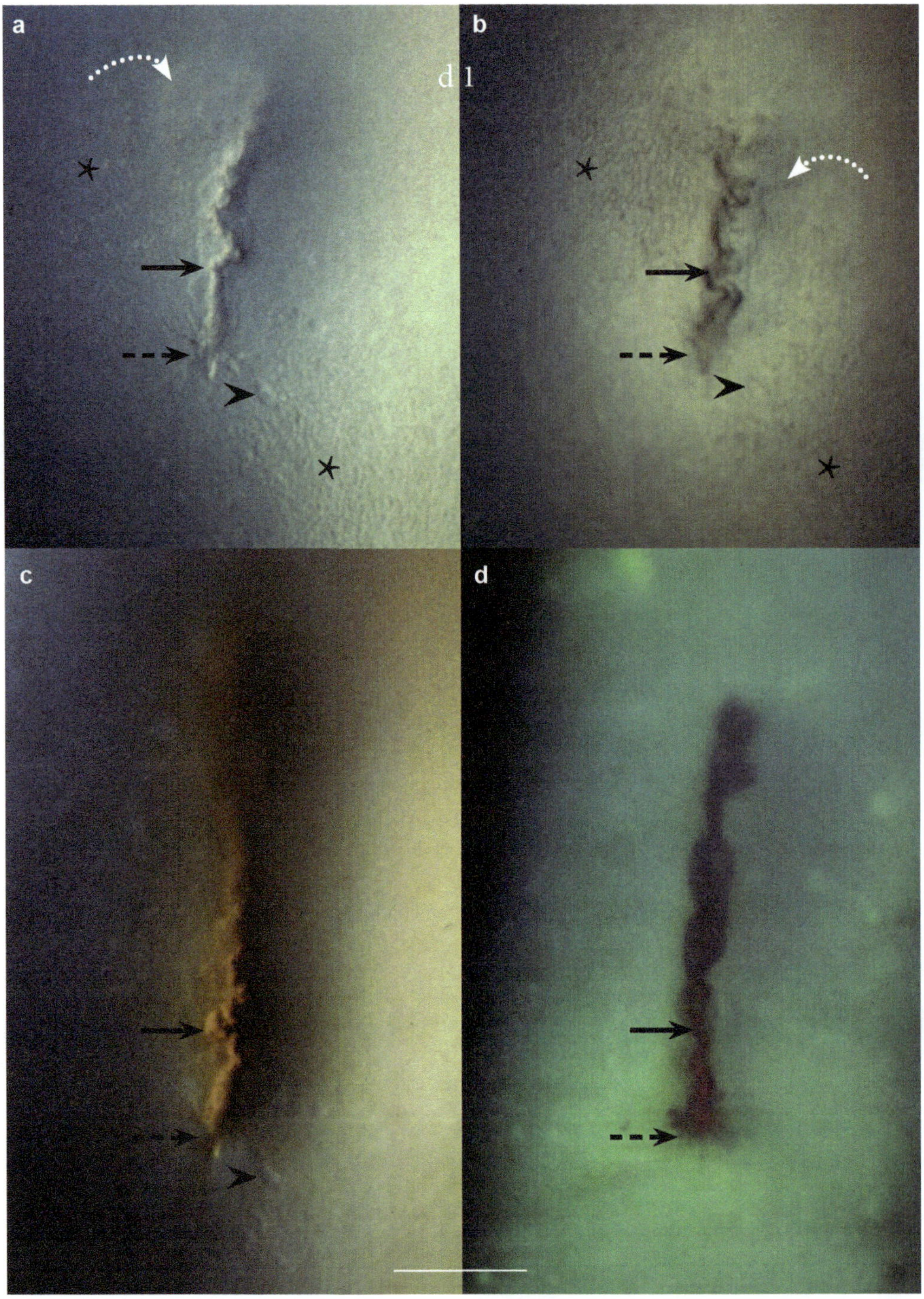

Fig. 7.35 (a, b) This slender filament, attached (*dashed arrows*) to the upper part of the cornea, shows a thick central thread (*plain arrows*) with attached mucus layer (*bowed arrows*), (c) yellow fluorescein and (d) red rose bengal staining. The *arrowheads* indicate a cystic space and the *asterisks* a fine texture of basal epithelial oedema. In (d) is visible fluorescein diffusion into the tissues (green). (The straight arrows are placed in corresponding locations; a Adapted from [4])

Case 5: Filaments After Herpes Zoster Ophthalmicus (cont.)

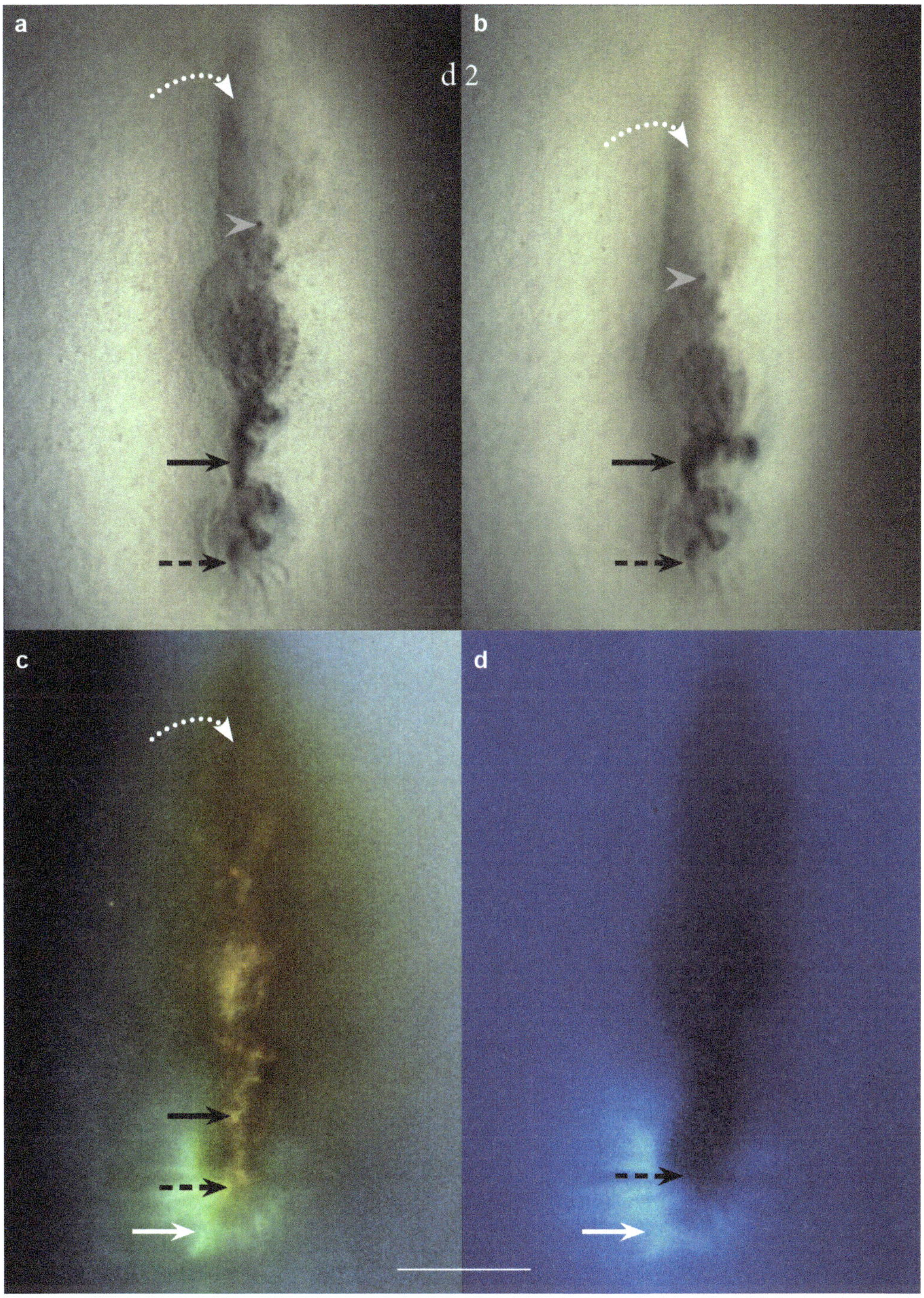

Fig. 7.36 (a–d) A filament attached (*dashed arrows*) to the upper part of the cornea shows a thick, coiled central thread (*plain black arrows*) carrying mucus (*bowed arrows*); its contents are partly granular (*arrowheads*). In (c) is visible non-fluorescent (yellow-brown) staining of the filament and a fluorescent one (green, *white arrow*) around its attachment. (d) shows the same with the blue filter. (The dashed arrows are placed in corresponding locations)

Case 5: Filaments After Herpes Zoster Ophthalmicus (cont.)

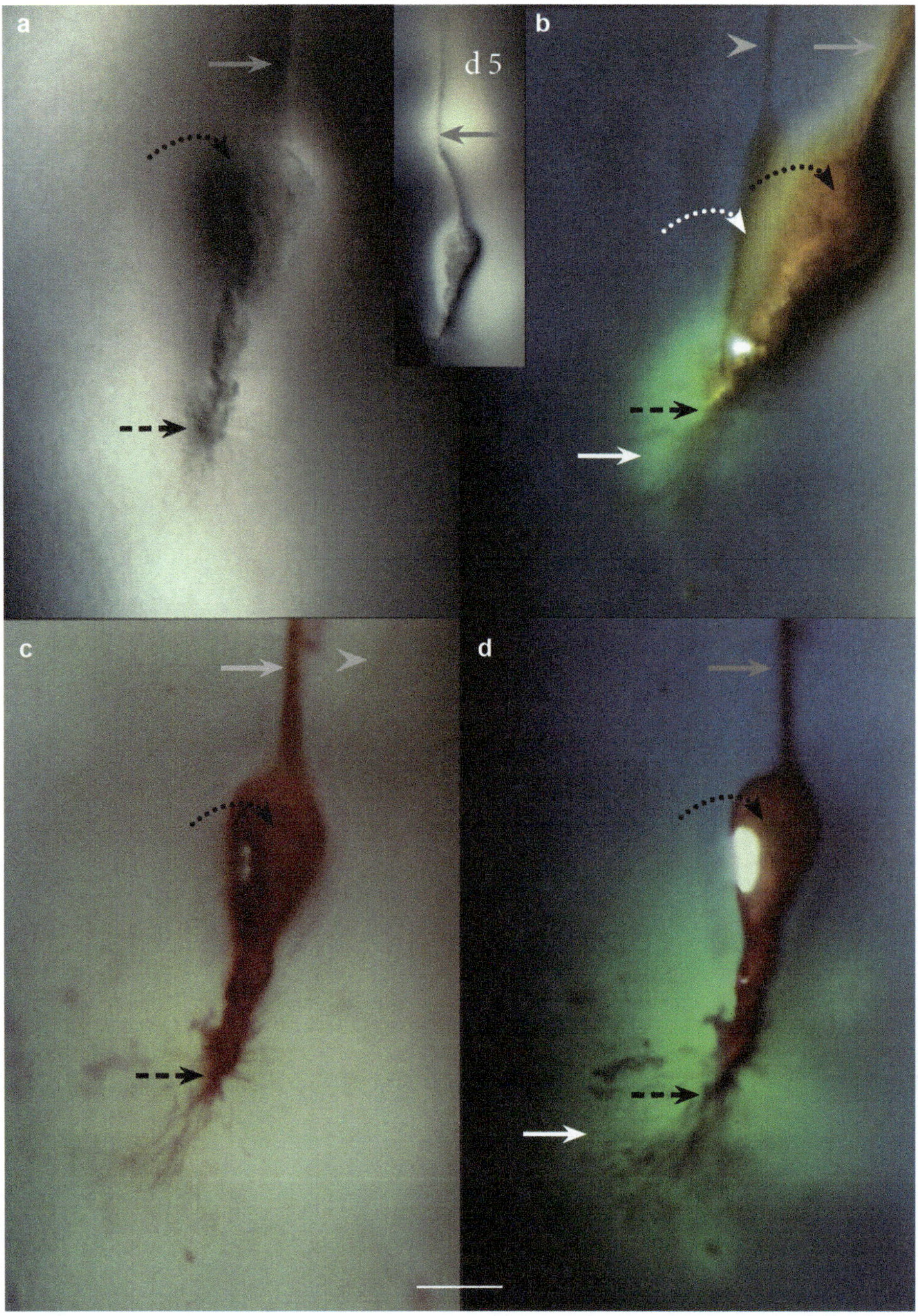

Fig. 7.37 (a–b) A filament present in the upper part of the cornea; the *dashed arrows* indicate its attachment point, the *white arrows* fluorescein diffusion into the tissues around it, the *black bowed arrows* its body and the *grey arrows* a long strand protruding from its upper end. The filament stains yellow with fluorescein and red with rose bengal. In (b) the filament seems enveloped by a sticky, elastic material which, with movements, partly remains in contact with the surface (*bowed white arrow*); the strand leaves imprints on the surface (b and c, *arrowheads*). Cf. Fig. 7.38

Case 5: Filaments After Herpes Zoster Ophthalmicus (cont.)

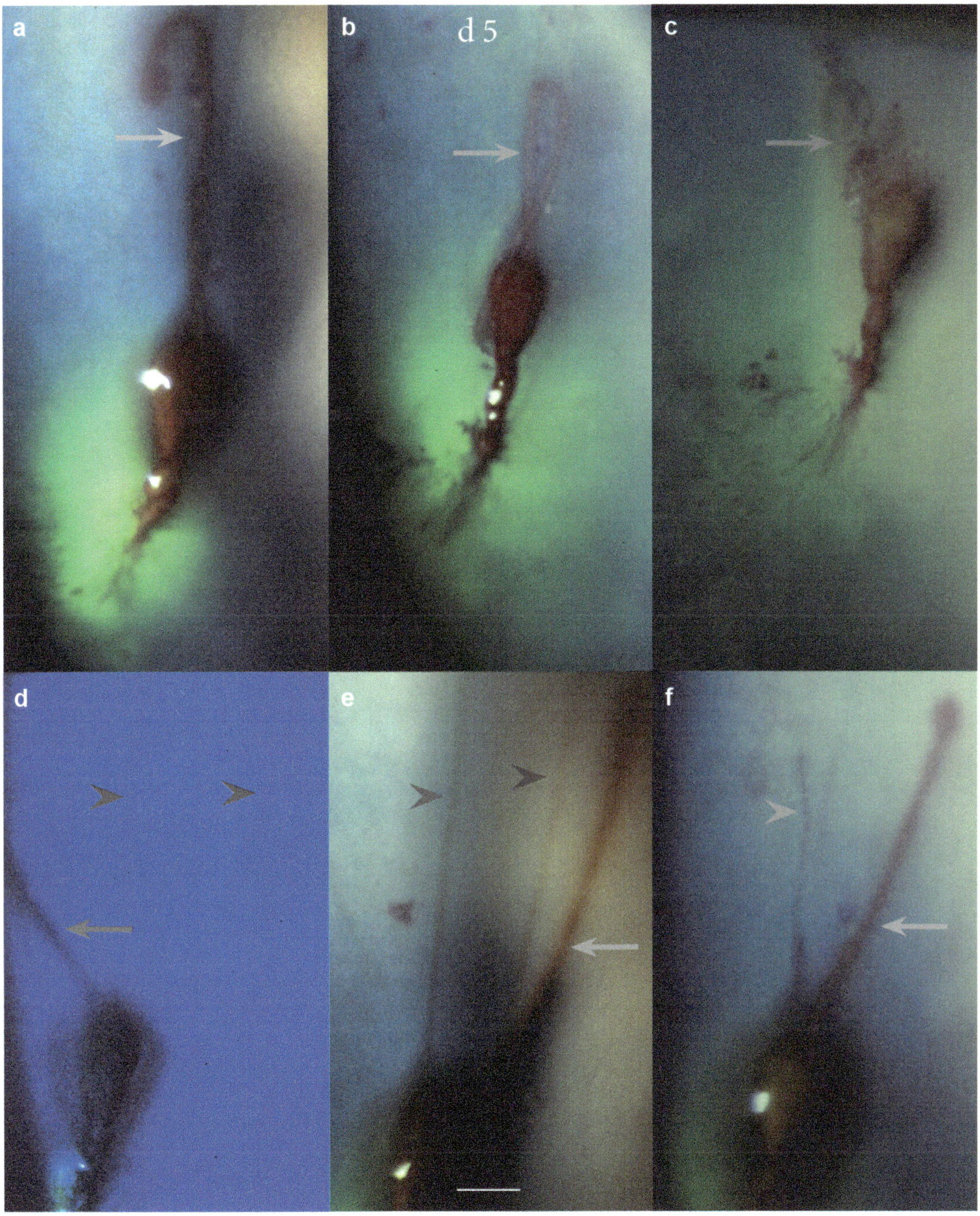

Fig. 7.38 The same filament as in Fig. 7.37. (a–c) show movements with blinks of a long mucus strand (*arrows*) attached to its free end: in (a) it is stretched upwards, in (b) partly wrapped around the filament body and in (c) apparently collapsed; the filament body stays in place. In (d, e) the strand (*arrows*) seems sticky; *arrowheads* indicate its imprints left behind on the surface (cf. also (a) and (f)). (d: blue filter)

Cases 6, 7, and 8: Filaments in Epithelial Oedema

Case Reports

Patient A: an 82-year-old woman with corneal endothelial dystrophy and stromal and epithelial oedema.

Patient B: a 75-year-old woman with KCS and recurrent herpes simplex keratitis.

Patient C: a 73-year-old man with glaucoma and a history of recurrent erosions in the right eye repeatedly treated with acyclovir because of presumed herpes simplex. At presentation, the epithelial defect was healed but the epithelium showed cystic oedema.

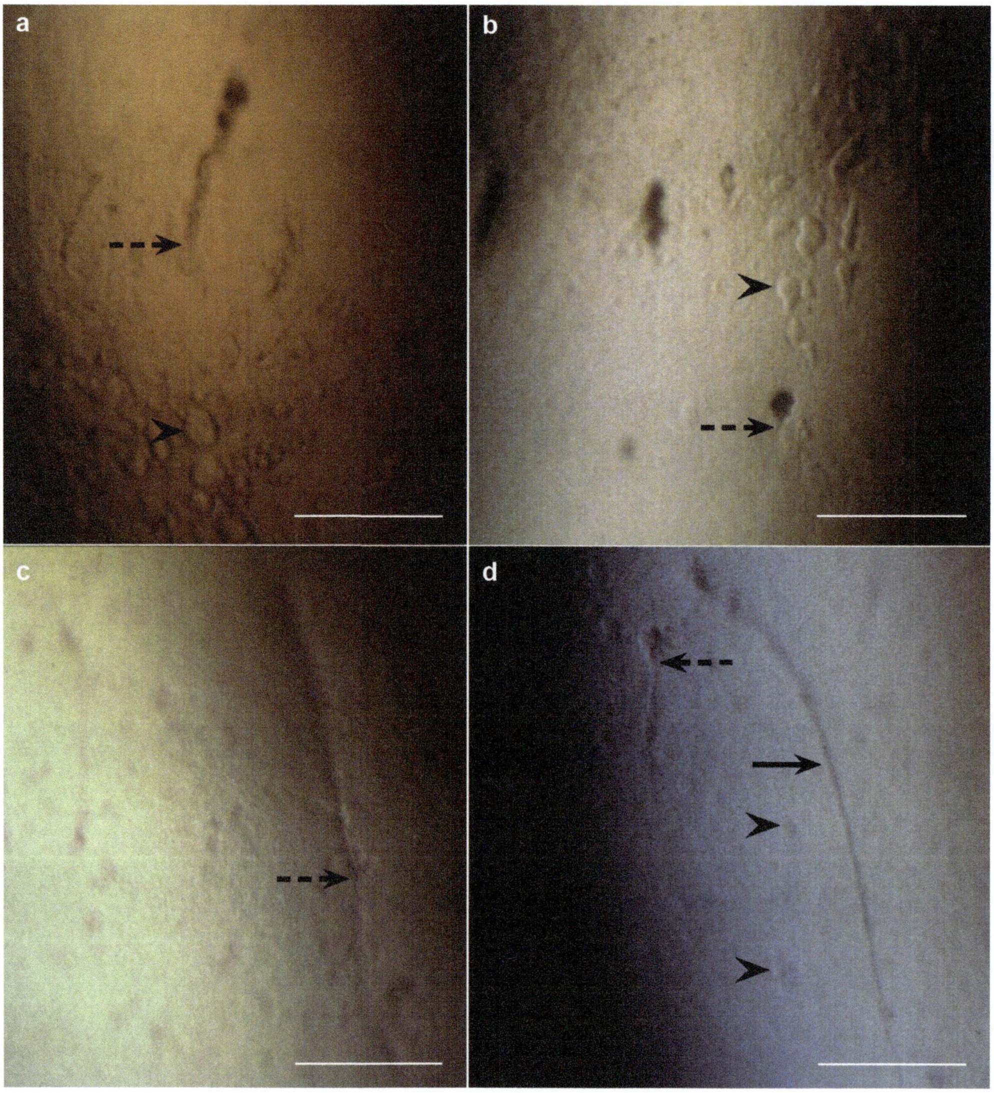

Fig. 7.39 (**a, b**) In patients A and B, the epithelium shows cystic spaces (*arrowheads*) and small filaments (*arrows*). (**c, d**) In patient C are visible small filaments attached to the surface (*dashed arrows*), a long mucus thread (**d**, *plain arrow*) and cystic spaces (**d**, *arrowheads*)

Case 9: Filaments in Diplopia

Case Report

A 37-year-old man presented with irritation in the right eye, which he had kept closed for several days because of sudden diplopia caused by a nerve palsy. The cornea showed several small filaments close to the upper limbus.

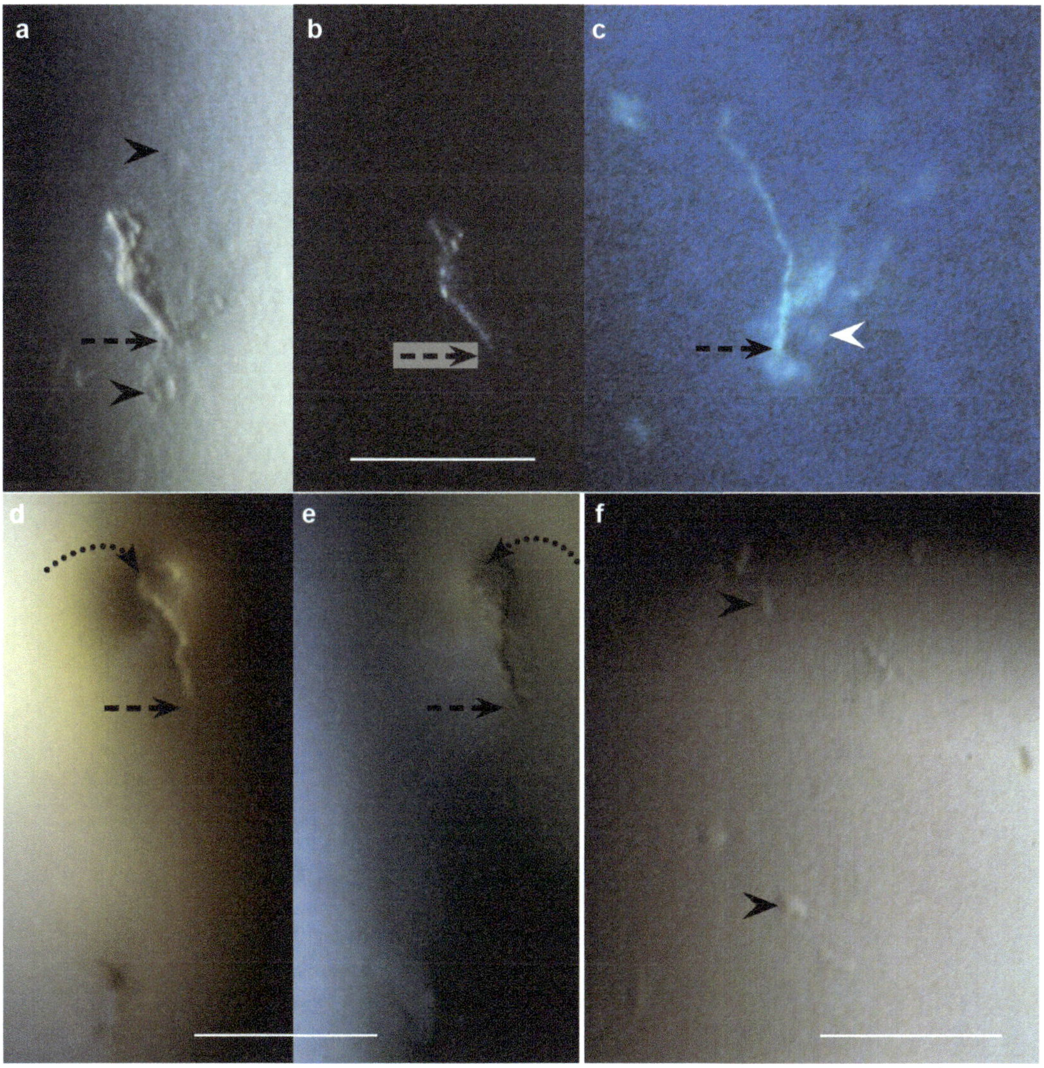

Fig. 7.40 (a–c) A light-reflecting mucus thread attached at one end to the surface (*arrows*), (a, b) coiling and (c) stretching with blinks. The surrounding epithelium shows a few cystic spaces (*black arrowheads*) and damaged surface cells (c, *white arrowhead*). (d, e) show a small filament; the *dashed arrows* indicate its attachment point and the *bowed arrows* its body. In (f) are visible epithelial cystic spaces (*arrowheads*)

Case 10: Filaments in Keratitis Photoelectrica

Case Report

A 48-year-old man helping a friend with welding did not use protective goggles but kept his left eye closed. About 16 h later, he presented with irritation and redness in the right eye. The eye was injected and the cornea showed cystic epithelial oedema and several filaments.

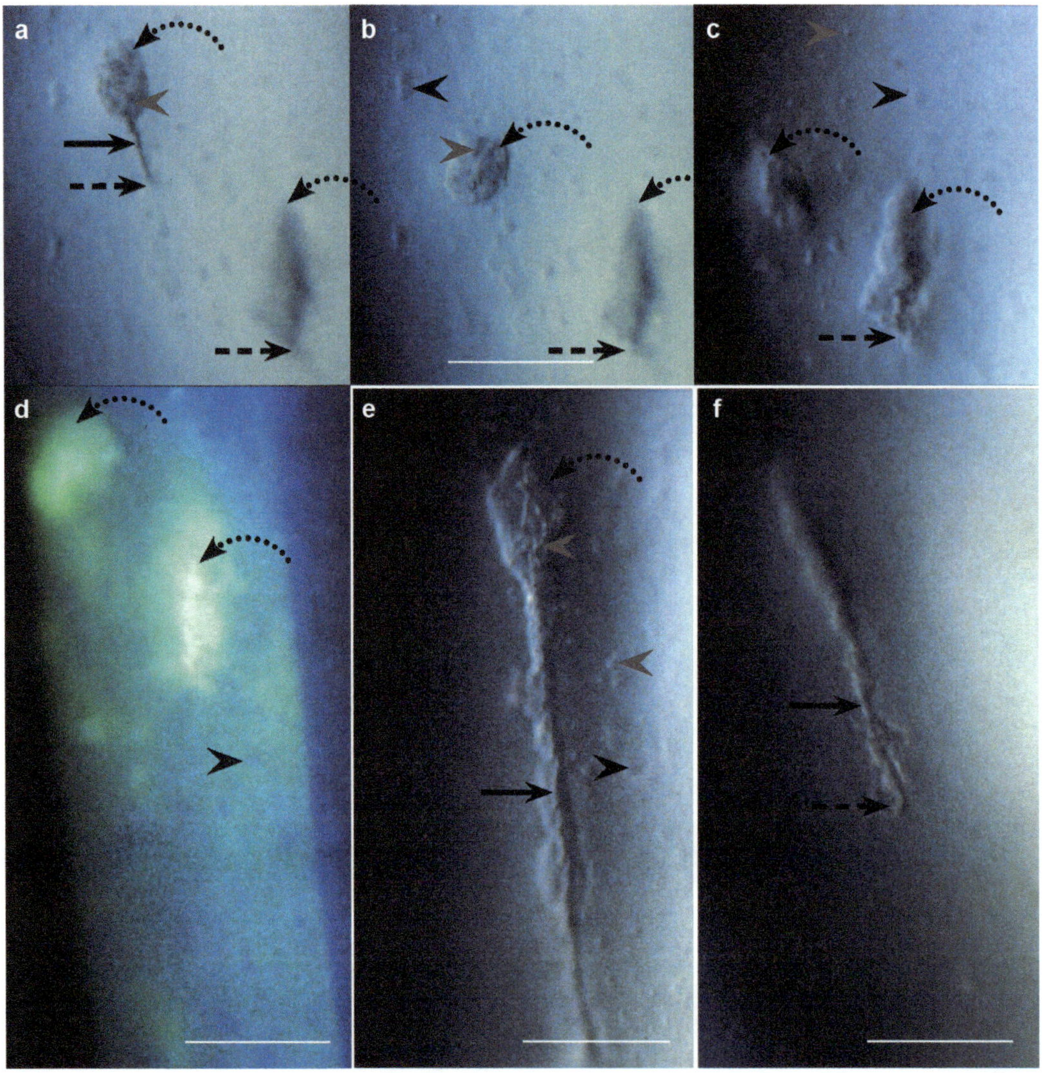

Fig. 7.41 (a–d) Two filaments. The *dashed arrows* indicate their attachment points, the *bowed arrows* their bodies, the *plain arrow* the central thread of the left filament and the *black arrowheads* cystic spaces. Rounded bodies (*grey arrowheads*) are present within and outside the filaments. In (b) and (c) is visible that the left filament has flipped over its attachment. (d) shows that both filaments are light reflecting (*arrows*); epithelial cystic spaces (*black arrowhead*) appear dark in the tear film stained green with fluorescein. (e, f) Two slender filaments with well discernible central threads (*plain arrows*). The *grey arrowheads* in (e) point to rounded bodies present within the filament (*bowed arrow*) and outside it, and the *dashed arrow* in (f) to the filament's attachment point

Case 11: Filaments in Subtarsal Foreign Body

Case Report

A 65-year-old man presented with foreign body sensation in the left eye. A small subtarsal foreign body was removed. The upper part of the cornea showed epithelial defects, corresponding to the position of the foreign body, and a filament.

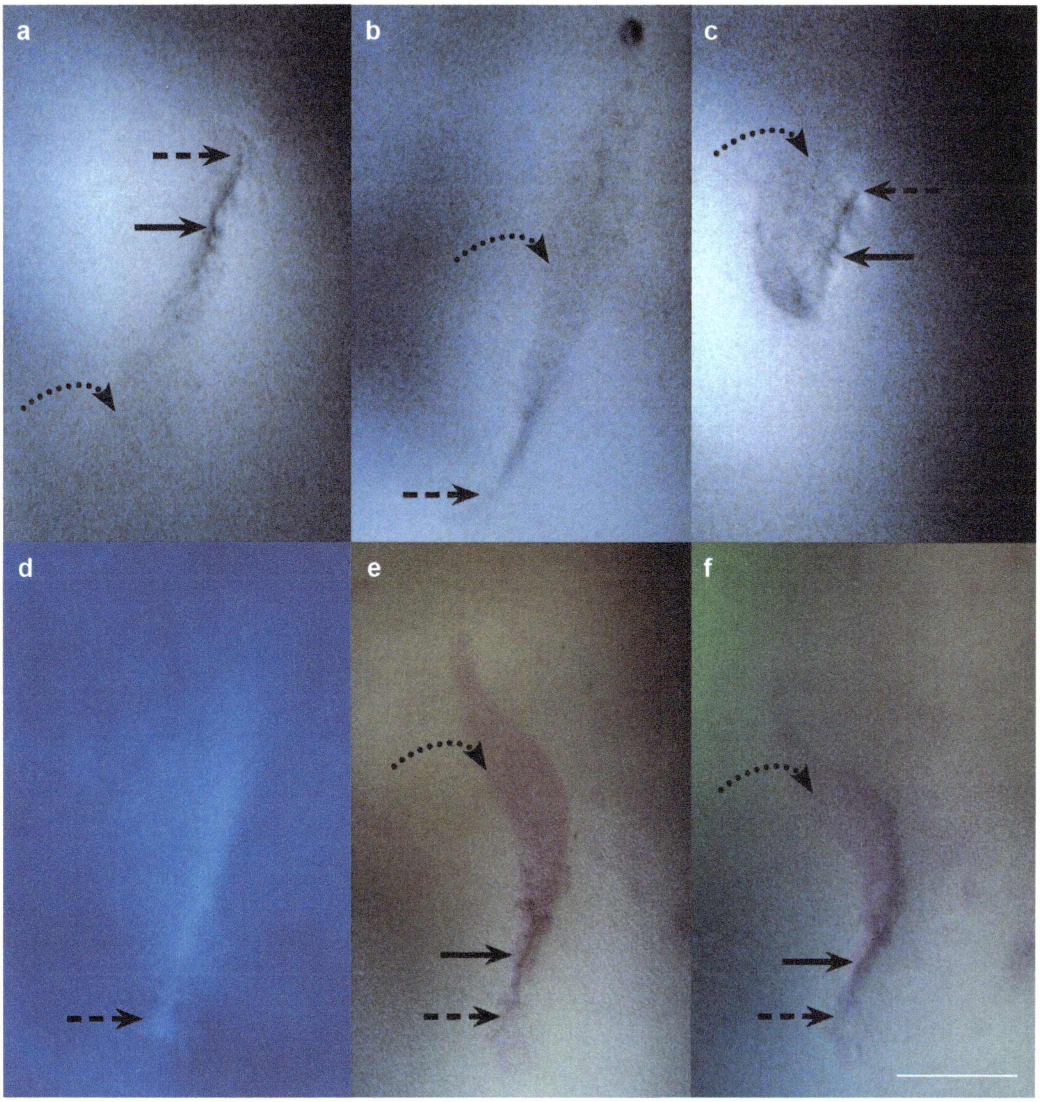

Fig. 7.42 (a–f) In this filament is visible attachment point (*dashed arrows*), central thread (*plain arrows*) and attached mucus (*bowed arrows*) that shows (d) bright fluorescein and (e, f) red rose bengal staining. In (a–c) are additionally visible its up and down movements occurring with blinks. (The dashed arrows are placed in corresponding locations; a, c and e Adapted from [4])

Case 12: A Filament in Trichiasis

Case Report

A 50-year-old woman with foreign body sensation in the left eye. Eyelashes sweeping the cornea caused epithelial scratches; a filament was present in the same area.

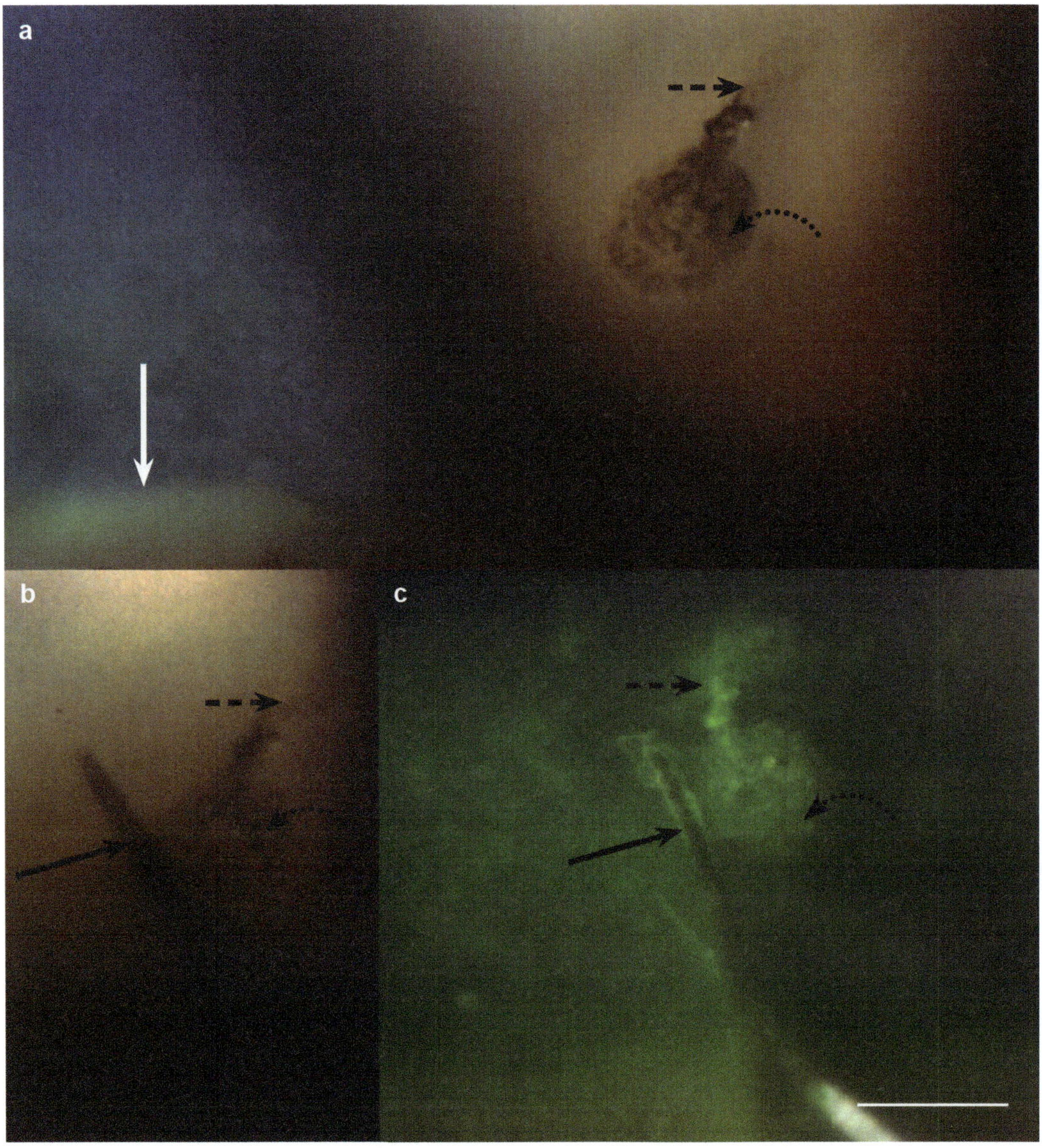

Fig. 7.43 (a–c) A filament (*bowed arrows*) attached (*dashed arrows*) to the lower part of the cornea. The *white arrow* indicates the lower tear meniscus and the *black arrows* the offending eyelashes. (The dashed arrows are placed in corresponding locations)

Case 13: A Filament for Causes Unknown

Case Report

A 44-year-old woman with psoriasis presented with a sudden irritation in both eyes. The right eye showed 2 epithelial erosions and the left one a long filament at the upper limbus. The causes remained unknown. Three years later, the right upper cornea showed basal membrane dystrophy.

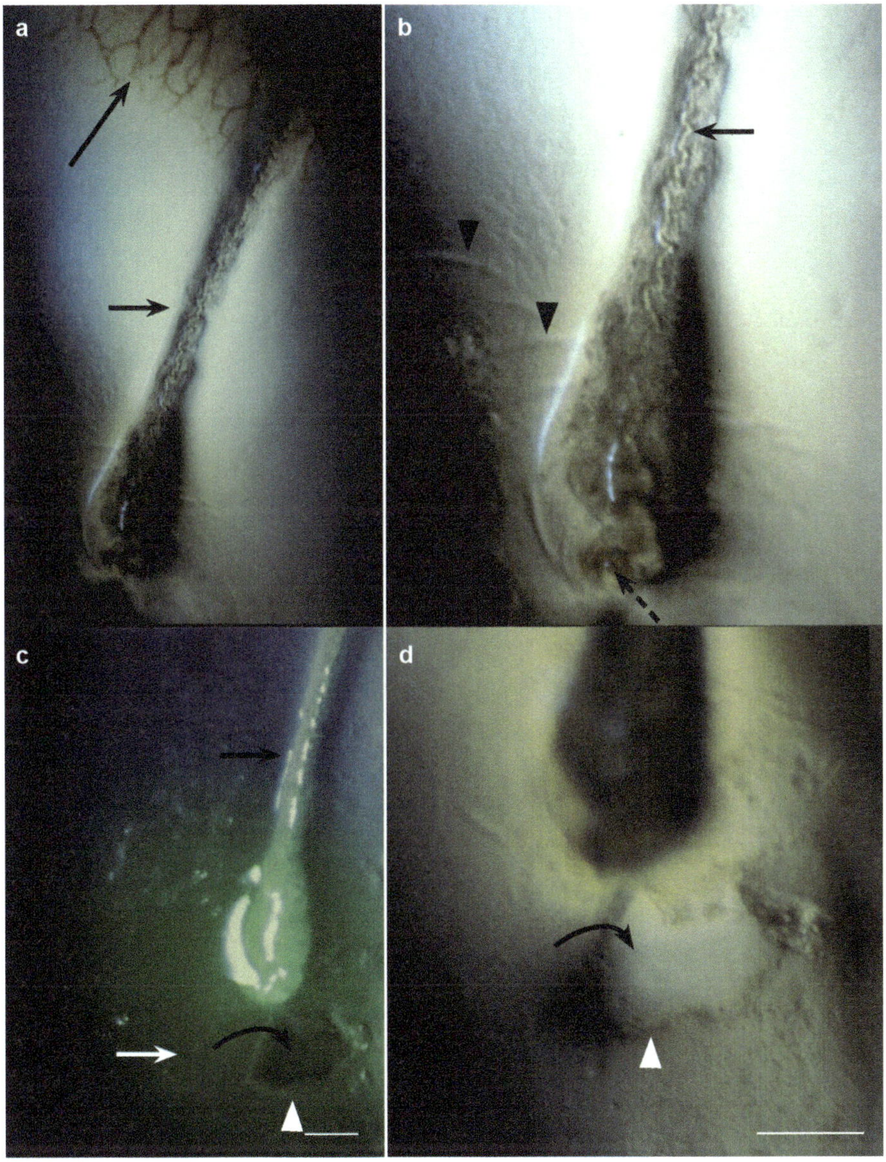

Fig. 7.44 (a, b) Lower part of a long filament (*short arrow*), avulsed from the epithelium and lying on the surface close to the upper limbus (*long arrow*); (b) at its base is visible an epithelial erosion (*bowed arrow*) and fluorescein diffusion into the tissues (green, *white arrow*). In (c) the *plain arrow* indicates the central thread of the filament of which the attachment (*dashed arrow*) is torn off; the *arrowheads* indicate folds in the surrounding epithelium. (d) shows the erosion (*arrow*) at the filament base; the underlying stroma is clear. The *white arrowheads* in (b) and (d) point to the edge of the erosion

Addendum. Pseudofilaments (1)

The images in Figs. 7.45 and 7.46 originate in patients who presented 1–2 years after cataract operation with a sudden onset of foreign body sensation in the operated eye. The cause was a suture at the upper limbus, left in situ after the operation; its rupture resulted in protrusions of variously long bits of nylon threads.

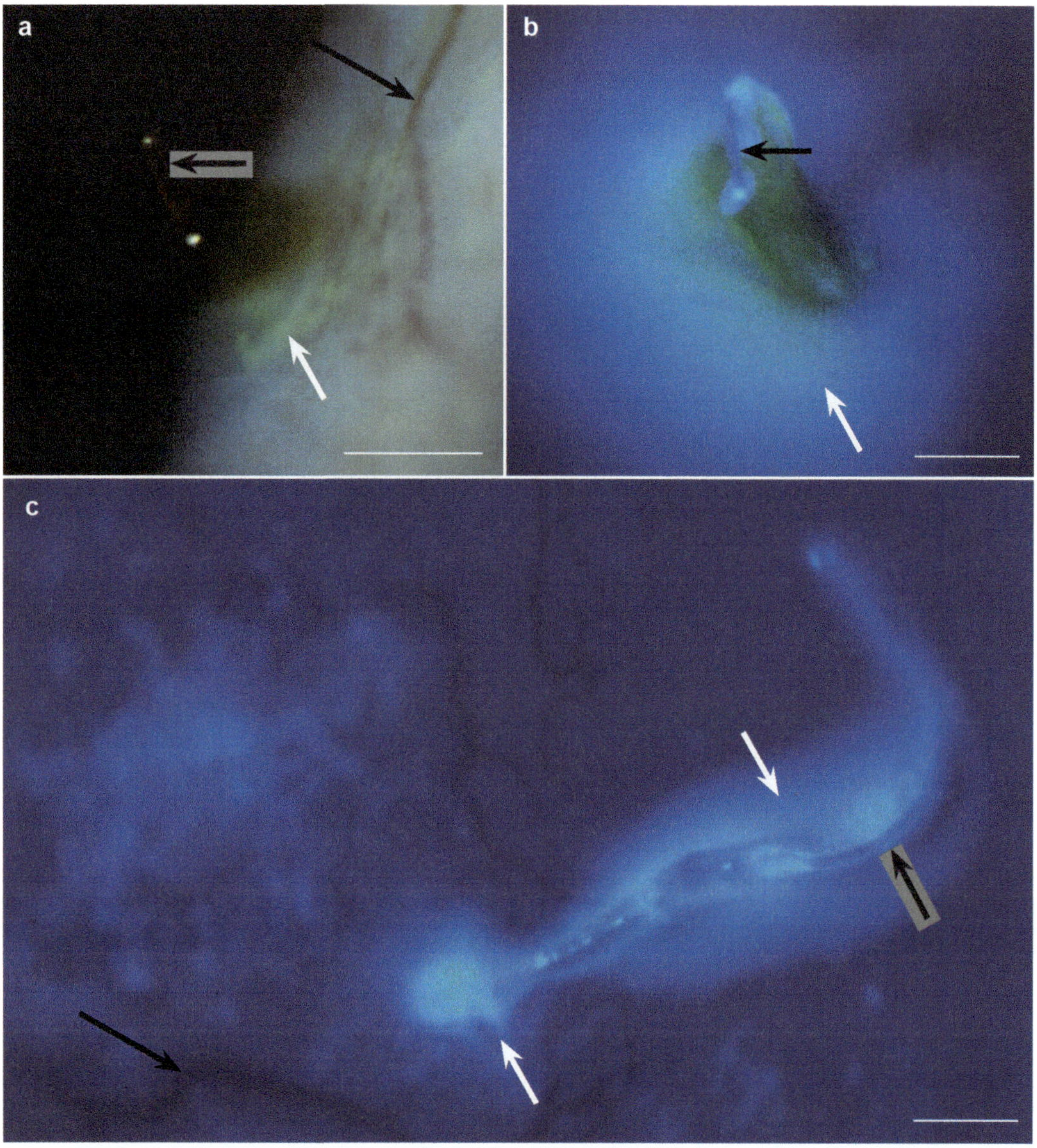

Fig. 7.45 (a, b) Short bits of ruptured nylon threads (*short black arrows*); fluorescein is pooling around their exits from the tissues (brownish-green) and diffuses into them (brilliantly green in (a) and bright with the blue filter in (b), *white arrows)*. (c) A longer bit of nylon thread (*black arrow*) sweeping the surface. The bright fluorescein staining (*white arrows*) indicates fluorescein diffusion into the tissues around its exit *(left white arrow*) and visualises mucus accumulated around the thread (*right white arrow*). The *long black arrows in* (a) and (c) point to vessels present in the area

Pseudofilaments (2)

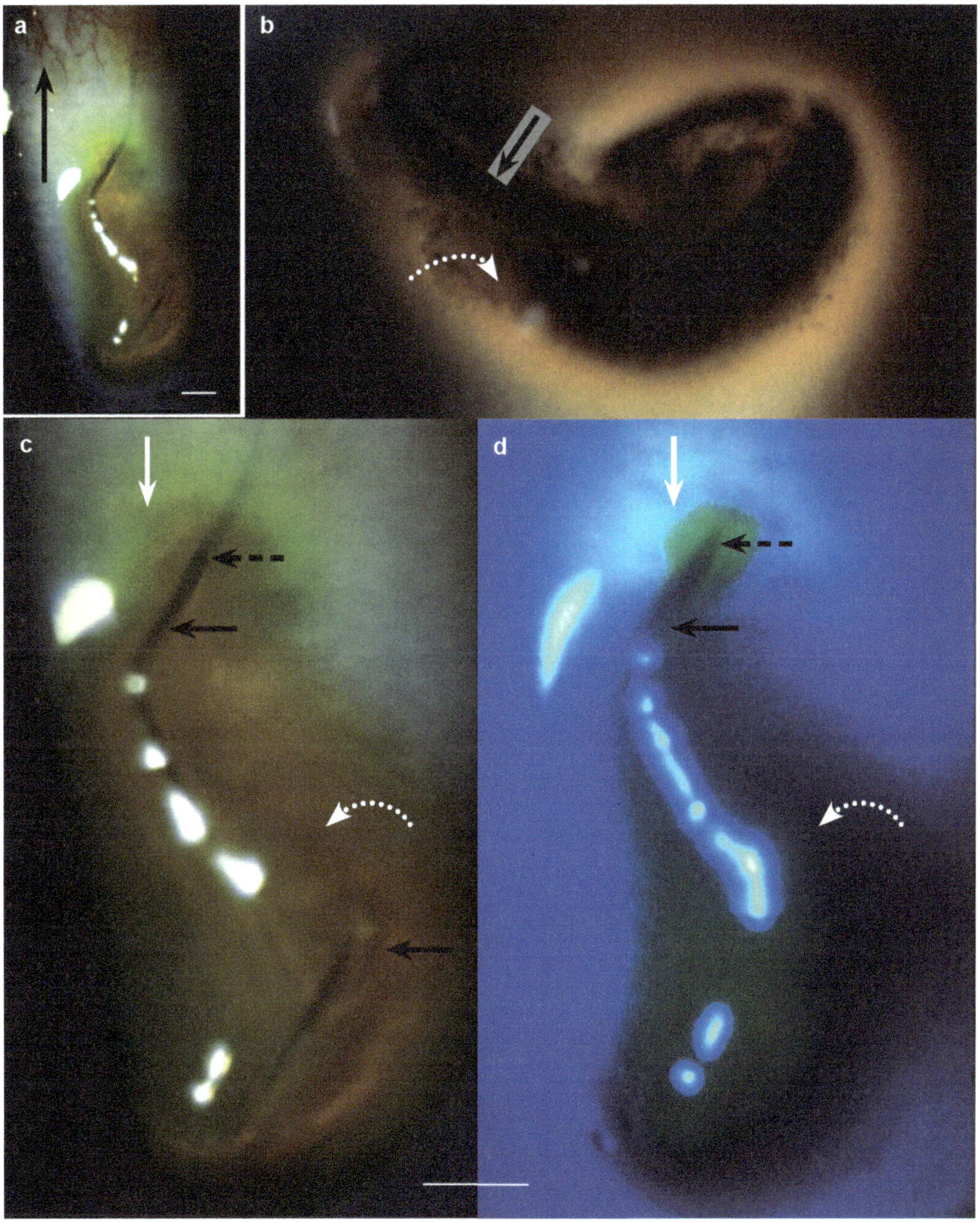

Fig. 7.46 A long piece of protruding nylon thread close to the upper limbus (*arrow*). (a) Survey. (b) shows the thread (*straight arrow*) coiled upon the surface and surrounded by mucus (*bowed arrow*). In (c) and (d) the mucus (*bowed arrows*) is visualised with fluorescein: the *plain black arrows* indicate the thread, the *dashed arrows* indicate its exit onto the surface and the *white arrows* fluorescein diffusion into the tissues. (The markers in c and d are placed in corresponding locations; d: blue filter)

Comment

The various hues of fluorescein are the result of a very complex interplay between the inherent properties of the dye, medium in which it is dissolved, and illuminating conditions.

Final Remark

Keratoconjunctivitis sicca (KCS) is a very common disease, mostly mild but in many individuals severe and disabling. Although at present neither curative treatment nor means of prevention are available, the diagnosis is very important, perhaps mainly because it may result in a reasonable suspicion of underlying systemic disease. But there is more to it. Patients disappointed by new eyeglasses or dissatisfied with the result of cataract operation despite excellent vision, patients repeatedly presenting with presumed foreign bodies or repeatedly treated with antibiotics because of presumed infections – does it sound familiar? It might because these are some typical, and common, examples of patients with undiagnosed KCS.

From clinical point of view, the absence of consensus on KCS criteria reflex the complexity of the disease: symptoms might not parallel findings; there might be a mismatch between surface changes and test results (one extreme being a patient with KCS symptoms, no detectable surface changes but a clearly abnormal Schirmer 1 test and the other a patient with minimal or even no symptoms, a clearly diseased surface but Schirmer 1 test well above the cut-off value); and both symptoms and findings might fluctuate without any apparent cause. All this does not make the diagnosis easier.

The in vivo captured images presented in this book show a broad spectrum of ocular surface changes occurring in KCS (as defined), in the first line detected with *fluorescein sodium*. As a screening means, fluorescein is superior to rose bengal partly because its application is painless and harmless and partly because it not only reveals diseased surface cells but also the diagnostically important surface disruptions. In the absence of fluorescein staining, there is little point in proceeding with rose bengal as no changes will be disclosed with that dye either (save for a new damage occurring before its application, for example such as caused by the paper strip used in the Schirmer test). On a deranged surface, however, *rose bengal* is superior to fluorescein in revealing some details; whether or not this supplementary information might serve clinical purposes such as estimations of the surface condition in the sense of judging the severity of the disease, treatment effects, and perhaps also in differentiating the causes is at present unclear. On the other hand, the knowledge on which phenomena disclosed with that dye may be an expression of KCS is very useful in differential diagnostics of ocular surface diseases, particularly in those superimposed. Epitheliopathy after *herpes zoster ophthalmicus* (HZO) (below) is an example how features diverging from KCS can be highlighted by rose bengal. (In this disease, theoretically, a disappearance of the particular features might serve as indicator of recovery of the corneal sensibility.)

One phenomenon deserves a special comment. It is generally agreed that KCS is a multifactorial disease and in many cases an inflammatory one. Inflammatory cells are well discernible with the present method, and with the slit lamp, when present in an optically clear medium (such as inflammatory cells on the endothelium in anterior uveitis) but, as mentioned in Chap. 2, they cannot be identified if diffusely spread in a deranged epithelium in which many other similarly appearing changes are possible. Concentrated in small areas,

H.M. Tabery, *Keratoconjunctivitis Sicca and Filamentary Keratopathy*,
DOI 10.1007/978-3-642-31028-7, © Springer-Verlag Berlin Heidelberg 2012

not light-reflecting but otherwise reminiscent of epithelial infiltrates in adenovirus infections or Thygeson's superficial punctate keratitis (Figs. 2.36 and 2.37), such 'rounded bodies' (as I have chosen to term them all) might represent inflammatory cells, but in KCS such lesions seem rather rare. In the more common enlarging green (fluorescent) flecks, in which some areas imply heaped-up rounded cells but others show a fine granularity more suggestive of incipient basal cell oedema, the doubts on their nature remain; possibly, both are present. Hence, the *green* (fluorescent) *flecks*, coming and going, are a puzzling phenomenon perhaps expressing a result of inflammatory activity, but their in vivo morphology offers no clear-cut proof. Nevertheless, they are a very useful clinical sign strongly suggestive of KCS, very often in combination with an autoimmune disease (personal observation).

Finally, it seems almost strange that patients with a severe KCS ocular surface derangement such as shown here were not prone to infections, epithelial break-downs resulting in stromal denudation, or corneal stromal involvement. Obviously, the natural defensive forces work despite the epithelial disturbance, and its causes, and it is probable that stromal infiltrates are just another manifestation of the patient's autiommune propensity rather than a sequela of epithelial disease.

Corneal epitheliopathy occurring as a *sequela of HZO* is not very common. The four patients presented in this book shared a severe HZO and an epitheliopathy resembling a severe KCS but, at a higher magnification level, showing peculiar changes occasionally perhaps hinted at but never that pronounced in KCS. Additional links were impaired corneal sensitivity (three patients tested) and a bilateral KCS (three patients tested). The role of a preexisting KCS in the resulting morphology is unclear, but it seems reasonable to assume that the well-known untoward effect of impaired corneal sensitivity on the epithelium should be the same whatever the causes. An example of that could have been a patient with combination of impaired corneal sensitivity after stroke and KCS (Chap. 4, Case 9) if not for the fact that the epitheliopathy, diverging from KCS but in places reminiscent of that captured after HZO (without rose bengal), had developed suddenly several years after the stroke. Lacking explanation, it is tempting to speculate that the stroke could have been caused by HZ (sine herpete) with cerebral involvement, which is a real possibility, but although HZ is an insidious disease an interpretation of the bout of epitheliopathy as HZ-related would be purely speculative. Nevertheless, I have included this case because it is diagnostically challenging.

In the four patients with post-HZO epitheliopathy, similarly to KCS, the most pronounced changes were located within the interpalpebral area. Despite the severe epithelial disturbance, no infections or stromal complications occurred during the observation period, fortunately, because HZO is unpredictable and recurrences may be more common than suspected. The exact mechanisms behind post-HZO epitheliopathy cannot be derived from their morphology but their divergence from the common KCS corneal surface changes indicate additional factors presumably relatable to impaired corneal sensitivity.

Corneal filaments have been proposed to originate from material adhering to the surface, from the corneal epithelium, and from the corneal stroma. It seems clear that their composition reflects material present in the tear film and on the surface (i.e. mucus and cell debris), and that their actual appearance is partly related to relative amounts of such material available, and partly to friction between two firm surfaces (such as the corneal and the conjunctival tarsal epithelia) occurring with blinks; in fact, conjunctival filaments are extremely rare. Some sequential photographs (Figs. 7.2, 7.39 and 7.40) clearly show that there is an affinity between the filament bodies and the surface, a phenomenon probably mediated by the same component that cements the material together, presumably the amorphous mucus. It is, however, unclear why large filaments appear in bouts in patients with a diseased surface visibly promoting mucus adherence. Actually, surface properties allowing or promoting attachments of mucus threads are difficult to point out because filaments occur in a large variety of surface diseases but are not a regular feature in any of them. These diseases seem to have in common epithelial oedema but what additional factor(s) are operating in each case is unclear. Hence, while the filament composition supplemented by their dynamics elucidates their nature, the exact mechanisms behind the bonds forming between mucus threads and the surface remain obscure.

Bibliography

1. Tabery HM (2004) Corneal surface changes in Thygeson's superficial punctate keratitis: a clinical and non-contact photomicrographic in vivo study in the human cornea. Eur J Ophthalmol 14:85–93
2. Tabery HM (2003) Corneal surface changes in kerato-conjunctivitis sicca. Part I: the surface propper. A non-contact photomicrographic in vivo study in the human cornea. Eye 17:482–487
3. Tabery HM (2003) Corneal surface changes in kerato-conjunctivitis sicca. Part II: the mucus component. A non-contact photomicrographic in vivo study in the human cornea. Eye 17:488–491
4. Tabery HM (2003) Filamentary keratopathy: a non-contact photomicrographic in vivo study in the human cornea. EJO 13(7):599–605
5. Tabery HM (2000) Morphology of epithelial keratitis in herpes zoster ophthalmicus. A non-contact photomicrographic study in the human cornea. Acta Ophthalmol Scand 78:651–655
6. Tabery HM (1998) Toxic effect of rose bengal dye on the living human corneal epithelium. Acta Ophthalmol Scand 76:142–145
7. Tabery HM (1997) Micropunctate staining of the human corneal surface: microerosions or cystic spaces? A non-contact photomicrographic in vivo study. Acta Ophthalmol Scand 75:134–136
8. Tabery HM (1995) Morphology of herpes simplex dendritic keratitis. A non-contact photomicrographic study in the human cornea. Herpes 2:55–57
9. Tabery HM (1992) Dual appearance of fluorescein staining in vivo of diseased human corneal epithelium. A non-contact photomicrographic study. Br J Ophthalmol 76:43–44
10. Tabery HM, Holm O (1987) Photography in vivo of epithelial lesions in the human cornea. Acta Ophthalmol (Kbh) 65:513–514
11. Tabery HM (2010) Herpes simplex virus epithelial keratitis: in vivo morphology in the human cornea. Springer, Berlin/Heidelberg
12. Tabery HM (2011) Varicella-zoster virus epithelial keratitis in herpes zoster ophthalmicus: in vivo morphology in the human cornea. Springer, Berlin/Heidelberg
13. Tabery HM (2012) Adenovirus epithelial keratitis and Thygeson's superficial punctate keratitis: in vivo morphology in the human cornea. Springer, Berlin/Heidelberg

Index

H.M. Tabery, *Keratoconjunctivitis Sicca and Filamentary Keratopathy*,
DOI 10.1007/978-3-642-31028-7, © Springer-Verlag Berlin Heidelberg 2012